T0259507

Clinical Cytogenetics

Guest Editor

CAROLINE ASTBURY, PhD, FACMG

CLINICS IN LABORATORY MEDICINE

www.labmed.theclinics.com

Consulting Editor
ALAN WELLS, MD, DMSc

December 2011 • Volume 31 • Number 4

SAUNDERS an imprint of ELSEVIER, Inc.

W.B. SAUNDERS COMPANY
A Division of Elsevier Inc.

1600 John F. Kennedy Boulevard • Suite 1800 • Philadelphia, Pennsylvania 19103-2899

http://www.theclinics.com

CLINICS IN LABORATORY MEDICINE Volume 31, Number 4
December 2011 ISSN 0272-2712, ISBN-13: 978-1-4557-7985-7

Editor: Katie Hartner
Developmental Editor: Donald Mumford

© 2011 Elsevier Inc. All rights reserved.

This journal and the individual contributions contained in it are protected under copyright by Elsevier, and the following terms and conditions apply to their use:

Photocopying
Single photocopies of single articles may be made for personal use as allowed by national copyright laws. Permission of the Publisher and payment of a fee is required for all other photocopying, including multiple or systematic copying, copying for advertising or promotional purposes, resale, and all forms of document delivery. Special rates are available for educational institutions that wish to make photocopies for non-profit educational classroom use. For information on how to seek permission visit www.elsevier.com/permissions or call: (+44) 1865 843830 (UK)/(+1) 215 239 3804 (USA).

Derivative Works
Subscribers may reproduce tables of contents or prepare lists of articles including abstracts for internal circulation within their institutions. Permission of the Publisher is required for resale or distribution outside the institution. Permission of the Publisher is required for all other derivative works, including compilations and translations (please consult www.elsevier.com/permissions).

Electronic Storage or Usage
Permission of the Publisher is required to store or use electronically any material contained in this journal, including any article or part of an article (please consult www.elsevier.com/permissions). Except as outlined above, no part of this publication may be reproduced, stored in a retrieval system or transmitted in any form or by any means, electronic, mechanical, photocopying, recording or otherwise, without prior written permission of the Publisher.

Notice
No responsibility is assumed by the Publisher for any injury and/or damage to persons or property as a matter of products liability, negligence or otherwise, or from any use or operation of any methods, products, instructions or ideas contained in the material herein. Because of rapid advances in the medical sciences, in particular, independent verification of diagnoses and drug dosages should be made.

Although all advertising material is expected to conform to ethical (medical) standards, inclusion in this publication does not constitute a guarantee or endorsement of the quality or value of such product or of the claims made of it by its manufacturer.

Reprints. For copies of 100 or more, of articles in this publication, please contact the Commercial Reprints Department, Elsevier Inc., 360 Park Avenue South, New York, New York 10010-1710. Tel. (212) 633-3813, Fax: (212) 462-1935, E-mail: reprints@elsevier.com.

Clinics in Laboratory Medicine (ISSN 0272-2712) is published quarterly by Elsevier Inc., 360 Park Avenue South, New York, NY 10010-1710. Months of issue are March, June, September, and December. Business and Editorial offices: 1600 John F. Kennedy Blvd., Suite 1800, Philadelphia, PA 19103-2899. Periodicals postage paid at New York, NY and additional mailing offices. Subscription prices are $240.00 per year (US individuals), $382.00 per year (US institutions), $128.00 (US students), $291.00 per year (Canadian individuals), $483.00 per year (foreign institutions), $176.00 (foreign students). Foreign air speed delivery is included in all *Clinics* subscription prices. All prices are subject to change without notice. POSTMASTER: Send address changes to *Clinics in Laboratory Medicine*, Elsevier Health Sciences Division, Subscription Customer Service, 3251 Riverport Lane, Maryland Heights, MO 63043. **Customer Service: 1-800-654-2452 (US). From outside of the US and Canada, call 1-314-447-8871. Fax: 1-314-447-8029. E-mail: journalscustomerservice-usa@elsevier.com (for print support) or journalsonlinesupport-usa@elsevier.com (for online support).**

Clinics in Laboratory Medicine is covered in EMBASE/Exerpta Medica, MEDLINE/PubMed (Index Medicus), Cinahl, Current Contents/Clinical Medicine, BIOSIS and ISI/BIOMED.

Printed and bound by CPI Group (UK) Ltd, Croydon, CR0 4YY

Transferred to Digital Print 2011

Contributors

CONSULTING EDITOR

ALAN WELLS, MD, DMSc
Department of Pathology, University of Pittsburgh, Pittsburgh, Pennsylvania

GUEST EDITOR

CAROLINE ASTBURY, PhD, FACMG
Associate Director, Cytogenetics and Molecular Genetics Laboratory, Department of Pathology and Laboratory Medicine, Nationwide Children's Hospital; Associate Director, Children's Oncology Group Acute Lymphoblastic Leukemia, Neuroblastoma and Wilms Tumor Molecular Reference Laboratories; Assistant Professor (Clinical), Department of Pathology, The Ohio State University College of Medicine, Columbus, Ohio

AUTHORS

INA AMARILLO, PhD
Clinical Cytogenetics Fellow & SRA, Clinical and Molecular Cytogenetics Laboratories, Department of Pathology and Laboratory Medicine, David Geffen School of Medicine, University of California Los Angeles, Los Angeles, California

JOHN ANASTASI, MD
Associate Professor of Pathology, Hematopathology and Clinical Hematology Laboratory, and the Comprehensive Cancer Center, University of Chicago, Chicago, Illinois

CAROLINE ASTBURY, PhD, FACMG
Associate Director, Cytogenetics and Molecular Genetics Laboratory, Department of Pathology and Laboratory Medicine, Nationwide Children's Hospital; Associate Director, Children's Oncology Group Acute Lymphoblastic Leukemia, Neuroblastoma and Wilms Tumor Molecular Reference Laboratories; Assistant Professor (Clinical), Department of Pathology, The Ohio State University College of Medicine, Columbus, Ohio

ADAM BAGG, MD
Professor, Director of Hematology, Medical Director of Clinical Cancer Cytogenetics, Director of Minimal Residual Disease Resource Laboratory, Department of Pathology and Laboratory Medicine, University of Pennsylvania, Philadelphia, Pennsylvania

MICHELLE M. LE BEAU, PhD
Professor of Medicine, Section of Hematology/Oncology, and the Comprehensive Cancer Center, University of Chicago, Chicago, Illinois

LAURA K. CONLIN, PhD
Department of Pathology and Laboratory Medicine, The Children's Hospital of Philadelphia, Philadelphia, Pennsylvania

BHAVANA J. DAVE, PhD, FACMG
Professor, Departments of Pediatrics, Pathology/Microbiology and Pediatrics, and Munroe Meyer Institute for Genetics and Rehabilitation, University of Nebraska Medical Center, Omaha, Nebraska

KRISTEN L. DEAK, PhD, FACMG
Department of Pathology, Duke University, Durham, North Carolina.

CHRISTINE J. HARRISON, PhD, FRCPath
Professor of Childhood Cancer Cytogenetics, Leukaemia Research Cytogenetics Group, Northern Institute for Cancer Research, Newcastle University, Newcastle-upon-Tyne, United Kingdom

SARAH R. HORN, PhD
Department of Pathology, Duke University, Durham, North Carolina.

COLLEEN JACKSON-COOK, PhD, FACMG
Professor and Director of Cytogenetics, Departments of Pathology and Human & Molecular Genetics, Virginia Commonwealth University, Richmond, Virginia

HUTTON M. KEARNEY, PhD
Fullerton Genetics Center, Mission Health System, Asheville, North Carolina

JOSEPH B. KEARNEY, PhD
Fullerton Genetics Center, Mission Health System, Asheville, North Carolina

ALLEN N. LAMB, PhD, FACMG
Medical Director, Cytogenetics and Genomic Microarray Laboratory, ARUP Institute for Clinical and Experimental Pathology; Associate Professor (Clinical), Department of Pathology, University of Utah Health Sciences Center, Salt Lake City, Utah

XU LI, MD, PhD
ABMG, Director of Cytogenetics Laboratory, Department of Genetics, Kaiser Permanente, San Jose Medical Center, San Jose, California

DANIEL MERTENS, PhD
Department of Internal Medicine III, University of Ulm, Ulm, Germany

JENNIFER J.D. MORRISSETTE, PhD, FACMG
Assistant Professor, Director of Clinical Cancer Cytogenetics, Department of Pathology and Laboratory Medicine, University of Pennsylvania, Philadelphia, Pennsylvania.

GOURI NANJANGUD, PhD
Clinical Cytogenetics Fellow & SRA, Clinical and Molecular Cytogenetics Laboratories, Department of Pathology and Laboratory Medicine, David Geffen School of Medicine, University of California Los Angeles, Los Angeles, California

MARILU NELSON, MS, CG, MB (ASCP)^{CM}
Human Genetics Laboratories, Munroe Meyer Institute for Genetics and Rehabilitation, University of Nebraska Medical Center, Omaha, Nebraska

OLATOYOSI ODENIKE, MD
Assistant Professor of Medicine, Section of Hematology/Oncology, and the Comprehensive Cancer Center, University of Chicago, Chicago, Illinois

ROBERT E. PYATT, PhD
Assistant Director, Cytogenetics and Molecular Genetics Laboratory, Department of Pathology and Laboratory Medicine, Nationwide Children's Hospital, and Department of Pathology, The Ohio State University College of Medicine, Columbus, Ohio

P. NAGESH RAO, PhD, FACMG
Chief, Clinical and Molecular Cytogenetics Laboratories, Professor, Pathology and Laboratory Medicine, David Geffen School of Medicine, University of California Los Angeles, Los Angeles, California

CATHERINE W. REHDER, PhD, FACMG
Department of Pathology, Duke University, Durham, North Carolina

JANET D. ROWLEY, MD, FACMG
Blum Riese Distinguished Service Professor of Medicine, Molecular Genetics & Cell Biology, and Human Genetics, Section of Hematology/Oncology, The University of Chicago, Chicago, Illinois

WARREN G. SANGER, PhD, FACMG
Human Genetics Laboratories, Munroe Meyer Institute for Genetics and Rehabilitation, University of Nebraska Medical Center, Omaha, Nebraska

ANDREA SCHNAITER, MD
Department of Internal Medicine III, University of Ulm, Ulm, Germany

STUART SCHWARTZ, PhD, FACMG
Strategic Director, Cytogenetics, Cytogenetics Laboratory, Laboratory Corporation of America, North Carolina

MARILYN L. SLOVAK, PhD, FACMG
Senior Technical Director, Cytogenetics Laboratory, Quest Diagnostics Nichols Institute, Chantilly, Virginia

SARAH T. SOUTH, PhD
Cytogenetics, Genomic Microarray, Genetic Processing at ARUP Laboratories; Department of Pediatrics and Pathology, University of Utah, Salt Lake City, Utah

STEPHAN STILGENBAUER, MD
Department of Internal Medicine III, University of Ulm, Ulm, Germany

KAREN D. TSUCHIYA, MD
Associate Professor of Laboratory Medicine, University of Washington School of Medicine; Director of Cytogenetics, Seattle Children's Hospital, Seattle, Washington

YANMING ZHANG, MD
Associate Professor, Department of Pathology, Feinberg School of Medicine, and Medical Director, Cytogenetics Laboratory, Northwestern Memorial Hospital, Northwestern University, Chicago, Illinois

Contents

cytogenetics, FISH remains indispensible. While array technology provides a high resolution screen of the entire genome for gains and
losses, it does not allow for visualization of the genomic structure of
gains. Thus, FISH continues to be useful as an adjunct to arrays. FISH
also continues to be widely used in conjunction with banded chromosome analysis, and as a stand-alone technique for the detection of
genomic alterations in neoplastic disorders.

Several new microdeletion and microduplication syndromes have been
discovered in a genotype-first approach. Many of these disorders are
caused by nonallelic homologous recombination between blocks of
segmental duplication. The authors describe 9 regions for which copy
number alteration is proposed to cause an abnormal phenotype. Some
of these disorders have been observed in affected individuals and
individuals lacking a clearly abnormal phenotype. These deletions and
duplications are thought to be contributory, but not always sufficient, to
elicit an abnormal outcome. Additional studies are necessary to further
evaluate the penetrance and delineate the clinical spectrum associated
with many of these newly described disorders.

Many copy number alterations (CNA) currently interpreted as variants of
unknown significance (VUS) will ultimately be determined to be benign;
however, their classification requires a more extensive characterization
of the human genome than currently exists. There is no definitive set of
rules or level of evidence required to define a CNA as benign. The
information needed to accurately assess the pathogenic impact of CNA
is beginning to be assembled. Although the lack of understanding of the
human genome can make clinical array-comparative genomic hybridization interpretation frustrating, it is precisely why clinical human
genetics is an exciting arena in which to work.

Detection of chromosomal abnormalities has evolved over the past 30
years. Microarray analysis allows for the detection of abnormalities at a
level of resolution 100 times greater than chromosomal analysis. In this
article, one specific array, a single nucleotide polymorphism array, is
reviewed. This array not only allows for increased resolution to detect copy
number changes, but the genotyping aspect of the array allows copy
neutral detection (for both uniparental disomy and consanguinity). Additionally, use of this array in constitutional postnatal, prenatal, and products
of conception studies is reviewed along with the use of the array in
oncology studies.

Acute myeloid leukemia (AML) is a complex group of hematologic neoplasms characterized by distinctive morphologic, immunophenotypic, and genetic abnormalities. However, it has become evident that genetic aberrations are central to the genesis of AML and have assumed an increasingly relevant role in the classification of AML. Here we discuss hallmark recurrent translocations that define specific World Health Organization (WHO) entities and other frequently encountered genetic aberrations that do not (yet) define specific entities. Additionally, we discuss emerging technologies and their application to the discovery of new abnormalities and to their potential role in the future diagnosis and classification of AML.

Chronic myeloid leukemia (CML), characterized by the t(9;22) and BCR/ABL1 fusion, is a disease model for studying the mechanisms of genetic abnormalities in leukemogenesis. The detection of the t(9;22), characterization of the BCR/ABL fusion, and the discovery of imatinib have elegantly reflected the success of our research efforts in CML. However, genomic instabilities that lead to the formation of the BCR/ABL1 fusion are not fully understood. It is important to understand how various genes that are involved in regulating the signaling pathway and epigenetic deregulation cooperate with the BCR/ABL1 fusion in the initiation and progression of CML.

Multiple myeloma (MM) is a malignancy of terminally differentiated plasma cells characterized by complex genetic aberrations and heterogeneous outcomes. Over the past 25 years, cytogenetic analysis has played a key role in the diagnosis and management of MM. This article reviews the conventional cytogenetics, molecular cytogenetics, and genomic diagnostics of MM and highlights a few recent clinical trials that demonstrate the impact of genetic risk stratification on the treatment of this plasma cell malignancy.

Lymphomas are a heterogeneous group of neoplasms with distinct morphologic, immunologic, and cytogenetic characteristics. Overlapping morphologic and immunophenotypic features often makes accurate diagnosis difficult. Cytogenetics helps simplify the diagnostic complexities presented in transforming and progressive lymphoid malignancies. Genetic studies using technical advances such as fluorescence in situ hybridization and the newer approaches of array comparative genomic hybridization and gene expression profiling play a critical and often defining role in the diagnosis, progression, prognosis, and therapeutic stratification. This article reviews characteristic cytogenetic abnormalities in specific subtypes of lymphomas at diagnosis, disease progression, and prognosis.

The myelodysplastic syndromes are a diverse group of clonal stem cell disorders characterized by ineffective hematopoiesis, peripheral cytopenias, and an increased propensity to evolve to acute myeloid leukemia. The molecular pathogenesis of these disorders is poorly understood, but recurring chromosomal abnormalities occur in approximately 50% of cases and are the focus of much investigation. The availability of newer molecular techniques has allowed the identification of additional genetic aberrations, including mutations and epigenetic changes of prognostic and potential therapeutic importance. This review focuses on the key role of cytogenetic analysis in myelodysplastic syndromes in the context of the diagnosis, prognosis, and pathogenesis of these disorders.

Conventional cytogenetics in conjunction with Fluorescence in Situ Hybridization (FISH) continues to remain an important and integral component in the diagnosis and management of solid tumors. The ability to effectively detect the vast majority of clinically relevant chromosomal aberrations with a rapid-to-acceptable turnaround time makes them the most cost-effective screening/detection tool currently available in modern pathology. In this review, we describe a representative set of solid tumors in which chromosomal analysis and/or FISH plays a significant role in the routine clinical management of solid tumors.

THE CLINICS ARE NOW AVAILABLE ONLINE!

Access your subscription at:
www.theclinics.com

Preface

Cytogenetics

It has been a great pleasure to serve as guest editor for the Clinical Cytogenetics edition of *Clinics in Laboratory Medicine*. For this issue, I have recruited authors who are experts in their field, from both academic and commercial clinical laboratories, and, while the majority of the authors reside in the United States, an international flavor is supplied by contributions from both the United Kingdom and Germany. I am extremely grateful to all of the authors for their time, effort, and expertise: the importance of clinical cytogenetics continues to be felt in the prenatal, postnatal, and oncological arenas, and the information obtained from analyzing chromosomes remains vital to patients and their physicians.

The first illustrations of chromosomes ("colored bodies") were published in the 1880s. From those early days of chromosome studies to the current clinical techniques for banding and analysis, chromosomes have held an intrinsic beauty for those who study them. The field of cytogenetics has evolved enormously: first with the discovery of the correct number of chromosomes in humans (Tijo and Levan, 1956), to the discovery that nonrandom chromosome rearrangements are a hallmark of many cancers (Nowell and Hungerford, 1960), to the discovery of different stains that revealed the presence of differential banding along each chromosome pair (Caspersson, 1970), to the development of fluorescence in situ hybridization (FISH) techniques (~1986), comparative genomic hybridization (~1992), and microarray technologies, from bacterial artificial chromosome (BAC) to oligonucleotide to single-nucleotide polymorphism (SNP) arrays.

Although some traditional cytogenetic techniques have been superseded by the newer technologies, there is still a basic need for technologists to sit at a microscope and to count and analyze metaphase chromosomes. The article on sex chromosomes and sex chromosome abnormalities by Dr Li emphasizes this fact; the best way to diagnose abnormalities involving the X and Y chromosomes is initially via banded analysis. In addition, chromosome analysis is the most important tool when investigating autosomal aneuploidy and mosaicism, as detailed by Dr Jackson-Cook in her article on "Constitutional and Acquired Autosomal Aneuploidy." While the first microdeletion syndromes to be described (Cri-du-Chat syndrome and Wolf-Hirschhorn syndrome) were readily identified by chromosome analysis, the use of FISH and microarray technologies have expanded the number of contiguous gene syndromes, as reviewed by Dr Rehder and coauthors in their article on the evolving picture of microdeletion/microduplication syndromes. Again, while microarray analysis has become the recommended initial diagnostic tool in patients with certain phenotypic findings such as developmental delay, autism, or unexplained mental retardation, there is still a need for analysis of chromosomes in tandem. This topic is detailed by Dr South in her article discussing cytogenomic technologies to elucidate chromosomal structural rearrangements and the

Clin Lab Med 31 (2011) xiii–xv
doi:10.1016/j.cll.2011.08.017
labmed.theclinics.com
0272-2712/11/$ – see front matter © 2011 Elsevier Inc. All rights reserved.

common mechanisms that lead to phenotypically important imbalances. The utilization and benefits of FISH are referenced in almost every article in this issue of *Clinics in Laboratory Medicine*; Dr Tsuchiya provides a comprehensive and illustrative review of its various applications.

The impact of microarray technologies on the field of clinical cytogenetics cannot be overemphasized. Dr Schwartz summarizes the various clinical applications of SNP-based microarrays. Dr Lamb discusses the issues associated with designing, running, and reporting prenatal microarrays, while Dr Pyatt and I summarize the interpretation of copy number alterations detected by oligoarray in postnatal analyses in our laboratory. Dr Kerney and coauthors discuss some of the diagnostic implications of SNP-based microarrays, focusing on consanguinity, uniparental disomy, and recessive single-gene mutations.

The articles on acquired chromosomal abnormalities cover the majority of hematological tumors. There is a broad theme to each of these articles, in that specific chromosomal rearrangements are frequently associated with specific types of cancer and have diagnostic, prognostic, and therapeutic implications. Professor Harrison describes the impact cytogenetics has had on the outcome and long-term survival of children with acute lymphoblastic leukemia. Drs Zhang and Rowley discuss chronic myelogenous leukemia, a disease that has served as an excellent model for our understanding of the mechanisms of genetic abnormalities in leukomogenesis. The discovery of specific genes that are involved in the initiation and progression of many cancers has led to the development of successful targeted drug therapies. Dr Schnaiter and coauthors describe the key genes associated with chronic lymphocytic leukemia, as well as the prospective applications of SNP arrays and Next Gen Sequencing in the clinical setting. Drs Morrissette and Bagg discuss conventional cytogenetics, FISH, and moleculocentric methodologies as applied to acute myeloid leukemia, summarizing the multifaceted approach to its diagnosis and treatment. The theme of combined chromosome analysis with FISH and array technologies is continued in the comprehensive article on myelodysplastic syndromes (MDS) by Dr Le Beau and colleagues; the authors emphasize the fact that cytogenetic analysis in MDS is critical for therapeutic decision-making in this disease. The article on multiple myeloma by Dr Slovak also points to the importance of the analysis of cytogenetic alterations in clonal plasma cells to enable ultimately genetic risk stratification. Dr Dave and coauthors' article on lymphomas describes the role cytogenetics has played in categorizing the various subtypes of this disease, which has led to a greater understanding of the genetic changes which have prognostic implications. All of these articles emphasize the importance of elucidating the pathogenesis of these diseases, so as to guide therapeutic targets and risk stratification and to tailor specific treatments to individuals.

Last, Dr Rao and colleagues discuss the cytogenetics of specific solid tumors, such as sarcomas, gliomas, and lung and bladder cancer, among others. In conjunction with cytology, histology, and morphology, conventional karyotyping in association with FISH has become an essential tool in the diagnosis, classification, and prognosis of these tumors.

In conclusion, by the time there is another issue of *Clinics in Laboratory Medicine* dedicated to the topic of Clinical Cytogenetics, it may be that whole genome sequencing or other as yet unidentified technologies will be the primary clinical tool in diagnosing a child with Down syndrome, or identifying the couple carrying a balanced translocation, or determining the specific mutation that leads to a relapsed acute myelogenous leukemia. Although new technologies have enhanced and broadened the field of clinical cytogenetics, I believe that there will always be a need for someone, be it a technologist, director, or pathologist, to look at colored bodies/ chromosomes and to report on their fascinating findings.

Caroline Astbury, PhD
Cytogenetics and Molecular Genetics Laboratory
Department of Pathology and Laboratory Medicine
Nationwide Children's Hospital, 700 Children's Drive
Columbus, OH 43205, USA

Department of Pathology
The Ohio State University College of Medicine
129 Hamilton Hall, 1645 Neil Avenue
Columbus, OH 43210, USA

E-mail address:
caroline.astbury@nationwidechildrens.org

Sex Chromosomes and Sex Chromosome Abnormalities

Xu Li, MD, PhD

KEYWORDS
- Sex chromosome • Sex chromosome abnormalities
- X-inactivation • Mosaicism • X-linked mental retardation

The X and Y chromosomes are the two sex chromosomes in humans. Females have two X chromosomes, whereas males have one X and one Y chromosome. It is believed that the X was named by earlier researchers as unknown and the Y was named alphabetically after X. Compared with the 22 pairs of autosomes in humans, the pair of the sex chromosomes is unique in many aspects.

- The X chromosome is much larger and more gene-rich than the Y chromosome. The X chromosome is 2.6 times the size of the Y chromosome, containing 155.27 Mb or 5% of the total genome of 3.10 billion base pairs (bp), whereas the Y chromosome contains 59.37 Mb or 1.9% of the total genome. There are 1965 genes in an X chromosome compared with 421 genes in the Y chromosome. The gene density in the X chromosome is 17.8-fold higher than the Y chromosome, 1 gene per 7901 bp in X versus 1 gene per 141,029 bp in Y (**Table 1**).[1]
- Unlike the X chromosome, the main function of the Y chromosome is in male sexual development. The presence of the Y chromosome, specifically the gene *SRY* (sex-determining region Y) or TDF (testis-determining factor) located at Yp11.3, determines a male gender, whereas the absence of the *SRY* gene results in a female phenotype. However, many other genes located on the X chromosome and autosomes are also involved in sex determination and development. The other Y-specific genes also play a role in spermatogenesis.
- Pairing and recombination between the X and the Y chromosomes during male meiosis only occurs between homologous segments located on both ends of the X and the Y chromosomes, the so-called *pseudoautosomal regions* (PAR). The ends of the Xp/Yp, or PAR1 region, are 2.64 Mb in size with 24 genes and transcripts, and the ends of the Xq/Yq, or PAR2 region, are 330 kb in size with 8 genes and transcripts (**Fig. 1**).[1] The genes in the PAR regions act like genes in the autosomes and do not follow sex-linked inheritance. The suppression of X-Y recombination through evolution prevents sex-determining genes on the Y

The author has nothing to disclose.
Department of Genetics, Kaiser Permanente, San Jose Medical Center, San Jose, CA 95123, USA
E-mail address: xu.li@kp.org

Table 1
X and Y chromosome statistics

	X	Y
Length (bp)	155,270,560	59,373,566
Known protein-coding genes	825	47
Novel protein-coding genes	27	12
Pseudogene	762	318
MicroRNA genes	128	15
Ribosomal RNA genes	22	7
Small nuclear RNA genes	85	17
snoRNA genes	64	3
Miscellaneous RNA genes	52	2
Total genes	1965	421
Single-nucleotide polymorphisms	1,342,023	273,615

Data from Human Genome Build 19, UCSC, Ensembl release 61—Feb 2011. http://may2009.archive. ensembl.org/Homo_sapiens/Location/Chromosome?r=X:1-154913754 and http://may2009.archive. ensembl.org/Homo_sapiens/Location/Chromosome?r=Y. Accessed April 15, 2011.

chromosome moving to the X chromosome. However, the repairing function for accumulated mutations on the Y chromosome relies on its unusual abundant segmented duplications organized in palindrome structures.[2,3]

- The huge difference in size and gene content between the X and the Y chromosomes has created an "inequality" between the two sexes. To compensate, one X chromosome in females is inactivated and forms a Barr body during early embryogenesis. X-inactivation, or lyonization, is regulated by the gene called inactive X (Xi)-specific transcript (*XIST*) located at the X-inactivation center on the proximal long (q) arm of the X chromosome (Xq13.2) (see **Fig. 1**). Normally, X-inactivation occurs in a random fashion in female somatic cells and results in somatic mosaicism. X-inactivation may happen nonrandomly or skewed as a mechanism to minimize harm when there are structural abnormalities involving an X chromosome such as deletions, duplications, and translocations. For this reason a female carrier may be phenotypically normal but a male is affected or will not survive even though he has the same X chromosome abnormality. Incomplete skewed X-inactivation is often the basis for various degrees of manifestation of phenotypes in females with X chromosome abnormalities. Genes in the PAR regions are not subject to X-inactivation. Many genes on the X chromosome, most of them on the short (p) arm, escape from inactivation. Dosage imbalance of the genes in PAR regions and genes that escape X-inactivation contribute to the phenotypes in females with an X chromosome anomaly.[4,5]

- Although mosaicism is not unique in sex chromosome abnormalities, the consequences are not as straightforward as in autosomes. This is particularly true in external genital appearance, which may vary from female ambiguous external genitalia, male of hermaphroditism depending on the type, level, and distribution of the mosaicism. The presence of a cell line with the Y chromosome (SRY locus) in females or the presence of a 45,X cell line in males has the greatest influence on gender appearance and sexual development.

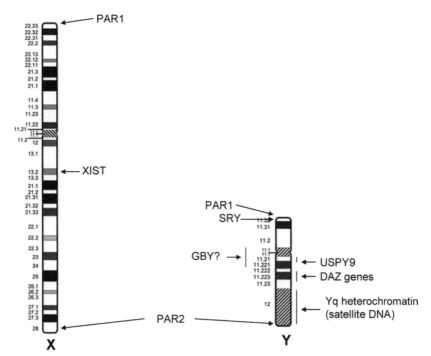

Fig. 1. X and Y chromosomes. (Idiograms are from International System for Human Cytogenetic Nomenclature (ISCN) 2009, *Data from* Nussbaum R, McInnes RR, Willard HF. Thompson & Thompson Genetics in Medicine. 6th edition. Saunders: Elsevier; 2004.)

SEX CHROMOSOME ABNORMALITIES

From the point of view of clinical cytogenetics, this article focuses on constitutional sex chromosome abnormalities detected by conventional cytogenetics and fluorescence in situ hybridization (FISH). To simplify, sex chromosome abnormalities are classified into numerical and structural abnormalities, each further divided into the presence or absence of the Y chromosome as well as involvement of both the X and Y chromosomes by genotype (karyotype).

Sex Chromosome Numerical Abnormalities

Klinefelter syndrome (47,XXY) is the most common sex chromosome numerical abnormality in males, occurring in 1 in 1000 males. It is often diagnosed by chromosome analysis following a referral for infertility or gynecomastia. The 47,XYY syndrome is another common abnormality in males, also occurring in 1 in 1000 males. It is often an accidental finding in chromosome analysis or observed in individuals referred to cytogenetics as part of laboratory tests to rule out fragile X syndrome because of behavioral problems. Some rare forms of sex chromosome numerical aberrations in males have been reported, including 48,XXYY, 48,XXXY, 49,XXXXY, and 49,XYYYY. A chromosome number over 50 with 6 or more sex chromosomes has never been reported and is likely lethal. For every extra X chromosome the IQ decreases about 15 to 16 points, with language most affected.[6] All these patients have global developmental delay in gross motor, fine motor, and speech and language. Males with 48,XXYY have a higher IQ and adapt better in daily living skills compared with 48,XXXY and 49,XXXXY males, but all seem equally problematic with regard to communication and socialization skills.[7] The intellectual deficiency in males with poly Y, such as 49,XYYYY, is not as proportional as in poly X.[8] Height seems to be increased with the gain of an extra Y chromosome but decreased with the gain of an extra X chromosome.

Turner syndrome, or 45,X, is one of the most common sex chromosome numerical aberrations in females, occurring in 1 in 5000 females. The great majority of nonmosaic 45,X conceptions do not survive to term. It is still debatable whether all the surviving individuals with a nonmosaic 45,X karyotype found in amniotic fluid or a peripheral blood sample are actually mosaic in other types of tissues. The 47,XXX syndrome is seen in 1 in 5000 females and is often found by accident rather than because of a specific clinical indication. The majority of individuals with 47,XXX are not diagnosed. Although the clinical phenotype is usually mild, recent reviews suggest that many clinical issues need to be addressed.[9–11] As in males, some rare forms of polysomy for the X chromosome, 48,XXXX[12] and 49,XXXXX[13,14] will result in severe developmental delay, mental retardation, and behavioral problems.

Mosaicism in sex chromosome abnormalities can present in a variety of combinations and potentially with different degrees of mosaicism in different tissues. This presents a great challenge in the clinical assessment of phenotypes, in particular when found in prenatal samples. Phenotypes are usually milder when there is a normal cell line, male or female, present, such as mosaic Turner syndrome or Klinefelter syndrome.[15] However, gender or sexual development can range from male to female to ambiguous when there is a mixture of cell lines with or without the Y chromosome (**Table 2**).

Some rare forms of mosaicism have been reported, such as Klinefelter variant with a 46,XX cell line[20,21] or mosaic 45,X/47,XYY or 45,X/46,XY/47,XYY.[22,23] Mosaicism may be present in as many as 4 or 5 different cell lines.[24,25] Whether the patient has a Turner syndrome phenotype largely depends on the percentage and the distribution of the 45,X cell line, and whether the patient has male external genitalia depends on the presence in the gonads of a Y chromosome containing cell line. Caution should be taken when interpreting a low percentage of X chromosome aneuploidy in advanced aged women, usually referred to cytogenetics with recurrent miscarriages. The most common karyotypes are 45,X/46,XX and 45,X/47,XXX/46,XX. X chromosome aneuploidy is usually under 10%. These women usually do not have a Turner syndrome phenotype, and there is no evidence that the finding is associated with miscarriages.[15,17–19] However, if the woman is younger and/or the X chromosome aneuploidy level is higher than expected for her age, careful clinical evaluation is warranted (**Table 3**).[26]

Sex Chromosome Structural Abnormalities

Y chromosome

The Y chromosome contains genes in the pseudoautosomal regions, which are also present on the X chromosome, as well as genes involved in sexual development. Deletions of Yp cause short stature (*SHOX*) and XY females (*SRY*), whereas deletions of Yq, including ring Y, results in infertility.[15,27,29] Y chromosome structural rearrangements with intellectual deficiency have been reported,[28] but it is unclear whether it was a coincidental finding. An isochromosome of Yp or i(Yp) has two copies of Yp including the PAR1 and the *SRY* gene. Isodicentric Y or idic(Y) contains two copies of Yp and proximal Yq. Infertility is inevitable in i(Yp) and likely in idic(Y), because the *DAZ* genes are usually deleted. Patients may have phenotypes resembling 47,XYY.

Table 2
Sex chromosome numerical abnormalities

Karyotype	Gender	Disorder	Phenotype
			Presence of the Y Chromosome
47,XXY	Male	Klinefelter syndrome	Tall, infertile, hypogonadism, small testicles, breast enlargement, learning difficulty in some including speech and language, motor skills, and educational achievement[9]
47,XYY	Male	XYY syndrome	Tall, normal sexual development, normal intelligence, behavioral problems are common, some have deficiency in speech and language, motor skills, and educational achievement[9]
48,XXYY	Male	XXYY syndrome	Similar to 47,XXY, tall stature, gynecomastia, hypergonadotropic hypogonadism, infertility but with more severe neurodevelopmental and psychological features including developmental delay, learning disabilities and behavioral problems, attention deficit hyperactivity disorder, autism spectrum, and mood, psychotic, and tic disorders. Other medical problems include allergies and asthma, congenital heart defects, radioulnar synostosis, inguinal hernia and/or cryptorchidism, seizures, intention tremor, and type 2 diabetes. IQs range from 60 to 80, with 10% having an IQ above 80[6,7,16]
48,XXXY	Male	Poly X	Average to tall stature with hypertelorism, flat nasal bridge, small penis and testicles, infertility, and gynecomastia (due to hypergonadotropic hypogonadism), and global developmental delay in gross motor, fine motor, and speech and language, IQ = 40–60[6,7]
49,XXXXY	Male	Poly X	Coarse face with microcephaly, ocular hypertelorism, flat nasal bridge, and upslanting palpebral fissures. Bifid uvula and/or cleft palate and skeletal abnormalities including radioulnar synostosis, genu valgum, pes cavus, or clinodactyly may be present. Most have short stature with hypotonia and hyperextensible joints. Genitalia are underdeveloped with hypergonadotropic hypogonadism. IQ = 20–60[6,7]
49,XYYYY	Male	Poly Y	Minor facial anomalies, cardiac and urinary tract abnormalities, hypogonadism, tall stature, delayed or disassociated bone development, mental retardation, and behavior problems[8]

(continued on next page)

Table 2
(continued)

Karyotype	Gender	Disorder	Phenotype
			Absence of the Y Chromosome
45,X	Female	Turner syndrome	Short stature, gonadal failure with infertility, IQ can be in normal range but reduced compared with siblings. Vulnerable in social adaptation. Diminished abilities in visual-spatial and perceptual skills[15]
47,XXX	Female	Trisomy X	Tall stature, in young girls motor and language delay are common, normal fertility but premature ovarian failure may be more common. IQ levels are 20 points below that of controls, and verbal IQ is lowest[9–11]
48,XXXX	Female	48,XXXX syndrome	Tall stature is common. Minor facial dysmorphic features. Skeletal anomalies include clinodactyly and radioulnar synostosis. Genitalia are usually normal, but development of secondary sex characteristics can be incomplete. About 50% have menstrual dysfunction. Mental retardation is characteristic with an average IQ of 60. Behavioral problems are common[6,12]
49,XXXXX	Female	Pentasomy X syndrome	Dysmorphic feature similar to Down syndrome with mental retardation and developmental delay, craniofacial, skeletal, and cardiovascular anomalies[6,13,14]
			Mosaicism (with or without the Y chromosome)
45,X/46,XX 45,X/47,XXX 45,X/47,XXX/46,XX	Female	Mosaic Turner syndrome	Milder Turner phenotypes.[15] NOTE: When found in <10% of cells in advanced aged women it is likely age-related with no clinical significance[15,17–19]

(continued on next page)

Table 2
(continued)

Karyotype	Gender	Disorder	Phenotype
45,X/46,XY 45,X/46,XY/47,XYY 45,X/47,XYY	Male/ female/ ambiguous	Sex chromosome aneuploidy	May have short stature. External genitalia may present as male, female, or ambiguous.[15,20,21]
47,XXY/46,XY	Male	Mosaic Klinefelter	Milder Klinefelter phenotype.[15]
47,XXY/46,XX 47,XXY/46,XY/ 46,XX or other combinations	Male	Klinefelter variant	Milder but variable Klinefelter phenotype. Hypergonadotropic hypogonadism. Normal average stature and have normal secondary sexual male features with small testes; sterile. Testicular histopathology reveals atrophy of the testes with no spermatogenesis and absence of germ cells.[20,21]

Table 3
Sex chromosome structural abnormalities

Karyotype	Gender	Disorder	Phenotype
		Y Chromosome	
del(Yp)	Male/female	Yp deletion	Deletion of *SRY* results in a XY female. Presence of a 45,X cell line is possible[15]
del(Yq)	Male	Yq deletion	Infertility, intellectual deficiency?, nonobstructive azoospermia and oligozoospermia. AZFa = USP9Y, AZFc = DAZ genes, AZFb = overlapped with AZFc? (OMIM 415000). Presence of a 45,X cell line is possible[27,28]
r(Y) and marker Y	Male/female	Deletion of Yp and/or Yq	Depends on the breakpoints on Yp and Yq (see Yp and Yq deletion)[15,29]
i(Y)(p10)	Male/female/ambiguous	Two copies of Yp and deletion of Yq	Infertile, hypospadias, testicular defect, may have similar phenotypic findings as seen in XYY, presence of a 45,X cell line is common[15]
idic(Y)(q11.21-q12)	Male/female/ambiguous	Two copies of Yp and proximal Yq and partial deletion of Yq	May be infertile depending on the breakpoint in Yq, may have similar phenotypic findings as seen in XYY, presence of a 45,X cell line is common, most as male (>20%) but can be female or ambiguous[20–32]
t(Y;A)	Male	Y;autosome translocation	Infertile[15]
t(Y;Y)	Male/ambiguous	Y;Y translocation	May have infertility, a 45,X cell line may present[22,33,34]
Yqs	Male	Y;acrocentric chromosome translocation	der(15)t(Y;15)(q12;p12) or der(22)t(Y;22)(q12;p12) are most common. Normal variants with no clinical significance[15]

(continued on next page)

Table 3
(continued)

Karyotype	Gender	Disorder	Phenotype
		X Chromosome	
del(Xp)	Female/male	Contiguous deletion syndromes in males/Turner variant in females	X-linked idiopathic short stature (*SHOX*) in both males and females. Contiguous deletion syndromes in males: Leri-Weill dyschondrosteosis (*SHOX*), chondrodysplasia punctata (*ARSE*), mental retardation (*NLGN4*), ichthyosis (*STS*), Kallmann syndrome (KAL1), ocular albinism (*GPR143*), congenital adrenal hypoplasia (*DAX1*), glycerol kinase deficiency (*GK*), and Duchenne muscular dystrophy (*DMD*)[35-38](OMIM 300002, OMIM 300697)
del(Xq)	Female/male	Xq deletions/Infertility POF	Male: few survive, certain regions lethal, MR and/or multiple congenital anomalies.[39-42] Female: POF, infertility, regions in Xq are critical for ovarian development[15,40,43]
46,XY,dup(X)(p21)	Female	Xp21 duplication including *DAX1*	Male-to-female sex reversal (OMIM 30018).
dup(Xq)	Female/male	Xq duplications	Male: variable depending on genes involved, including MR, short stature, microcephaly, hemihyperplasia, and digital anomalies[41-44] Female: asymptomatic or mild phenotype[45]

(continued on next page)

Table 3
(continued)

Karyotype	Gender	Disorder	Phenotype
rec(X)	Female/male	Deletion and duplication of Xp/Xq	Recombinant from a parental pericentric inversion. Deletion of one end of X and duplication of the other end. Males have a phenotype consistent with deletions/duplications of Xp/Xq[46]
idic(Xp)	Female only	Xq deletions	Always contains proximal part of Xq including the XIST locus?, otherwise lethal[32,47]
i(Xq)	Female only	Monosomy for Xp and trisomy for Xq, Turner variant	Turner syndrome phenotype[15]
r(X)/marker X	Female only	Xp/Xq deletions	Resemble deletions of Xp and Xq depending on the breakpoints. Mental retardation if XIST is not included
t(X;A)	Female	X;autosome translocation	POF and/or infertility may be the only phenotypic finding even in unbalanced forms, but may have mild MR if X-inactivation is not completely skewed to the normal X chromosome
t(X;X)	Female	X;X translocation	Increased risk for infertility or POF
Micro del(X), dup(X)	Female/male	Microdeletion/microduplication	X-linked MR, not detected by conventional cytogenetics but by aCGH. See discussion in text

(continued on next page)

Table 3
(continued)

Karyotype	Gender	Disorder	Phenotype
		X:Y Translocation[15]	
46,X,der(X)t(Xp;Yq)	Female	Partial monosomy for Xp and additional Yq material	Most cases are familial; short or normal stature, normal intelligence, fertile, history of SAB. Predominant activation of t(X;Y) is associated with hypoplastic internal genitalia and polycystic ovaries. Increased risk for gonadoblastoma?
46,Y,der(X)t(X;Y)(p22.3;q12)	Male	Nullisomic for Xp and partial disomy for Yq	Most cases are familial; infertile, males may have one or more of contiguous deletions syndromes depending on the breakpoints (see Xp deletion)[48]
46,X,der(X)t(X;Y)(p22.3;p11.3)	Male	SRY gene translocated to Xp	Sporadic. Accounts for 80% of 46,XX males
46,X,der(Y)t(X;Y)(p21;p11.3)	Female	Sex reversal	SRY+; duplication of DAX1. MR, hypotonia, dysmorphic facial features, and sex reversal[49]
46,X,der(Y)t(Xq;Yq)	Male	Yq monosomy (heterochromatin) and Xq disomy	Sporadic. Phenotypic findings minimal
Karyotype	Gender	**Mosaicism** Disorder	Phenotype
45,X/der(Y)	Female	Mosaic Turner with visible or cryptic derivative Y	Risk for gonadoblastoma, refer to guideline[50] whether to perform FISH and/or PCR to rule out a cryptic derivative Y chromosome in Turner patients
45,X/der(X)	Female	Turner variants with a rearranged X	Turner phenotype

Abbreviations: aCGH, array comparative genomic hybridization; MR, mental retardation; PCR, polymerase chain reaction; POF, premature ovarian failure; SAB, spontaneous abortion.

More significantly, a mosaic karyotype with a 45,X cell line is very common, in particular in patients with idic(Y).[51,52] This is because the idic(Y) cell line is unstable and often lost during mitosis. If conventional chromosome analysis does not reveal a 45,X cell line, interphase FISH is warranted. The patient's gender may present as male, female, or ambiguous. The factors that affect gender may include the percentage and distribution of the 45,X cell line, the timing of the mitotic loss of the idic(Y) during gonadal ontogenesis, and the proportion of *SRY*-positive pre-Sertoli cells in the gonad.[30–32] Translocations between the Y chromosome and an autosome may cause infertility. Y;Y translocations are rare. Infertility and the presence of a 45,X cell line with mixed gonadal dysgenesis have been reported.[22,33,34]

X chromosome

Obviously, any genomic imbalances, deletions, or duplications of an X chromosome have a much more severe impact on males than females. Actually, males can only tolerate or survive larger deletions in certain regions of the X chromosome, 10 to 11 Mb from the terminal Xp region[35–37] and Xq26-X27.3 region including the *FMR1* gene.[38] The largest reported Xq deletion in males is about 13 Mb.[39] Therefore, idic(Xp), i(Xq), small r(X), and marker X are only observed in live-born females. Partial deletions of Xp in males result in contiguous gene deletion syndromes including Leri-Weill dyschondrosteosis (*SHOX*), chondrodysplasia punctata (*ARSE*), mental retardation (*NLGN4*), ichthyosis (*STS*), Kallmann syndrome (*KAL1*), ocular albinism (*GPR143*), congenital adrenal hypoplasia (*DAX1*), glycerol kinase deficiency (*GK*), and Duchenne muscular dystrophy (*DMD*).[35–38] Deletions in Xq26-q27 cause severe mental retardation and multiple congenital anomalies.[39,40] Duplications may also cause severe phenotypes in males, such as sex reversal (Xp21 including *DAX1*) (OMIM 30018), hemihyperplasia and digital anomalies (Xq25),[41] mental retardation (*MECP2* at Xq28)[42] and other congenital anomalies (Xq21-q25).[44] The clinical consequences for females are more difficult to predict. A large deletion of Xq in a female was reported to have a normal phenotype.[45] Most females with X chromosome imbalances have no to variable phenotypes. The manifestation of certain phenotypes in females is most likely because of the inability of or incomplete skewed X-inactivation.[40] Isochromosome Xp without proximal Xq or including the *XIST* locus is likely lethal.[32,47] Ring X and marker X in females may cause mental retardation if the *XIST* locus is not included because the abnormal X cannot be inactivated. In general, a karyotype with a deletion of Xp including the *SHOX* gene will have Turner syndrome phenotypic findings, including short stature. A deletion of part of Xq or an interruption of Xq (translocations or inversions) will have an increased risk for malfunction of the ovaries, such as premature ovarian failure (POF) or infertility. A female with an unbalanced t(X;18) translocation had diminished ovarian reserve, but her mother with the same unbalanced translocation had normal fertility. X-inactivation studies on peripheral blood samples showed skewed inactivation of the normal X in both mother and daughter. Therefore, there are likely other genes that act as a modifier for the variable expression of the phenotypes.[43] The presence of a 45,X cell line is very common in individuals with X chromosome structural rearrangements, such as del(Xp), idic(Xp), i(Xq), and r(X). These patients have mosaic karyotypes as Turner syndrome variants.

The presence of Y chromosome material in Turner patients increases the risk for gonadoblastoma (GBY) in phenotypic females, especially with dysgenetic gonads.[53] Whether to rule out the presence of cryptic Y material by FISH or polymerase chain reaction in Turner patients has not yet become standard practice. A laboratory

Table 4
Hermaphroditism and chimerism

Karyotype	Gender	Disorder	Comment
46,XX/46,XY	Ambiguous external genitalia	Chimerism or mosaicism	Fusion of twin XX and XY embryos or postzygotic loss of the X and the Y in separate cells of a 47,XXY conception
46,XX	Ambiguous genitalia	True hermaphroditism	Cryptic mosaicism of *SRY*+ cell line in gonads or mutations of other genes involved in sexual development
46,XY	Ambiguous genitalia	True hermaphroditism	*SRY* gene mutation or mutations of other genes involved in sexual development
46,XX	Male	XX male	Xp;Yp translocation with the *SRY* gene to Xp is most common; rare case with 45,X karyotype and a t(Y;A) has been observed
46,XY	Female	XY female	1. XY pure gonadal dysgenesis. 2. X-linked/autosomal recessive. A mutation in an X-linked/autosomal gene controlling a later event in the testis developmental pathway. 3. Y-linked. A mutation in *SRY*. 4. Complete androgen insensitivity syndrome (testicular feminization) X-linked recessive. Mutations in the androgen receptor gene (Xq11-13). 5. XY female with extragonadal defects: campomelic dysplasia with sex reversal: mutations in the *SOX9* gene (17q24.3-q25.1) and dosage sensitive sex reversal: duplication of *DSS* gene at Xp21.3. Steroid enzyme deficiencies: autosomal recessive

From Gardner RJM, Sutherland GR. Chromosome abnormalities and genetic counseling. 3rd edition. New York: Oxford University Press; 2004.

guideline has been published by the American College of Medical Genetics Laboratory Quality Assurance Committee.[50]

Hermaphroditism, chimerism, XX males, and XY females

True hermaphroditism, defined as the presence of both ovarian and testicular tissue and ambiguous external genitalia, with a chimeric karyotype 46,XX/46,XY, is extremely rare. The likely mechanisms are either fusion of twin XX and XY embryos or postzygotic loss of the X and the Y chromosomes in separate cells of an 47,XXY conception.[15] True hermaphroditism can also have a 46,XX and 45,X/46,XX karyotype with cryptic mosaicism for an *SRY*-positive cell line in the gonads[54] or a 46,XY karyotype with an *SRY* gene mutation or mutations of other genes involved in the sexual development pathway.[55] Overreaction to the presence of a 46,XX/46,XY karyotype in a prenatal chromosome analysis should be avoided. In almost all cases, the 46, XX cell line is due to maternal cell contamination. Although in theory one of the cell lines is from an absorbed or vanishing twin, it is difficult to prove clinically. Ultrasonography can be offered to assure there are no ambiguous external genitalia. Molecular tests for maternal cell contamination can be used for further assurance if needed.

The Xp;Yp translocation involving the *SRY* gene is the most common cause for an XX male. A rare case with a 45,X karyotype and a cryptic t(Yp;18p) translocation has been observed (X.L, unpublished observation, 2002). Causes for XY females are usually not chromosomal but are mainly due to mutations in the *SRY* gene or in genes involved in sexual determination and development pathways, such as androgen insensitivity syndrome (**Table 4**).[56]

Submicroscopic X chromosome abnormalities and future perspectives

The merging of technologies in recent years has blurred the line between conventional cytogenetics and molecular genetics in a clinical laboratory. Chromosomal microarray analysis or array comparative genomic hybridization (aCGH) has greatly increased the resolution in the detection of chromosome imbalances. Array CGH can also define the breakpoints much more precisely and provides information about genes involved for phenotype prediction and genotype-phenotype correlation. Hundreds of syndromes have been associated with genes located on the X chromosome, and at least 95 nonsyndromic X-linked mental retardation (XMR) loci (OMIM) have been mapped to the X chromosome. Many of the microdeletion and microduplication syndromes and XMR have been detected by aCGH in recent years. Furthermore, XMR panels have been developed recently using a combination of aCGH and next-generation whole genome sequencing technologies for clinical diagnosis.[57] The data are accumulating at a very rapid pace, and the topic is beyond the scope of this review.

REFERENCES

1. Human Genome Build 19, UCSC, Ensembl release 61—Feb 2011. http://may2009.archive.ensembl.org/Homo_sapiens/Location/Chromosome?r=X:1-154913754 and http://may2009.archive.ensembl.org/Homo_sapiens/Location/Chromosome?r=Y. Accessed April 15, 2011.
2. Skaletsky H, Kuroda-Kawaguchi T, Minx PJ, et al. The male-specific region of the human Y chromosome is a mosaic of discrete sequence classes. Nature 2003;423: 825–37.
3. Rozen S, Skaletsky H, Marszalek JD, et al. Abundant gene conversion between arms of palindromes in human and ape Y chromosomes. Nature 2003;423:873–6.

4. Carrell L, Willard HF. X-inactivation profile reveals extensive variability in X-linked gene expression in females Nature 2005;17:400–4.
5. Payer B, Lee JT. X chromosome dosage compensation: how mammals keep the balance. Annu Rev Genet 2008;42:733–72.
6. Linden MG, Bender BG, Robinson A. Sex chromosome tetrasomy and pentasomy. Pediatrics 1995;96:672–82.
7. Tartaglia N, Ayari N, Howell S, et al. Behavioral phenotype of sex chromosome aneuploidies: 48,XXYY, 48,XXXY, and 49,XXXXY. Acta Paediatr 2011;10:1651–2227.
8. Shanske A, Sachmechi I, Patel DK, et al. An adult with 49,XYYYY karyotype: case report and endocrine studies. Am J Med Genet 1998;80(2):103–6.
9. Leggett V, Jacobs P, Nation K, et al. Neurocognitive outcomes of individuals with a sex chromosome trisomy: XXX, XYY, or XXY: a systematic review. Dev Med Child Neurol 2010;52:119–29.
10. Maarten O. Triple X syndrome: a review of the literature. Eur J Hum Genet 2010;18: 265–71.
11. Tartaglia NR, Howell S, Sutherland A, et al. Review of trisomy X (47,XXX). Orphanet J Rare Dis 2010;11:5:8.
12. Rooman RP, Van Driessche K, Du Caju MV. Growth and ovarian function in girls with 48,XXXX karyotype--patient report and review of the literature. J Pediatr Endocrinol Metab 2002;15(7):1051–5.
13. Kassai R, Hamada I, Furuta H, et al. Penta X syndrome: a case report with review of the literature. Am J Med Genet 1991;40:51–6.
14. Cho YG, Kim DS, Lee HS, et al. A case of 49,XXXXX in which the extra X chromosomes were maternal in origin J Clin Pathol 2004;57:1004–6.
15. Gardner RJM, Sutherland GR. Chromosome abnormalities and genetic counseling. 3rd edition. New York: Oxford University Press; 2004.
16. Tartaglia N, Davis S, Hench A, et al. A new look at XXYY syndrome: medical and psychological features. Am J Med Genet A 2008;15:1509–22.
17. Guttenbach M, Koschorz B, Bernthaler U, et al. Sex chromosome loss and aging: in situ hybridization studies on human interphase nuclei. Am J Hum Genet 1995;57: 1143–50.
18. Russell LM, Strike P, Browne CE, et al. X chromosome loss and ageing. Cytogenet Genome Res 2007;116:181–5.
19. Bukvic N, Gentile M, Susca F, et al. Sex chromosome loss, micronuclei, sister chromatid exchange and aging: a study including 16 centenarians. Mutat Res 2001;15;498(1–2):159–67.
20. Velissariou V, Christopoulou S, Karadimas C, et al. Rare XXY/XX mosaicism in a phenotypic male with Klinefelter syndrome: case report. Eur J Med Genet 2006;49(4): 331–7.
21. Mark HF, Bai H, Sotomayor E, et al. A variant Klinefelter syndrome patient with an XXY/XX/XY karyotype studied by GTG-banding and fluorescence in situ hybridization. Exp Mol Pathol 1999;67(1):50–6.
22. Hsu LYF. Phenotype/karyotype correlations of Y chromosome aneuploidy with emphasis on structural aberrations in postnatally diagnosed cases. Am J Med Genet 1994;53:108-40.
23. Pettenati MJ, Wheeler M, Bartlett DJ, et al. 45,X/47,XYY mosaicism: clinical discrepancy between prenatally and postnatally diagnosed cases. Am J Med Genet 1991; 39:42–7.
24. Al-Awadi SA, Teebi AS, Krishna Murthy DS, et al. Klinefelter's syndrome, mosaic 46,XX/46,XY/47,XXY/48,XXXY/48,XXYY: a case report. Ann Genet 1986;29(2): 119–21.

25. Zamora L, Espinet B, Salido M, et al. Report of 46,XX/46,XY/47,XXY/48,XXYY mosaicism in an adult phenotypic male. Am J Med Genet 2002;111(2):215–7.

26. Homer L, Le Martelot MT, Morel F, et al. 45,X/46,XX mosaicism below 30% of aneuploidy: clinical implications in adult women from a reproductive medicine unit. Eur J Endocrinol 2010;162(3):617–23.

27. Krausz C, Forti G, Mcelreavey K. The Y chromosome and male fertility and infertility. Int J Androl 2003;26:70–5.

28. Tyson C, Dawson AJ, Bal S. Molecular cytogenetic investigation of two patients with Y chromosome rearrangements and intellectual disability. Am J Med Genet A 2009; 149A(3):490–5.

29. Lin YH, Lin YM, Lin YH, et al. Ring (Y) in two azoospermic men. Am J Med Genet A 2004;128A(2):209–13.

30. Xu J, Siu VM. Is there a correlation between the proportion of cells with isodicentric Yp at amniocentesis and phenotypic sex? Prenat Diagn 2010;30(9):839–44.

31. Shinawi M, Cain MP, Vanderbrink BA, et al. Mixed gonadal dysgenesis in a child with isodicentric Y chromosome: does the relative proportion of the 45,X line really matter? Am J Med Genet A 2010;152A(7):1832–7.

32. Dalton P, Coppin B, James R, et al. Three patients with a 45,X/46,X,psu dic(Xp) karyotype. J Med Genet 1998;35(6):519–24.

33. Butler MG, Sanger WG, Walzak MP. A unique Y/Y translocation in an infertile male. Cytogenet Cell Genet 1981;31(3):175–7.

34. Parcheta B, Skawin'ski W, Wis'niewski L. DNA content and the size of Y chromosome in a patient with mixed gonadal dysgenesis and 45,X/46,Xt(Y;Y) (pter leads to q12::q12 leads to q11) karyotype]. Ginekol Pol 1982;53(12):889–95 [In Polish].

35. Lonardo F, Parenti G, Luquetti DV, et al. Contiguous gene syndrome due to an interstitial deletion in Xp22.3 in a boy with ichthyosis, chondrodysplasia punctata, mental retardation and ADHD. Eur J Med Genet 2007;50(4):301–8.

36. Melichar VO, Guth S, Hellebrand H, et al. A male infant with a 9.6 Mb terminal Xp deletion including the OA1 locus: limit of viability of Xp deletions in males. Am J Med Genet A 2007;143(2):135–41.

37. van Steensel MA, Vreeburg M, Engelen J, et al. Contiguous gene syndrome due to a maternally inherited 8.41 Mb distal deletion of chromosome band Xp22.3 in a boy with short stature, ichthyosis, epilepsy, mental retardation, cerebral cortical heterotopias and Dandy-Walker malformation. Am J Med Genet A 2008;146A(22):2944–9.

38. Stanczak CM, Chen Z, Zhang YH, et al. Deletion mapping in Xp21 for patients with complex glycerol kinase deficiency using SNP mapping arrays. Hum Mutat 2007; 28(3):235–42.

39. Parvari R, Mumm S, Galil A, et al. Deletion of 8.5 Mb, including the FMR1 gene, in a male with the fragile X syndrome phenotype and overgrowth. Am J Med Genet 1999;83(4):302–7.

40. Wolff DJ, Gustashaw KM, Zurcher V et al. Deletions in Xq26.3-q27.3 including FMR1 result in a severe phenotype in a male and variable phenotypes in females depending upon the X inactivation pattern. Hum Genet 1997;100(2):256–61.

41. Ricks CB, Masand R, Fang P, et al. Delineation of a 1.65 Mb critical region for hemihyperplasia and digital anomalies on Xq25. Am J Med Genet A 2010;152A(2): 453–8.

42. Jezela-Stanek A, Ciara E, Juszczak M, et al. Cryptic x; autosome translocation in a boy–delineation of the phenotype. Pediatr Neurol 2011;44(3):221–4.

43. Fusco F, Paciolla M, Chen E, et al. Genetic and molecular analysis of a new unbalanced X;18 rearrangement: localization of the diminished ovarian reserve disease locus in the distal Xq POF1 region. Hum Reprod 2011. [Epub ahead of print].

44. Cheng SF, Rauen KA, Pinkel D, et al. Xq chromosome duplication in males: clinical, cytogenetic and array CGH characterization of a new case and review. Am J Med Genet A 2005;135(3):308–13.
45. Vaglio A, Greif G, Bernal M, et al. Prenatal and postnatal characterization of a de novo Xq22.1 terminal deletion. Genet Test 2006;10(4):272–6.
46. Kokalj-Vokac N, Marcun-Varda N, Zagorac A, et al. Subterminal deletion/duplication event in an affected male due to maternal X chromosome pericentric inversion. Eur J Pediatr 2004;163(11):658–63.
47. Uehara S, Hanew K, Harada N, et al. Isochromosome consisting of terminal short arm and proximal long arm X in a girl with short stature. Am J Med Genet 2001;99(3): 196–9.
48. Bukvic N, Carri VD, Di Cosola ML, et al. Familial X;Y translocation with distinct phenotypic consequences: characterization using FISH and array CGH. Am J Med Genet A 2010;152A(7):1730–4.
49. Ashton F, O'Connor R, Love JM, et al. Molecular characterisation of a der(Y)t(Xp;Yp) with Xp functional disomy and sex reversal. Genet Mol Res 2010;9(3):1815–23.
50. Wolff DJ, Van Dyke DL, Powell CM, et al. Working Group of the ACMG Laboratory Quality Assurance Committee. Laboratory guideline for Turner syndrome. Genet Med 2010;12(1):52–5.
51. Stankiewicz P, Hélias-Rodzewicz Z, Jakubów-Durska K. Cytogenetic and molecular characterization of two isodicentric Y chromosomes. Am J Med Genet 2001;101(1): 20–5.
52. Tuck-Muller CM, Chen H, Martínez JE. Isodicentric Y chromosome: cytogenetic, molecular and clinical studies and review of the literature. Hum Genet 1995;96(1): 119–29.
53. Tsuchiya K, Reijo R, Page DC, et al. Gonadoblastoma: molecular definition of the susceptibility region on the Y chromosome. Am J Hum Genet 1995;57:1400–7.
54. Modan-Moses D, Litmanovitch T, Rienstein S, et al. True hermaphroditism with ambiguous genitalia due to a complicated mosaic karyotype: clinical features, cytogenetic findings, and literature review. Am J Med Genet A 2003;116A(3):300–3.
55. Chen CP, Chern SR, Sheu JC, et al. Prenatal diagnosis, sonographic findings and molecular genetic analysis of a 46,XX/46,XY true hermaphrodite chimera. Prenat Diagn 2005;25(6):502–6.
56. Jorgensen PB, Kjartansdóttir KR, Fedder J. Care of women with XY karyotype: a clinical practice guideline. Fertil Steril 2010;94(1):105–13.
57. Ambry genetics. Available at: http://www.ambrygen.com/X-Linked-Intellectual-Disabilities.html. Accessed April 30, 2011.

Constitutional and Acquired Autosomal Aneuploidy

Colleen Jackson-Cook, PhD*

KEY WORDS
- Aneuploidy • Mosaicism
- Acquired chromosomal aneuploidy • Epigenetics • Trisomy
- Age-related aneuploidy • Chromosomal instability

The consequences of chromosomal abnormalities have been noted "from the earliest stages of life well through the reproductive years, and even beyond."[1(p7)] These chromosomal imbalances can result from numerical or structural anomalies. The numerical chromosomal abnormalities are often referred to as aneuploid conditions. The Greek translation of the word aneuploidy is "not a good set." Thus, aneuploidy refers to a chromosomal number that is not an exact multiple of the haploid complement (ie, in humans 45 or 47 chromosomes per cell). Aneuploidy can arise in gametes/embryonic cells (constitutional) or in differentiated somatic cells (acquired) and can involve autosomes (chromosomes 1–22), as well as gonosomes (chromosomes X or Y). This article focuses on the occurrence of constitutional and acquired **autosomal** aneuploidy in humans.

CONSTITUTIONAL AUTOSOMAL ANEUPLOIDY
Frequency of Aneuploidy

The earliest cytogenetic studies, which were completed in liveborns, showed aneuploidy involving only 3 of the 22 autosomes, with only trisomy (no monosomy) conditions being seen.[2,3] Although cytogenetic methodology has advanced, the results of these pioneering investigations have remained relatively unchanged. The most frequently occurring autosomal aneuploidy condition noted in newborns is trisomy 21, which is seen in approximately 1 in 830 livebirths[2,3] (**Table 1**). The other autosomal trisomies that are seen in newborns include trisomy 18 (observed in

This work was supported, in part, by a grant from the National Institute of Environmental Health (R01 ES12074). Its contents are solely the responsibility of the author and do not necessarily represent the official views of the NIEHS, NIH.

Departments of Pathology and Human & Molecular Genetics, Virginia Commonwealth University, Richmond, VA 23298, USA

* Corresponding author. Department of Pathology, Virginia Commonwealth University, PO Box 980662, Richmond, VA 23298.

E-mail address: ccook@mcvh-vcu.edu

Clin Lab Med 31 (2011) 481–511
doi:10.1016/j.cll.2011.08.002
0272-2712/11/$ – see front matter © 2011 Elsevier Inc. All rights reserved.

Table 1
Frequencies of constitutional autosomal aneuploidy at different developmental timepoints

Chromosome	Liveborn[a]	Percent of Trisomy (Disomy in sperm)		Sperm[c] Disomy
		First Trimester Spontaneous Abortuses[b]	Mosaicism	
1	—	Case report	—	0.08
2	—	5.6	P/L[e]	0.09
3	—	0.8	P/L	0.20
4	—	2.5	P/L	0.08
5	—	0.1	P[f]	—
6	—	0.3	P/L	0.04
7	—	4.5	P/L	0.06
8	—	3.7	P/L	0.03
9	—	2.8	P/L	0.16
10	—	1.9	P/L	—
11	—	0.2	P	—
12	—	0.8	P/L	0.14
13	0.004	5.7	0.0002[g]	0.12
14	—	4.2	P/L	—
15	—	7.3	P/L	0.10
16	—	32.4	P/L	0.07
17	—	0.7	P/L	—
18	0.013	5.1	0.00065[h]	0.06
19	—	0.1	P/L	—
20	—	2.7	0.009[i]	0.12
21	0.120	8.3	0.006[j]	0.17
22	NA[d]	10.1	P/L	0.47

[a] Data from Hook[2] and Jacobs et al.[3]
[b] Data from Bond and Chandley.[5]
[c] Data from Templado et al[10] and presented as disomy frequencies.
[d] Case reports have been described, but the frequency is too rare to be estimated accurately.
[e] Mosaicism for this autosome has been reported through prenatal testing (P) and in liveborns (L), but is too rare for accurate frequencies to be estimated.
[f] Mosaicism for this autosome has been reported through prenatal testing (P), but is too rare for accurate frequencies to be estimated.
[g] Data from Magenis et al. based on liveborns.[19]
[h] Data from Carey based on liveborns.[20]
[i] Data from Hsu et al based on amniotic fluid specimens.[22]
[j] Data from Hook based on liveborns.[18]

approximately 1 in 7500 livebirths), trisomy 13 (approximately 1 in 22,700 livebirths), and very rare cases of trisomy 22.[2–4] Soon after the discovery of these autosomal aneuploidy conditions, cytogeneticists conjectured that the incidence of aneuploidy in humans was not limited to primarily three chromosomes (13, 18, and 21), but could occur for all autosomes, with the clinical consequences of aneuploidy for the other autosomes being incompatible with life. To test this hypothesis, investigations were initiated to determine if autosomal aneuploidy was present in spontaneous abortus tissue.[5] Chromosomal analyses of products of conception (primarily first trimester)

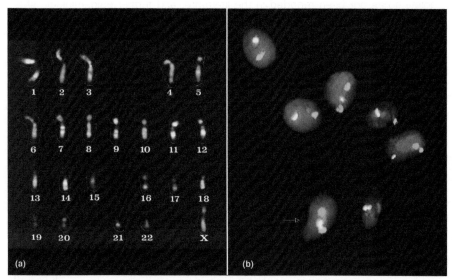

Fig. 1. Methods for evaluating sperm chromosomal complements. Hamster-egg/human sperm in vitro culture methodology allows one to directly observe chromosomes, as illustrated in (*a*), which shows QFQ-banded chromosomes from a sperm having a female haploid complement (23, X). Studies using FISH methodology on sperm nuclei allow for estimation of aneuploidy frequencies based on targeted loci (usually pericentromeric sequences). (*b*) Sperm nuclei after FISH with probes for chromosomes X (DXZ1: *green*); Y (DYZ3: *red*); 17 (D17Z1: *yellow*); and 18 (D18Z1: *aqua*). This field shows two sperm with a female complement, four sperm with a male complement, and one sperm (*arrow*) having an extra sex chromosome (inferred to be 24,XY). [Part (*b*) was prepared by Nurcan Gursoy.]

showed the presence of trisomies involving nearly all autosomes. Interestingly, trisomy for chromosome 16 accounted for approximately a third of all autosomal trisomic first-trimester abortuses[5] (see **Table 1**). Other autosomes that were observed to have increased frequencies of trisomy in first-trimester abortus tissue included chromosomes 2, 7, 8, 18 and the acrocentric chromosomes (13, 14, 15, 21, and 22; see **Table 1**). Explanations for these observed interchromosomal differences included (but were not limited to): (1) a true difference in the propensity for a chromosome to undergo malsegregation; or (2) a selection bias that reflected the differential viability of imbalances involving different chromosomes, or both. To distinguish between these plausible explanations, aneuploidy data were collected directly from gametes.

The earliest of the gametic aneuploidy studies directly analyzed metaphase chromosomes from oocytes or sperm (**Fig. 1**). More recently, researchers have completed these investigations using DNA-based methods (primarily fluorescence in situ hybridization [FISH], but also comparative genomic hybridization techniques).[6–8] Collectively, the results of these gametic studies have shown that humans have a relatively high frequency of gametic aneuploidy compared to the frequencies seen in other species.[9] Moreover, the frequency of sperm aneuploidy has been shown to differ between chromosomes (see **Table 1**), suggesting that at least a portion of the observed variation in autosome-specific frequencies of aneuploidy reflects true differences in autosomal malsegregation, rather than being limited solely to selective growth pressures.[6,10] Gender differences have also been noted in gametic aneuploidy frequencies, with oocytes having higher levels of aneuploidy than sperm.[6–8]

However, technical challenges have thwarted investigators' abilities to provide unbiased, chromosome-specific estimates of autosomal aneuploidy present in oocytes.[11,12] One factor that is thought to contribute to the observed overall increased frequency of aneuploidy in oocytes compared to spermatocytes in humans is their means of ascertainment. The majority of oocytes available for study are ones found unsuitable for transfer from assisted reproductive procedures (such as in vitro fertilization), thus leading to biases associated with maternal age (see later) or with the presence of morphologic anomalies.[8] However, studies of nonhuman mammals, which are not limited by these ascertainment biases, have also shown significant increases in the frequency of aneuploidy in oocytes compared to spermatocytes.[13,14] Etiologic factors that have been suggested to contribute to the higher incidence of aneuploidy in oogenesis include (but are not limited to) (1) the disruption of the meiotic division in prophase I (with the division starting prenatally, but not commencing until ovulation, which may occur decades later); (2) differences in meiotic checkpoint permissiveness for errors in males compared to females; (3) differences in the frequency and chromosomal location of meiotic recombinational events (see discussion of etiology later); and (4) epigenetic differences in response to environmental/stressor exposures.

Mosaicism for Autosomal Aneuploidy

Mosaicism for aneuploidy is defined as the presence of two or more distinct cell lines that are derived from a single zygote but differ from one another because of nondisjunction (or mutation).[15] The use of interphase FISH techniques has allowed for improvements in the ability to detect autosomal mosaicism because thousands of interphase nuclei from a variety of different tissues can be evaluated (not limited only to viable cells that can be successfully cultured in vitro to produce metaphase spreads).[16,17] Mosaicism for nearly all of the autosomes has been identified in either liveborns (usually ascertained because of health/developmental concerns) or in fetuses through prenatal testing (asymptomatically or due to ultrasound aberrations; see Table 1).[18-22] Given that most of the instances of trisomic mosaicism in liveborns are case reports, unbiased estimates of the frequency of mosaicism for all of the autosomes are not available. However, mosaicism for trisomy 21, which is thought to be one of the most frequent autosomal mosaicism conditions in liveborns, is seen in only 2% to 5% of all people with Down syndrome (or approximately 1 in 16,670–41,670 livebirths).[18] A caution to be noted when estimating frequencies of mosaic conditions in liveborns is that there is likely to be a bias toward studying only individuals who have clinical consequences resulting from their mosaicism. Thus, the estimates based on case reports/clinical studies are likely to be underestimates of the true frequency of constitutional autosomal mosaicism in humans.

The overall frequencies of true autosomal mosaicism (not pseudomosaicism) observed through prenatal testing is approximately 0.2% after amniocentesis and 1% to 2% after chorionic villi sampling (CVS), with the latter figure including both mosaic complements and nonmosaic complements from direct preparations that differed from those of the fetus (indicating confined placental mosaicism).[22,23] Chromosome-specific differences in the frequency of prenatally diagnosed autosomal mosaicism have been identified, with trisomies involving chromosomes 13, 18, 20, and 21 being seen most frequently in amniocytes.[24,25]

One means for gaining insight regarding the frequency of mosaicism in humans has been to study early embryos, which were obtained after assisted reproductive procedures. These embryos have shown an unexpectedly high frequency of mosaicism, with the majority (50%–91%) of early (day 4) embryos having mosaicism involving single or multiple (sometimes referred to as chaotic embryos) chromosomes.[26,27] Chromosomal mosaicism has also been observed in fetal (30%–35% of cells) and adult (10%) brains cells[28,29]; liver cells (approximately 3% in adults)[30]; and other tissues,[31] including germline mosaicism, which, if present, could have reproductive consequences.[32] These observations have led investigators to postulate that mosaicism may occur as a "normal" or global biological process in early human development, with tissue-specific selection leading to loss of most aneuploid cells in the early stages of development, but with some tissues "normally" retaining mosaicism.[31] Iourov and colleagues[31] further speculate that mosaicism (often undetected) may contribute to the development of several conditions (including autism, schizophrenia, autoimmune diseases, and Alzheimer disease), with a latent, age-related influence of mosaicism being conjectured for a portion of these conditions.

Phenotypic Findings Associated with Constitutional Mosaicism

As expected, because individuals with trisomy for chromosomes 13, 18, or 21 in every cell can survive to term, fetuses having mosaicism for these conditions can also survive. The phenotype of these individuals ranges from near normal to the demonstration of a subset (or in some cases all) of the phenotypic traits that have been well characterized in people having Patau, Edward, or Down syndrome.[16,33,34] Individuals with mosaicism for trisomy 21 have phenotypic variation that appears to be influenced by the proportion of cells having a trisomic (compared to a euploid) complement, as well as tissue-specific effects.[16] However, positive karyotype–phenotype correlations have not consistently been seen in people having mosaicism involving other trisomic conditions.[33,34] As a result, the percentage of trisomic cells present in an individual having mosaicism cannot be clearly used as a prognostic indicator.

Interestingly, many individuals having mosaicism (regardless of the chromosome involved) have skin pigmentary abnormalities, which may not be present until weeks or years after birth; intrauterine growth compromise; body/facial/limb asymmetry; and developmental delay. As a result of this phenotypic overlap, the term "general chromosomal mosaic syndrome" has been coined.[35] However, for a subset of these conditions, specific syndromic patterns have emerged (summarized in **Table 2**[4,16,21,23–25,33–75]), thereby facilitating the recognition of the chromosomal basis for these individual's health/developmental problems. The provision of genetic counseling after a prenatal diagnosis of autosomal mosaicism can be especially challenging. Genetic counseling concerns for these patients include (1) variation in phenotypic consequences ranging from the extremes of a normal outcome to a severely abnormal phenotype; (2) identification/confirmation/quantitation of the trisomic cell line, with fibroblasts (and placenta) tending to show the presence (or higher frequencies) of the trisomic line more often than blood; (3) an assessment of the possible presence of uniparental disomy in the euploid line, due to a trisomy (or monosomy) rescue mechanism (particularly in cases where mosaicism was detected through CVS and in cases where the trisomic [monosomic] chromosome is one known to have imprinted regions); (4) recognition that clinical outcome can vary based on the mode of ascertainment (eg, was the mosaicism detected through CVS [if so, is it confined placental mosaicism?] vs amniocentesis, or after birth [due to phenotypic findings]); and (5) the technical criteria that were used to define the mosaicism (true mosaicism vs pseudomosaicism).[22] For mosaic cases ascertained after prenatal testing, one may wish to recommend a fetal scan to potentially detect phenotypic abnormalities and to advise that follow-up confirmation chromosomal testing be completed (if CVS, then confirm through amniocentesis; if amniocentesis, then

Table 2
Phenotypic consequences of mosaicism for autosomal trisomies

Autosomal Mosaic Condition	Prenatal Ascertainment			Postnatal Ascertainment	
	Consistent Findings at Birth/Termination in Patients with Abnormal Outcome	Possibility of Normal Outcome	References[a]	Consistent Abnormalities Reported[b]	References[a]
Mosaicism for trisomy 2	IUGR; oligohydramnios; CHD including acardia; kidney anomalies	Yes (tend to lack confirmation of trisomic line) CVS detection associated with CPM	Sifakis et al[36] Hsu et al[24,*] Sago et al[37,*]	DD; CHD; small stature; hypertelorism; CFA; radio-ulnar hypoplasia; microcephaly; hypomelanosis of Ito; cleft lip or cleft palate; small penis, bilateral cryptorchidism, bilateral club foot; body and facial asymmetry, neural tube anomalies; Hirschsprung disease	Prontera et al[38,*]
Mosaicism for trisomy 3	IUGR; CHD; DD; oligohydramnios; bilateral cleft lip/palate; microphthalmia, vertebral anomalies, ear anomalies	Yes (tend to lack confirmation of trisomic line) CVS detection associated with CPM	Zaslav et al[39,*]; Hsu et al[24,*]	CHD; DD; CFA; short stature; coloboma; and hip dislocation	Metaxotou et al[40]; Kuhn et al[41]; DeKeyerser et al[42]
Mosaicism for trisomy 4	CFA; CHD; microcephaly; short neck; small stature; pigmentary abnormalities; facial asymmetry; ear anomalies; thumb aplasia and hypoplastic fingers; nail hypoplasia; variable DD	Yes (tend to lack confirmation of trisomic line)	Wieczorek et al[43]; Zaslav et al[44,*]; Hsu et al[24,*]	Small stature; pigmentary abnormalities; facial asymmetry; ear anomalies; thumb aplasia and hypoplastic fingers; nail hypoplasia; variable DD	Wieczorek et al[43]

(continued on next page)

Table 2
(continued)

Autosomal Mosaic Condition	Prenatal Ascertainment			Postnatal Ascertainment	
	Consistent Findings at Birth/Termination in Patients with Abnormal Outcome	Possibility of Normal Outcome	References[a]	Consistent Abnormalities Reported[b]	References[a]
Mosaicism for trisomy 5	IUGR; CHD; DD; CFA; growth delay	Yes (tend to lack confirmation of trisomic line)	Hsu et al[24,*]		
Mosaicism for trisomy 6	CHD; DD; growth delay; renal anomalies; cleft hand, syndactylies; overlapping toes; low-set ears; micrognathia	Yes (tend to lack confirmation of trisomic line)	Destree et al[45,*]; Hsu et al[24,*]	CHD; DD; growth delay; renal anomalies; cleft hand, syndactylies; overlapping toes; low-set ears; micrognathia	Destree et al[45,*]
Mosaicism for trisomy 7	DD; facial asymmetry; hypomelanosis of Ito; micrognathia; Russell–Silver syndrome and growth abnormalities in cases with uniparental disomy (trisomy rescue)	Yes (tend to lack confirmation of trisomic line)	Chen et al[46,*]; Hsu et al[24,*]	DD; CHD; renal abnormalities; radial hypoplasia; hypomelanosis of Ito; mental illness	Verghese et al[47]; Hsu et al[24,*]
Mosaicism for trisomy 8	Limited reports	Yes (confirmation of trisomic line in fibroblasts and blood for some cases)	Hsu et al[24,*]	Thick lips; deep-set eyes; prominent ears, deep plantar and palmar creases; CHD; skeletal anomalies; camptodactyly; clinodactyly mild to severe developmental delay (speech most affected); Marfanoid habitus; renal malformations	Hale and Keane[48]; Wisniewska and Mazurek[49]; Riccardi[50]

(continued on next page)

Table 2 (continued)

Autosomal Mosaic Condition	Prenatal Ascertainment			Postnatal Ascertainment	
	Consistent Findings at Birth/Termination in Patients with Abnormal Outcome[c]	Possibility of Normal Outcome	References[a]	Consistent Abnormalities Reported[b]	References[a]
Mosaicism for trisomy 9	IUGR; CHD; CFA; micrognathia, skeletal malformations; low-set ears; urogenital anomalies	Yes (confirmation of trisomic line in fibroblasts and blood for some cases)	Chen et al[51]; Schwendemann et al[52]; Hsu et al[24,*]	Low-set ears; microcephaly; CHD; deep set eyes; joint anomalies; small jaw; feeding/respiratory difficulties in infancy; kidney problems; variable DD	Bruns[53,*]
Mosaicism for trisomy 10	CFA; ear abnormalities; cleft lip/palate; rockerbottom feet; hand/finger deformities; cardiac anomalies		Hahnemann et al[54,*]	CHD; CFA; growth retardation; ear anomalies; cleft lip/palate; renal malformations; hand and foot abnormalities; eye anomalies	Hahnemann et al[54,*]
Mosaicism for trisomy 11	Acardia; renal anomalies; Potter syndrome facies[c]	Yes (tend to lack confirmation of trisomic line)	Balasubramanian[55,*]; Hsu et al[24,*]		
Mosaicism for trisomy 12	IUGR; CHD; skeletal anomalies; renal abnormalities	Yes (tend to lack confirmation of trisomic line)	Parasuraman et al[56,*]; Gentilin et al[57]; Staals et al[58]; Hsu et al[24,*]	Variable DD; CHD; CFA; microcephaly; scoliosis; short stature; pigmentary findings	DeLozier-Blanchet et al[59,*]; Hsu et al[19,*]

(continued on next page)

Table 2
(continued)

Autosomal Mosaic Condition	Prenatal Ascertainment			Postnatal Ascertainment	
	Consistent Findings at Birth/Termination in Patients with Abnormal Outcome	Possibility of Normal Outcome	References[a]	Consistent Abnormalities Reported[b]	References[a]
Mosaicism for trisomy 13	IUGR; CHD; DD; low-set ears; syndactyly/polydactyly; scalp defects; cleft lip/palate; small jaw	Yes (liveborns tend to lack confirmation of trisomic line)	Chen[60],*; Wallerstein et al[25],*	Mild to typical phenotype seen in trisomy 13, including CHD; ear anomalies; cleft lip/palate; phylloid hypomelanosis; variable DD	Griffith et al[33],*; Delatycki and Gardner[61],*
Mosaicism for monosomy 13				IUGR; CFA: CHD; microcephaly; hypertelorism; ptosis; eye anomalies including retinoblastoma; limb/finger abnormalities; renal, and dental anomalies	Golabi et al[62],*
Mosaicism for trisomy 14	Low-set ears; rockerbottom feet; hip anomalies; hydrocephaly	Yes (tend to lack confirmation of trisomic line)	Merritt and Natarajan[63]; Hsu et al[24],*	CFA; variable DD; CHD; small size; genital anomalies; body/limb asymmetry; pigmentary findings; short neck/redundant neck skin; micro/retrognathia	Shinawi et al[64],*; Von Sneidern and Lacassie[35],*
Mosaicism for trisomy 15	IUGR; CHD; CFA; renal and gastrointestinal anomalies; skeletal abnormalities; limb anomalies; CPM	Yes (tend to lack confirmation of trisomic line)	Hahnemann et al[23]; Zaslov et al[65],*; Hsu et al[24],*	CHD; IUGR; DD; CFA; skeletal anomalies; hypotonia; hydrospadius; neck abnormalities; limb anomalies	Zaslov et al[65],*; Hsu et al[24],*

(continued on next page)

Table 2
(continued)

Autosomal Mosaic Condition	Prenatal Ascertainment		Postnatal Ascertainment	
	Consistent Findings at Birth/Termination in Patients with Abnormal Outcome	Possibility of Normal Outcome	References[a]	Consistent Abnormalities Reported[b]	References[a]
Mosaicism for trisomy 16	IUGR; CHD; CFA; DD; renal, skeletal, and gastrointestinal anomalies; skin pigmentary abnormalities; microcephaly	Yes (tend to lack confirmation of trisomic line)	Langlois et al[75]; Benn[66],*; Hsu et al[24],*	IUGR; CHD; CFA[c]	Benn[66],*; Hsu et al[24],*
Mosaicism for trisomy 17	CFA; CPM	Yes (majority have normal phenotype; tend to lack confirmation of trisomic line)	Utermann et al[67],*; Genuardi et al[68]; Hsu et al[24],*	DD; growth delay; microcephaly; cerebellar malformations; limb/body asymmetry	Utermann et al[67],*; Hsu et al[24],*
Mosaicism for trisomy 18	IUGR; CFA; CHD	Yes (liveborns tend to lack confirmation of trisomic line)	Wallerstein et al[25],*	Mild to typical phenotype seen in trisomy 18, including CHD; variable DD; CFA; microcephaly; delayed bone age; brachydactyly; short stature; premature ovarian delay; ear/respiratory infections; high arched palate	Tucker et al [34],*
Mosaicism for trisomy 19		Yes[c] Limited to a single case	Hsu et al[24],*	CFA; neonatal death[c]	Hsu et al[24],*

(continued on next page)

Table 2
(continued)

Autosomal Mosaic Condition	Prenatal Ascertainment			Postnatal Ascertainment	
	Consistent Findings at Birth/Termination in Patients with Abnormal Outcome	Possibility of Normal Outcome	References[a]	Consistent Abnormalities Reported[b]	References[a]
Mosaicism for trisomy 20	IUGR; CFA; hypotonia; variable DD; seizures; renal anomalies	Yes (majority have normal phenotype; tend to lack confirmation of trisomic line)	Wallerstein et al[25],*; Hsu et al[24]	Hypomelanosis of Ito; variable development (normal to delay with learning disabilities in cases having normal intelligence); spinal abnormalities; hypotonia; lifelong constipation; sloped shoulders	Willis et al[21]; Bianca et al[69]
Mosaicism for trisomy 21	IUGR; CHD; facies consistent with Down syndrome	Yes (tend to lack confirmation of trisomic line)	Wallerstein et al[25],*	CHD; CFA including upslanting palpebral fissures and flat nasal bridge; variable DD; simian crease; ear/respiratory infections; eye findings; short hands/fingers; low set ears; hyperextensibility of joints; hypotonia	Papavassiliou et al[16]; Wallerstein et al[25],*
Mosaicism for monosomy 21	Holoprosencephaly; low-set ears; renal and lung anomalies; thumb abnormalities		Van der Kevie-Kersemaekers et al[70],*; Cheng et al[71]	IUGR; CHD; CFA; DD; microcephaly; seizures; eye and ear anomalies; cleft lip/palate; renal anomalies; low set ears; syndactyly; limited number of cases	Nguyen et al[72],*

(continued on next page)

Table 2
(continued)

Autosomal Mosaic Condition	Prenatal Ascertainment			Postnatal Ascertainment	
	Consistent Findings at Birth/Termination in Patients with Abnormal Outcome	Possibility of Normal Outcome	References[a]	Consistent Abnormalities Reported[b]	References[a]
Mosaicism for trisomy 22	IUGR; CHD; CFA; nuchal thickening; hydrocephaly; cleft lip; microcephaly; skeletal anomalies; facial asymmetry; finger anomalies; neonatal death	Yes (tend to lack confirmation of trisomic line)	Hsu et al[24,*]	CHD; variable DD; CFA; small stature; eye, ear, limb anomalies; facial/body asymmetry; microcephaly; epicanthal folds; hypoplastic nails; clinodactyly; dental anomalies; hearing loss; ovarian failure	Leclercq et al[73,*] Crowe et al[74,*]; Hsu et al[24,*]
Mosaicism for monosomy 22				IUGR; microcephaly; CFA	Wang[4]

Abbreviations: CFA, craniofacial anomalies; CHD, congenital heart defect; CPM, confined placental mosaicism; DD, developmental delay; IUGR, intrauterine growth retardation.

[a] When available, the reference(s) cited are review papers that summarize the findings of multiple investigators. These review papers are denoted by an asterisk.

[b] Represents a biased population presenting with phenotypic outcome (does not include people who might have mosaicism with a normal outcome).

[c] Based on a small number of cases, so not clear if these findings are indicative of a syndromic pattern or incidental observations.

confirm through percutaneous umbilical blood sampling [for cases in which the trisomic line can be seen in blood] or at termination/birth).[37]

In addition to mosaicism involving autosomal trisomy, patients having mosaicism for autosomal monosomy have also been described, including mosaic monosomies for chromosomes 13,[62] 21,[70,72] and 22[4] (see **Table 2**). However, these conditions are too rare to allow for the establishment of a distinct syndromic phenotype. On a cautionary note, when feasible, the presence of an apparent autosomal monosomic cell line should be confirmed using molecular cytogenetic approaches, as several patients reported to have monsomic cell lines on the basis of GTG-banding were subsequently determined to have cryptic structural abnormalities (not full monosomy).[72]

Etiology of Constitutional Autosomal Aneuploidy

Having well established that constitutional autosomal aneuploidy was a significant factor leading to morbidity and mortality in humans, investigators initiated studies to understand the underlying causes of aneuploidy and to understand the basis for the observed differences in aneuploidy frequencies between chromosomes. Despite years of study, the etiology of aneuploidy in humans remains largely enigmatic, as does the specific mechanism(s) whereby the observed imbalances (trisomy) result in phenotypic consequences involving multiple organs. Investigators completing epidemiologic studies have consistently shown that advanced maternal age correlates with an increased risk for having a child with trisomy 21 (as well as most other trisomic conditions). This association has been observed in women from all ethnic and geographic backgrounds.[76] Knowledge of other factors (or the mechanistic influence of maternal age) contributing to the propensity for human chromosomes to malsegregate in meiosis has come from studies of the parental origin of the extra chromosome in trisomic probands.[77] Investigations of nuclear families (mother, father, and trisomic child) have shown that the majority (93%–95%) of nondisjunctional events leading to a child having trisomy 21 occurred in oogenesis (primarily meiosis I).[77] Similar studies of nuclear families in which a child has Edward syndrome or Patau syndrome have also shown that gametic malsegregation occurred more often in oogenesis than in spermatogenesis. However, the malsegregational event that occurred in the gametes that resulted in the birth of a child with trisomy 18 occurred more frequently in meiosis II (58.7% of cases) than in meiosis I.[77] Studies of abortus tissue (and parental samples) have revealed variation in the parental and meiotic origin of the malsegregational events for the different autosomes.[77]

Attributes that have been conjectured to influence a chromosome's propensity to malsegregate include the presence of chromosomal heteromorphisms.[78,79] However, because the association of these heteromorphisms with aneuploidy has not been consistently observed, their influence on chromosomal segregation, if any, seems to be either minimal or to act via a mechanism that is not straightforward (eg, increased amounts of heterochromatin may have epigenetic effects that, in turn, influence aneuploidy).[79,80]

Based on information gained from studies of the DNA markers evaluated in parental origin studies, perturbations in recombination have been recognized to occur in gametes that resulted in aneuploidy offspring/conceptuses.[80] For trisomy 21, reductions in the number of chiasmata, as well as changes in their location, have been observed, with the results of more recent studies suggesting that these patterns may be influenced by age, as well as environmental factors.[14,81] One can speculate that a lack of recombination (achiasmate bivalents) could lead to distributive segregation of the chromosomes, which is a phenomenon that has been shown to arise in *Drosophila*, but has not been definitively observed in humans.[82] Simplistically, the

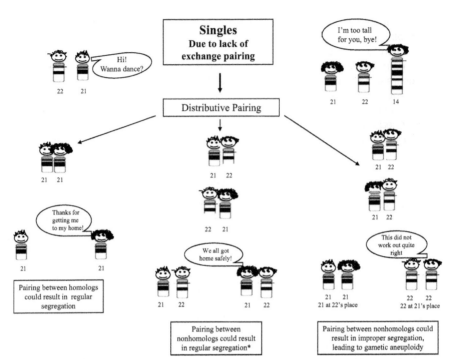

Fig. 2. Achiasmate chromosomes may engage in distributive pairing. In *Drosophila*, there is evidence that a lack of meiotic recombination leads to nonexchange pairing, with distributive pairing preferentially occurring between chromosomes that are similar in size. In humans it is not known if distributive pairing occurs, but one could speculate that the observed perturbations in recombination could result in distributive pairing. If this occurs between homologs (*left*), it could lead to a balanced gamete; if it occurs between nonhomologs, it could result in either a balanced, euploid gamete (*center*); or imbalances (*right*). *It should be noted that the nonhomologs can segregate in more combinations than the ones illustrated here, but for simplicity only one representative pattern is shown for balanced and unbalanced segregants. (*Adapted from* Grell RF. The meiotic process and aneuploidy. Basic Life Sci 1985;36:317–35.)

hypothesis of distributive pairing can be likened to a "singles' bar" (**Fig. 2**). In distributive pairing, the unpaired chromosome(s) are thought to be more likely to pair with chromosomes having a similar size. By chance, the unpaired homologs could pair with one another, leading to potentially normal segregation at meiosis. Alternatively, the achiasmatic chromosomes could pair with a nonhomologous chromosome. The segregation of these nonhomologous chromosomes could result in either a euploid or aneuploidy gamete (see **Fig. 2**). Aberrant localization of chiasmata between homologs can also lead to malsegregation, with a location that is too proximal resulting in entanglement whereas one too distal can result in unorganized, random segregation.[80]

The "trigger(s)" inducing perturbations in recombination, or other mechanisms contributing to the genesis of gametic aneuploidy, have not been clearly recognized, but are likely to include both genetic and environmental influences (**Fig. 3**). Although studies of nonhuman eukaryotic species have allowed for the recognition of many genes that contribute to the proper segregation of chromosomes in meiosis, the a

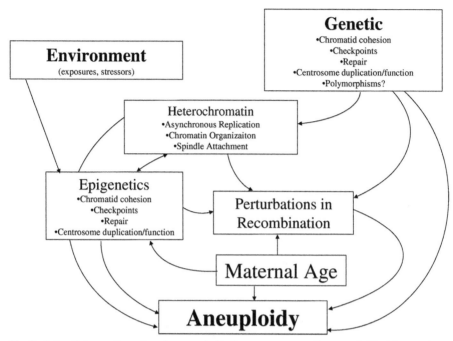

Fig. 3. Potential genetic and environmental influences on gametic aneuploidy. Maternal age has consistently been shown to be associated with an increased risk for gametic aneuploidy, with the mechanism for this association appearing to include aberrant recombination, as well as other factors. In humans, it is speculated that genetic and environmental components impact one's risk for producing aneuploid gametes, with epigenetic changes acquired over time potentially serving as a bridge for these influences. Genes that have been implicated to contribute to aneuploidy (either through mutation or epigenetic alterations) include those involved with chromatid cohesion, meiotic and spindle checkpoints; repair; centrosome function/duplication; and recombination. Chromatin organization (heterochromatin vs euchromatin) has been conjectured to influence a chromosome's propensity for gametic aneuploidy and may be influenced by epigenetic changes, but could also elicit epigenetic alterations (hence, the *two-headed arrow*). Heterochromatin may directly impact the frequency of aneuploidy (possibly by compromising the fidelity of the spindle attachments and replication/pairing processes), or its purported role may result from perturbations in recombination, which, in turn, could lead to aneuploidy.

priori recognition of genetic changes leading to an increased risk for gametic aneuploidy in humans is still lacking. Genes that have been identified as likely candidates contributing to gametic aneuploidy include (but are not limited to) those involved in meiotic/spindle checkpoints, centrosome formation/duplication, chromatid cohesion, and chromatin organization.[83–89] A "two-hit" model of aneuploidy has been proposed to integrate the maternal age influence with the effects from genetic and other potential etiologic factors that have been associated with aneuploidy in humans.[90,91] This model postulates that the "first hit" is the presence of a primary oocyte(s) having a susceptible meiotic configuration (such as perturbations in recombination). If these susceptible oocytes experience a "second hit," which could occur years later due to compromises in the functioning of key genes (noted previously), they could result in an aneuploid conceptus. Alternatively, the "second hit" could be related to environmental exposure(s).

The designation of specific environmental exposures as aneugens in humans has been problematic, with both supportive and nonsupportive data reported for a variety of toxins/lifestyle exposures.[92] In studies performed in mice, Hunt and colleagues[93] clearly showed an increase in aneuploidy frequencies in response to bisphenol A (BPA) exposure. BPA, which is a xenoestrogen that activates estrogen receptors, has been conjectured to elicit its aneugenic effect through perturbations in the function of the tubulin gene, thereby disrupting spindle organization.[94] BPA has also been shown to induce epigenetic changes in developing mammals that differ between species and vary with dosage.[95] Excitingly, the biological response of mice to BPA can be modulated with diet, suggesting that the impact of this chemical (and possibly the effects of other aneugens) may have biological plasticity/reversibility.[95,96]

The field of epigenetics, which investigates heritable alterations in gene expression or phenotype that are caused by mechanisms other than changes in the underlying DNA sequence (eg, methylation changes, histone alterations, microRNA expression), is an exciting area of study that may allow for improvements in the understanding of etiologic factors contributing to aneuploidy.[97] One can conjecture that epigenetic changes may explain, at least in part, the long recognized influence of advanced maternal age on chromosomal aneuploidy in humans. Epigenetic modifications could be acquired (over time) in gametes, leading to changes in the expression of genes that are involved in the resumption of meiosis I segregation or meiosis II segregation (including but not limited to genes involved in chromatid cohesion, meiotic/spindle checkpoints, centrosomes, spindle formation, DNA repair). These epigenetic modifications could result from a wide variety of "environmental" stressors (classic environmental exposures or social stresses) that may have occurred over many years, making their detection elusive (see **Fig. 3**). Their impact may also be modulated by diet or hormonal influences, thereby mimicking patterns consistent with those noted for complex diseases. Although the role of epigenetic changes on the initiation of chromosomal malsegregation is largely speculative, investigators have shown that epigenetic changes arise in response to trisomic imbalances and may also contribute to the variation in phenotypic findings present in people having chromosomal aneuploidy conditions.[98]

Studies of individuals having mosaicism may provide valuable insight about the causes of aneuploidy in humans. Although all cases of mosaicism require at least one postzygotic error, we (unpublished data) and other investigators[99,100] have shown that in the majority of individuals having mosaicism for trisomy 21, two chromosome malsegregational events occurred (both a meiotic and a mitotic error), with a "trisomy rescue" scenario giving rise to the normal cell line. Thus, it is feasible that the chromosomes in these individuals (which malsegregated twice) have a biological basis for a predisposition to aneuploidy. From a genetic counseling perspective, this observation is important to recognize because the recurrence risks for couples having a child with mosaicism for trisomy 21 may be comparable to those of couples having a child with "complete" trisomy 21, rather than being negligible, as has been suggested in the early literature (probably as a result of the rarity of this condition, which prohibited the collection of robust empiric risk data).

ACQUIRED AUTOSOMAL ANEUPLOIDY IN HEALTHY INDIVIDUALS

In addition to constitutional aneuploidy, chromosomal malsegregation can occur in differentiated somatic cells, resulting in acquired aneuploidy. In the first report of acquired chromosomal changes in somatic cells, Jacobs and colleagues[101] described an increase in numerical chromosomal abnormalities (primarily losses) in cultured lymphocytes from older, compared to younger, individuals. This observation has since been confirmed for the sex chromosomes by several investigators (with X chromosome loss seen most often in females and Y chromosome loss seen most frequently in males).[102–108] Although age-related sex chromosomal aneuploidy has been widely studied, much less is known about the frequency of acquired autosomal aneuploidy.

Frequency of Acquired Autosomal Aneuploidy

In contrast to findings in sex chromosomes, the potential association between the frequency of acquired autosomal abnormalities and age is **not** clear cut, with some investigators reporting an age effect[109,110] and others seeing no such influence.[106,111,112] The earliest studies of acquired autosomal aneuploidy, which were performed by evaluating metaphase spreads, showed an excess of chromosomal losses compared to gains.[105,108,112–115] To avoid potential biases for observing artifactual chromosomal losses that might arise due to cell disruption during harvest/slide making procedures, investigators have used FISH techniques on interphase nuclei to estimate acquired aneuploidy frequencies. Although few in number, the results of these interphase FISH studies have also shown losses (monosomy or nullisomy) to occur more often than gains (trisomy, tetrasomy, and similar abnormalities).[110,111,116] This consistent observation suggests that age-related, acquired aneuploidy may arise, at least in part, from a loss-specific mechanism(s) rather than a mitotic nondisjunctional event(s), the latter of which would be expected to result in equal frequencies of the reciprocal products of monosomy and trisomy.

Akin to the observations of constitutional aneuploidy, the frequencies of acquired somatic cell aneuploidy have been shown to vary among chromosomes. The nonrandom, chromosome-specific patterns observed by cytogeneticists studying metaphase spreads have shown the smaller chromosomes to have higher frequencies of acquired aneuploidy (primarily loss) than larger chromosomes.[117] However, this size correlation has not been universally observed,[118] and has not consistently been seen by investigators studying acquired aneuploidy frequencies in interphase nuclei using FISH methodology[110,111,116] (Rehder CW, Corey L, York TP, et al. Chromosome-specific and tissue-specific differences in acquired aneuploidy frequencies in uncultured lymphocytes and buccal mucosa cells: a twin study. Submitted for publication) **(Table 3)**. The FISH studies of cultured and/or uncultured interphase nuclei have shown **increased** frequencies of loss for autosomes 1, 2, 6, 9, 15, 16, 17, 18, and 21,[110,111,119] (Rehder CW, Corey L, York TP, et al. Chromosome-specific and tissue-specific differences in acquired aneuploidy frequencies in uncultured lymphocytes and buccal mucosa cells: A twin study. Submitted for publication) and **decreased** frequencies of loss for chromosome 3 in both cultured and uncultured cells[110,119] (see **Table 3**). Interestingly, six of the nine autosomes having the highest frequencies of loss are heterochromatin-rich chromosomes.[110,120,121]

Etiology of Autosomal Acquired Aneuploidy

The two primary hypotheses that have been proposed to explain chromosome-specific differences in acquired, somatic cell autosomal aneuploidy frequencies are (1) the selection hypothesis and (2) the nonrandom loss/gain hypothesis. The selection hypothesis states that the chromosome-specific differences in the frequency of acquired aneuploidy reflect the differential survival of the resultant imbalanced cells, with the loss (or gain) of a large chromosome that contains many actively transcribed genes having a more deleterious effect on a cell's survival (ultimately being eliminated from the cell population) than the loss of a small

Table 3
Distribution of acquired somatic cell autosomal aneuploidy in lymphocytes from healthy subjects

Chromosome	Cultured			Uncultured		
	Loss[a]	Gain[a]	No. of Subjects	Loss	Gain	No. of Subjects
1	2.7[b]	0.5	68	2.9[c]	0.7[c]	53
2	1.2	0.6	60	2.45[c,d]	0.11[c,d]	75
3	0.8	0.8	62	0.36[d]	0.7[d]	22
4	1.3	0.1	65	0.93[e]	0.03[e]	24
5	0.9	0.7	44	1.36[c]	0.41[c]	53
6	2.0	0.3	40	—	—	—
7	1.8	0.2	62	1.9[c,d]	0.16[c,d]	75
8	1.4	0.2	66	0.80[e]	0.05[e]	24
9	1.8	0.5	36	4.09[c]	0.32[c]	53
10	1.4	0.2	36	—	—	—
11	1.7	0.3	61	1.23[d]	0.11[d]	22
12	1.2	0.3	59	1.84[c,d]	0.34	75
13	1.4	0.6	58	1.50[c]	0.42[c]	53
14	1.6	0.5	65	0.64[e]	0.28[e]	24
15	2.5	0.6	33	—	—	—
16	2.9	0.4	43	4.68[c]	0.41[c]	53
17	1.5[b]	0.4	50	4.75[c,f]	0.25[c,d]	96
18	2.7	0.6	67	0.52[e]	0.08[e]	24
19	1.2	0.8	31	—	—	—
20	0.9	0.6	66	0.53[e]	0.04[e]	24
21	1.0	0.5	40	3.10[c]	0.60[e]	53
22	2.0	0.7	66	0.97[g]	0.03[g]	31

[a] Data from unpublished studies completed in our laboratory on males and females aged 7–85 years.
[b] Data from unpublished studies completed in our laboratory and from data published by Guttenbach et al,[111] who evaluated males and females aged 1 week to 93 years.
[c] Data from Rehder et al[119] on females aged 52–80 years.
[d] Data from Aboalela et al[120] on males aged 7–78 years and females aged 15–32 years.
[e] Data from Aboalela et al[120] on males aged 9–78 years and females aged 15–25 years.
[f] Data from Aboalela et al[120] on males aged 7–80 years.
[g] Data from Aboalela et al[120] on males aged 9–78 years and females aged 15–25 years.

chromosome (or a heterochromatin-rich chromosome). Alternatively, the nonrandom loss hypothesis postulates that different chromosomes have different propensities for abnormality occurrence and that the genetic makeup or structure of the chromosome (eg, the heterochromatin content of a chromosome) is the primary determining factor for its acquisition of abnormalities.[122]

To test these plausible hypotheses, investigators have studied the frequency of acquired somatic cell chromosomal abnormalities using a cytokinesis-blocked micronucleus assay, which provides information regarding the previous interphase/mitotic division of a somatic cell before the presence of selective pressure on the resultant daughter cells. A micronucleus is defined as a small structure that is

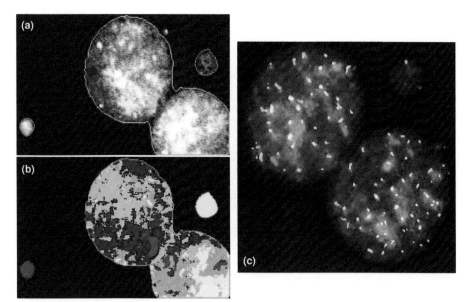

Fig. 4. Micronuclei as seen following spectral karyotyping (SKY) and FISH using a pantelo-meric/pancentromeric probe. The majority of micronuclei contain chromatin from a single chromosome, as shown in the spectral (a) and classified (b) images of a binucleate having two micronuclei, one containing chromatin from chromosome 1 (*yellow; right*) and one containing chromatin from chromosome 13 (*red; lower left*). The majority of micronuclei also contain telomeric (*red*) and centromeric (*green*) signals (c), suggesting that an intact chromosome/chromatid is present in the micronucleus. The micronucleus shown in (c) has two telomeric signals (*red*) and one centromeric (*green*) signal.

juxtaposed to the main daughter nuclei and is thought to contain chromatin (from one or more chromosomes) that was not incorporated into the daughter nuclei ("lagging" or "lost") after cell division[123] (**Fig. 4**). Micronuclei frequencies have been shown to correlate with age and gender, with older subjects (50 years of age or older) showing a higher level than young (younger than 30 years old) individuals,[109,124–130] and women showing a higher increase with age than men.[130] Through the use of FISH methodology, the chromatin present in spontaneously occurring micronuclei has been inferred and has been observed to have a nonrandom pattern, with sex chromatin being present most frequently.[109,125,126,128,129] FISH studies have also shown nonrandom patterns of autosomal chromatin in micronuclei, but these studies have involved only a targeted subset of autosomes rather than assessing all autosomes in a random manner.[131] Our studies, using spectral karyotyping (SKY) techniques,[132] have allowed for the identification of all chromatin that might be present in micronuclei (rather than being limited to a targeted subset of genomic regions as reported in the FISH assays). These SKY analyses have also shown a nonrandom pattern of autosomal exclusion into micronuclei, with chromatin from chromosomes 4, 8, and 9 being present in the micronuclei most frequently, and chromatin from chromosomes 17 and 22 being present least frequently.[133]

Thus, the results of the micronuclei studies support the nonrandom loss hypothesis, with innate differences in acquired aneuploidy frequencies appearing to be present for at least a subset of autosomes. As noted previously, one chromosomal attribute that has been suggested to result in an increased tendency for that

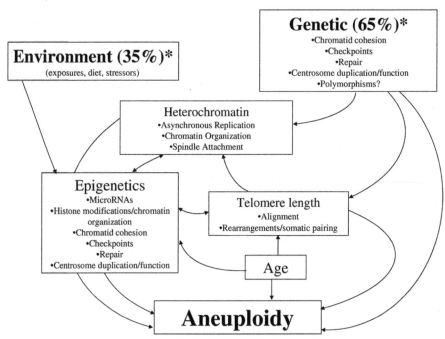

Fig. 5. Potential genetic and environmental influences on somatic aneuploidy. *Acquired aneuploidy frequencies reflect contributions from both genetic (65% of variance) and environmental (35% of variance) factors.[130] Genes that have been implicated to contribute to acquired aneuploidy (either through mutation or epigenetic alterations) are similar to those associated with constitutional aneuploidy and include genes influencing chromatid cohesion, meiotic and spindle checkpoint function; DNA repair; centrosome function/duplication; histone modification; and microRNAs. Heterochromatin-rich chromosomes have been reported to have increased frequencies of aneuploidy (primarily loss). The presence of heterochromatin in somatic cells has been speculated to be influenced by epigenetic changes, but changes in heterochromatin could also illicit epigenetic alterations (demonstrated with a *two-headed arrow*). Alterations in heterochromatin may directly impact the frequency of aneuploidy (potentially by compromising the fidelity of the spindle attachments and replication/pairing processes). Telomere attrition has also been suggested to lead to aneuploidy. Telomere shortening would reduce the amount of heterochromatin present in the telomeric region, and could lead to an epigenetic change by altering the chromatin conformation which, in turn, could allow for the expression of a gene(s) that would typically be silenced. Telomeres might also have a direct influence on aneuploidy which may be implemented through perturbations in alignment/somatic pairing/chromosomal rearrangements, as well as other potential mechanisms. In contrast to constitutional aneuploidy, the role of advancing age on autosomal acquired aneuploidy is uncertain. Age effects have been denoted for a subset of chromosomes, and, when present, may have direct influences on aneuploidy, or indirect influences (eg, increased age leads to telomere shortening, which, in turn, could predispose to aneuploidy).

chromosome to acquire aneuploidy (with age) is its heterochromatin content. However, the molecular basis for this observed correlation is not known (**Fig. 5**). It is feasible that variation in large blocks of heterochromatin between homologs could lead to asynchrony in their replication, which, in turn, may contribute to misalignment and malsegregation. Alternatively, epigenetic changes (primarily hypomethylation) may arise in pericentromeric heterochromatin (especially for autosomes 1, 9, 15, 16, and the acrocentric chromosomes), leading to changes in chromatin conformation that compromise the ability of the chromosomes to align, attach to mitotic spindle fibers, and separate.[97] Although this latter hypothesis has not yet been fully tested in healthy humans (studies are currently underway in our laboratory), it has been tested through analyses of hypomethylated cells obtained either (1) after in vitro induction (primarily using 5-azacytidine) or (2) as a result of mutation (cells from patients having immunodeficiency, centromeric heterochromatin instability, and facial anomalies [ICF] syndrome, who have a mutation in the DNA methyltransferase 3b gene). Collectively, the results of these studies have shown increases in the frequencies of somatic pairing among chromosomes 1, 9, and 16, with concomitant delays in centromere separation that led to the preferential exclusion of these chromosomes into micronuclei.[97,121,134–137] Given the observation of increased somatic pairing associated with hypomethylation, it is also feasible that the apparent increase of acquired aneuploidy for heterochromatin-rich chromosomes reflects its tendency to coalesce or "merge" in the interphase nuclei (rather than having true loss), with this effect being more pronounced with age.[137] Support for this conjecture comes from studies using multiple probes distributed along the length of heterochromatin-rich chromosomes. Although limited in number, investigations of this type have shown the "loss" or observation of single signals to be predominantly localized to the pericentromeric region of chromosomes in the majority of cells evaluated, with two signals (euploid number) being observed for the more distally located probes evaluated in a portion of the same cells.[138]

Another chromosome-specific attribute that has been correlated with acquired aneuploidy frequencies in humans is telomere length[121,139] (see **Fig. 5**). The mechanisms whereby alterations in telomere length predispose a chromosome to loss are not known, but have been speculated to involve a compromise in the localization of cohesin proteins in mitotic cells[140–142]; illegitimate somatic recombination or rearrangements leading to chromosome entanglement or misalignment[97,143]; differential gene expression (especially genes involved in spindle assembly, mitotic checkpoints/controls, or DNA repair); or asynchronous replication timing (which, in turn, could lead to misalignment).[144] The causes of the observed variation in telomere lengths among chromosomes also are not fully known,[145] but are thought to include heritable differences in the initial length of the repeats in the telomeres,[146,147] as well as differences in the rates of telomere attrition due to exposure history (including stress, toxins, oxidative stress, and other environmental factors).[148]

In addition to chromosome-specific variation in aneuploidy frequencies, individual-specific variation in acquired aneuploidy and micronuclei frequencies has been reported,[35,109,125,127,129,149,150] with both genetic (65% of variance) and environmental (35% of variance) factors being shown to influence these frequencies[92,129] (Rehder CW, Corey L, York TP, et al. Chromosome-specific and tissue-specific differences in acquired aneuploidy frequencies in uncultured lymphocytes and buccal mucosa cells: A twin study. Submitted for publication) (see **Fig. 5**). Environmental exposures that have been shown to increase the frequency of micronuclei include, but are not limited to, diet (especially folate deficiency),[130,151–154] hormone levels,[130,154] tobacco use, alcohol consumption, and occupational hazards[130] (Rehder CW, Corey L, York TP, et al. Chromosome-specific and tissue-specific differences in acquired aneuploidy frequencies in uncultured lymphocytes and buccal mucosa cells: A twin study. Submitted for publication).

As with constitutional aneuploidy in humans, the recognition of specific genes that predispose an individual to acquire aneuploidy in noncancerous somatic cells is lacking. Nonetheless, several genes have been implicated to play a contributory/causal role and include (but are not limited to) genes involved in (1) centrosomal structure/duplication,[155–157] (2) DNA repair,[158–160] (3) mitotic checkpoint maintenance,[161,162] (4) chromatid cohesion,[163] (5) chromatin organization,[164] and (6) the formation/function of the spindle and other components of the mitotic machinery[165,166] (see **Fig. 5**). Perturbations in genes involved in histone methylation or small interfering RNAs have also been noted to lead to disturbances in chromosomal malsegregation or kinetochore protein organization, respectively.[167,168]

Phenotypic Findings Reported in People with Acquired Aneuploidy

The clinical consequence(s) of acquired autosomal aneuploidy in normal somatic cells are not known, but are thought to range from no phenotypic effect to being a potential precursor for the development of a variety of diseases. Woida and Witt[169] noted that several of the autosomes that have been shown to have higher frequencies of acquired aneuploidy are chromosomes that harbor genes that play roles in cellular senescence or premature aging syndromes. Aviv and Aviv[170] have further speculated that the imbalances resulting from the acquired changes could be a prerequisite step for the development of cancer or other age-related conditions such as hypertension, non-insulin-dependent diabetes mellitus, atherosclerosis, and cancer.

SUMMARY

When reviewing our knowledge of autosomal aneuploidy in humans, one is reminded of a quote by Noam Chomsky which, paraphrased, asks, "How it is we have so much information, but know so little?"[171] When comparing constitutional to acquired aneuploidy one can detect both similarities and differences in their frequencies and purported etiologic mechanisms. Chromosome-specific differences in the frequencies of aneuploidy are observed in both abortus tissue (constitutional) and lymphocytes (acquired), with consistent increases in frequencies noted for chromosomes 15, 16, and 18 and consistent decreases in frequencies observed for chromosomes 3, 5, and 19. Although acquired aneuploidy frequencies have been shown to be more heavily influenced by genetic than by environmental factors, less is known about the impact of genetic versus environmental effects on gametic aneuploidy. Clear overlap in the genes contributing to somatic and gametic aneuploid is present (ie, genes involved in chromatid cohesion, meiotic/spindle checkpoints, DNA repair, centrosome formation/duplication). Nonetheless, strong influences that are unique to constitutional (ie, meiotic recombination) and acquired (ie, telomere attrition) aneuploidy have also been recognized. Technological advances have allowed for improvements in the understanding of the causes and consequences of aneuploidy, and it is anticipated that future improvements will continue to provide the necessary tools to better tease apart the biological basis of autosomal malsegregation. These anticipated advances (especially in the area of epigenetics, which may allow a means for bridging the knowledge gained from studies of environmental and genetic influences) allow one to be guardedly optimistic that we will expand our knowledge of the causes of aneuploidy in the near future. Exploitation of the knowledge gained from these future studies might allow for the development of screening tests to identify people who are most "at risk" for having offspring with aneuploid conditions and lead to improvements in our understanding and management of the role that aneuploidy plays in the aging process and acquisition of age-related diseases.

REFERENCES

1. Hook EB. The impact of aneuploidy upon public health: mortality and morbidity associated with human chromosome abnormalities. Basic Life Sci 1985;36: 7–33.
2. Hook EB. Chromosome abnormalities: prevalence, risks and recurrence. Edinburgh (Scotland): Churchill Livingstone; 1992.
3. Jacobs PA, Browne C, Gregson N, et al. Estimates of the frequency of chromosome abnormalities detectable in unselected newborns using moderate levels of banding. J Med Genet 1992;29(2):103–8.
4. Wang J-CC. Autosomal aneuploidy. In: Gersen SL, Keagle MB, editors. The principles of clinical cytogenetics. Totowa (NJ): Humana Press; 1999. p. 157–90.
5. Bond DJ, Chandley AC. Aneuploidy in man: the problem stated. In: Bond DJ, Chandley AC, editors. Aneuploidy. New York: Oxford University Press; 1983. p. 4–26.
6. Martin RH. Meiotic errors in human oogenesis and spermatogenesis. Reprod Biomed Online Apr 2008;16(4):523–31.
7. Pacchierotti F, Adler ID, Eichenlaub-Ritter U, et al. Gender effects on the incidence of aneuploidy in mammalian germ cells. Environ Res 2007;104(1):46–69.
8. Fragouli E, Wells D, Delhanty JD. Chromosome abnormalities in the human oocyte. Cytogenet Genome Res 2011;133(2–4):107–18.
9. Bond DJ, Chandley AC. Spontaneous aneuploidy in mammals other than man. In: Bond DJ, Chandley AC, editors. Aneuploidy. New York: Oxford University Press; 1983. p. 77–91.
10. Templado C, Vidal F, Estop A. Aneuploidy in human spermatozoa. Cytogenet Genome Res 2011;133(2–4):91–9.
11. Pellestor F, Andreo B, Anahory T, et al. The occurrence of aneuploidy in human: lessons from the cytogenetic studies of human oocytes. Eur J Med Genet 2006; 49(2):103–16.
12. Rosenbusch B. The incidence of aneuploidy in human oocytes assessed by conventional cytogenetic analysis. Hereditas 2004;141(2):97–105.
13. Hunt PA, Hassold TJ. Sex matters in meiosis. Science 2002;296(5576):2181–3.
14. Hunt PA, Hassold TJ. Human female meiosis: what makes a good egg go bad? Trends Genet 2008;24(2):86–93.
15. Nussbaum RL, McInnes RR, Willard HF. In: Nussbaum RL, McInnes RR, Willard HF, editors. Glossary Thompson & Thompson Genetics in Medicine. 7th edition. Philadelphia: Saunders Elsevier; 2007. p. 542.
16. Papavassiliou P, York TP, Gursoy N, et al. The phenotype of persons having mosaicism for trisomy 21/Down syndrome reflects the percentage of trisomic cells present in different tissues. Am J Med Genet A 2009;149A(4):573–83.
17. Vorsanova SG, Yurov YB, Iourov IY. Human interphase chromosomes: a review of available molecular cytogenetic technologies. Mol Cytogenet 2010;3:1.
18. Hook EB. Prevalence of chromosome abnormalities during human gestation and implications for studies of environmental mutagens. Lancet 1981;2(8239):169–72.
19. Magenis RE, Hecht F, Milham S Jr. Trisomy 13 (D1) syndrome: studies on parental age, sex ratio, and survival. J Pediatr 1968;73(2):222–8.
20. Carey JC. Trisomy 18 and trisomy 13 syndromes. In: Cassidy SB, Allanson J, editors. Management of genetic syndromes. 2nd edition. New York: Wiley-Liss; 2005. p. 555–68.
21. Willis MJ, Bird LM, Dell'Aquilla M, et al. Expanding the phenotype of mosaic trisomy 20. Am J Med Genet A 2008;146(3):330–6.

22. Hsu LY, Kaffe S, Jenkins EC, et al. Proposed guidelines for diagnosis of chromosome mosaicism in amniocytes based on data derived from chromosome mosaicism and pseudomosaicism studies. Prenat Diagn 1992;12(7):555–73.

23. Hahnemann JM, Vejerslev LO. European collaborative research on mosaicism in CVS (EUCROMIC)—fetal and extrafetal cell lineages in 192 gestations with CVS mosaicism involving single autosomal trisomy. Am J Med Genet 1997;70(2):179–87.

24. Hsu LY, Yu MT, Neu RL, et al. Rare trisomy mosaicism diagnosed in amniocytes, involving an autosome other than chromosomes 13, 18, 20, and 21: karyotype/phenotype correlations. Prenat Diagn 1997;17(3):201–42.

25. Wallerstein R, Yu MT, Neu RL, et al. Common trisomy mosaicism diagnosed in amniocytes involving chromosomes 13, 18, 20 and 21: karyotype-phenotype correlations. Prenat Diagn 2000;20(2):103–22.

26. Santos MA, Teklenburg G, Macklon NS, et al. The fate of the mosaic embryo: chromosomal constitution and development of day 4, 5 and 8 human embryos. Hum Reprod 2010;25(8):1916–26.

27. Daphnis DD, Delhanty JD, Jerkovic S, et al. Detailed FISH analysis of day 5 human embryos reveals the mechanisms leading to mosaic aneuploidy. Hum Reprod 2005;20(1):129–37.

28. Yurov YB, Iourov IY, Monakhov VV, et al. The variation of aneuploidy frequency in the developing and adult human brain revealed by an interphase FISH study. J Histochem Cytochem 2005;53(3):385–90.

29. Yurov YB, Iourov IY, Vorsanova SG, et al. Aneuploidy and confined chromosomal mosaicism in the developing human brain. PLoS One 2007;2(6):e558.

30. Wilkens L, Flemming P, Gebel M, et al. Induction of aneuploidy by increasing chromosomal instability during dedifferentiation of hepatocellular carcinoma. Proc Natl Acad Sci USA 2004;101(5):1309–14.

31. Iourov IY, Vorsanova SG, Yurov YB. Chromosomal mosaicism goes global. Mol Cytogenet 2008;1:26.

32. Delhanty JD. Inherited aneuploidy: germline mosaicism. Cytogenet Genome Res 2011;133(2–4):136–40.

33. Griffith CB, Vance GH, Weaver DD. Phenotypic variability in trisomy 13 mosaicism: two new patients and literature review. Am J Med Genet A 2009;149A(6):1346–58.

34. Tucker ME, Garringer HJ, Weaver DD. Phenotypic spectrum of mosaic trisomy 18: two new patients, a literature review, and counseling issues. Am J Med Genet A 2007;143(5):505–17.

35. von Sneidern E, Lacassie Y. Is trisomy 14 mosaic a clinically recognizable syndrome? Case report and review. Am J Med Genet A 2008;146A(12):1609–13.

36. Sifakis S, Staboulidou I, Maiz N, et al. Outcome of pregnancies with trisomy 2 cells in chorionic villi. Prenat Diagn 2010;30(4):329–32.

37. Sago H, Chen E, Conte WJ, et al. True trisomy 2 mosaicism in amniocytes and newborn liver associated with multiple system abnormalities. Am J Med Genet 1997;72(3):343–6.

38. Prontera P, Stangoni G, Ardisia C, et al. Trisomy 2 mosaicism with caudal dysgenesis, Hirschsprung disease, and micro-anophthalmia. Am J Med Genet A 2011;155(4):928–30.

39. Zaslav AL, Pierno G, Davis J, et al. Prenatal diagnosis of trisomy 3 mosaicism. Prenat Diagn 2004;24(9):693–6.

40. Metaxotou C, Tsenghi C, Bitzos I, et al. Trisomy 3 mosaicism in a live-born infant. Clin Genet 1981;19(1):37–40.

41. Kuhn EM, Sarto GE, Bates BJ, et al. Gene-rich chromosome regions and autosomal trisomy. A case of chromosome 3 trisomy mosaicism. Hum Genet 1987;77(3):214–20.
42. DeKeyerser F ME, DePaepe A, Verschraegen-Spae MR. Trisomy 3 mosaicism in a patient with Barter syndrome. J Med Genet 1988;25:358.
43. Wieczorek D, Prott EC, Robinson WP, et al. Prenatally detected trisomy 4 and 6 mosaicism — cytogenetic results and clinical phenotype. Prenat Diagn 2003;23(2): 128–33.
44. Zaslav AL, Blumenthal D, Willner JP, et al. Prenatal diagnosis of trisomy 4 mosaicism. Am J Med Genet 2000;95(4):381–4.
45. Destree A, Fourneau C, Dugauquier C, et al. Prenatal diagnosis of trisomy 6 mosaicism. Prenat Diagn 2005;25(5):354–7.
46. Chen CP, Su YN, Chern SR, et al. Mosaic trisomy 7 at amniocentesis: prenatal diagnosis and molecular genetic analyses. Taiwan J Obstet Gynecol 2010;49(3): 333–40.
47. Verghese S, Newlin A, Miller M, et al. Mosaic trisomy 7 in a patient with pigmentary abnormalities. Am J Med Genet 1999;87(5):371–4.
48. Hale NE, Keane JF Jr. Piecing together a picture of trisomy 8 mosaicism syndrome. J Am Osteopath Assoc 2010;110(1):21–3.
49. Wisniewska M, Mazurek M. Trisomy 8 mosaicism syndrome. J Appl Genet 2002; 43(1):115–8.
50. Riccardi VM. Trisomy 8: an international study of 70 patients. Birth Defects Orig Artic Ser 1977;13(3C):171–84.
51. Chen CP, Lin HM, Su YN, et al. Mosaic trisomy 9 at amniocentesis: prenatal diagnosis and molecular genetic analyses. Taiwan J Obstet Gynecol 2010;49(3): 341–50.
52. Schwendemann WD, Contag SA, Wax JR, et al. Sonographic findings in trisomy 9. J Ultrasound Med 2009;28(1):39–42.
53. Bruns D. Presenting physical characteristics, medical conditions, and developmental status of long-term survivors with trisomy 9 mosaicism. Am J Med Genet A 2011;155(5):1033–9.
54. Hahnemann JM, Nir M, Friberg M, et al. Trisomy 10 mosaicism and maternal uniparental disomy 10 in a liveborn infant with severe congenital malformations. Am J Med Genet A 2005;138A(2):150–4.
55. Balasubramanian M, Peres LC, Pelly D. Mosaic trisomy 11 in a fetus with bilateral renal agenesis: co-incidence or new association? Clin Dysmorphol 2011;20(1):47–9.
56. Parasuraman R, Mercer C, Bascombe L, et al. A case of trisomy 12 mosaicism presenting antenatally with fetal cardiomyopathy. J Obstet Gynaecol 2011;31(3): 261–3.
57. Gentilin B, Giardino D, Boschetto C, et al. Limited value of echography to predict true fetal mosaicism for trisomy 12. Prenat Diagn 2006;26(12):1186–9.
58. Staals JE, Schrander-Stumpel CT, Hamers G, et al. Prenatal diagnosis of trisomy 12 mosaicism: normal development of a 3 years old female child. Genet Couns 2003;14(2):233–7.
59. DeLozier-Blanchet CD, Roeder E, Denis-Arrue R, et al. Trisomy 12 mosaicism confirmed in multiple organs from a liveborn child. Am J Med Genet 2000;95(5): 444–9.
60. Chen CP. Prenatal diagnosis and genetic counseling for mosaic trisomy 13. Taiwan J Obstet Gynecol 2010;49(1):13–22.
61. Delatycki M, Gardner RJ. Three cases of trisomy 13 mosaicism and a review of the literature. Clin Genet 1997;51(6):403–7.

62. Golabi M, James AW, Good WV, et al. Tissue-limited mosaicism for monosomy 13. Am J Med Genet A 2010;152A(10):2634–9.
63. Merritt TA, Natarajan G. Trisomy 14 Mosaicism: a case without evidence of neuro-developmental delay and a review of the literature. Am J Perinatol 2007;24(9):563–6.
64. Shinawi M, Shao L, Jeng LJ, et al. Low-level mosaicism of trisomy 14: phenotypic and molecular characterization. Am J Med Genet A 2008;146A(11):1395–405.
65. Zaslav AL, Fallet S, Brown S, et al. Prenatal diagnosis of low level trisomy 15 mosaicism: review of the literature. Clin Genet 1998;53(4):286–92.
66. Benn P. Trisomy 16 and trisomy 16 Mosaicism: a review. Am J Med Genet 1998;79(2):121–33.
67. Utermann B, Riegel M, Leistritz D, et al. Pre- and postnatal findings in trisomy 17 mosaicism. Am J Med Genet A 2006;140(15):1628–36.
68. Genuardi M, Tozzi C, Pomponi MG, et al. Mosaic trisomy 17 in amniocytes: phenotypic outcome, tissue distribution, and uniparental disomy studies. Eur J Hum Genet 1999;7(4):421–6.
69. Bianca S, Boemi G, Barrano B, et al. Mosaic trisomy 20: considerations for genetic counseling. Am J Med Genet A 2008;146A(14):1897–8.
70. van der Kevie-Kersemaekers AM, Suijkerbuijk RF, Moll FC, et al. A live-born child with a mosaic chromosomal pattern of either monosomy 21 or trisomy 4 in different embryonal germ layers. Prenat Diagn 2010;30(1):86–8.
71. Cheng PJ, Shaw SW, Shih JC, et al. Monozygotic twins discordant for monosomy 21 detected by first-trimester nuchal translucency screening. Obstet Gynecol 2006;107(2 Pt 2):538–41.
72. Nguyen HP, Riess A, Kruger M, et al. Mosaic trisomy 21/monosomy 21 in a living female infant. Cytogenet Genome Res 2009;125(1):26–32.
73. Leclercq S, Baron X, Jacquemont ML, et al. Mosaic trisomy 22: five new cases with variable outcomes. Implications for genetic counselling and clinical management. Prenat Diagn 2010;30(2):168–72.
74. Crowe CA, Schwartz S, Black CJ, et al. Mosaic trisomy 22: a case presentation and literature review of trisomy 22 phenotypes. Am J Med Genet 1997;71(4):406–13.
75. Langlois S, Yong PJ, Yong SL, et al. Postnatal follow-up of prenatally diagnosed trisomy 16 mosaicism. Prenat Diagn 2006;26(6):548–58.
76. Hassold T, Hunt P. Maternal age and chromosomally abnormal pregnancies: what we know and what we wish we knew. Curr Opin Pediatr 2009;21(6):703–8.
77. Hassold T, Hall H, Hunt P. The origin of human aneuploidy: where we have been, where we are going. Hum Mol Genet 2007;16(Spec No. 2):R203–8.
78. Jackson-Cook CK, Flannery DB, Corey LA, et al. Nucleolar organizer region variants as a risk factor for Down syndrome. Am J Hum Genet 1985;37(6):1049–61.
79. Warburton D. Genetic factors influencing aneuploidy frequency. Basic Life Sci 1985;36:133–48.
80. Hassold T, Hunt P. To err (meiotically) is human: the genesis of human aneuploidy. Nat Rev Genet 2001;2(4):280–91.
81. Oliver TR, Feingold E, Yu K, et al. New insights into human nondisjunction of chromosome 21 in oocytes. PLoS Genet 2008;4(3):e1000033.
82. Grell RF. The meiotic process and aneuploidy. Basic Life Sci 1985;36:317–35.
83. Jones KT. Meiosis in oocytes: predisposition to aneuploidy and its increased incidence with age. Hum Reprod Update 2008;14(2):143–58.
84. Eichenlaub-Ritter U, Staubach N, Trapphoff T. Chromosomal and cytoplasmic context determines predisposition to maternal age-related aneuploidy: brief overview and update on MCAK in mammalian oocytes. Biochem Soc Trans 2010;38(6):1681–6.

85. Chiang T, Duncan FE, Schindler K, et al. Evidence that weakened centromere cohesion is a leading cause of age-related aneuploidy in oocytes. Curr Biol 2010; 20(17):1522–8.

86. Miao YL, Sun QY, Zhang X, et al. Centrosome abnormalities during porcine oocyte aging. Environ Mol Mutagen 2009;50(8):666–71.

87. van den Berg IM, Eleveld C, van der Hoeven M, et al. Defective deacetylation of histone 4 K12 in human oocytes is associated with advanced maternal age and chromosome misalignment. Hum Reprod 2011;26(5):1181–90.

88. Holt JE, Jones KT. Control of homologous chromosome division in the mammalian oocyte. Mol Hum Reprod 2009;15(3):139–47.

89. Dumont J, Oegema K, Desai A. A kinetochore-independent mechanism drives anaphase chromosome separation during acentrosomal meiosis. Nat Cell Biol 2010;12(9):894–901.

90. Hassold T, Sherman S. Down syndrome: genetic recombination and the origin of the extra chromosome 21. Clin Genet 2000;57(2):95–100.

91. Warren WD, Gorringe KL. A molecular model for sporadic human aneuploidy. Trends Genet 2006;22(4):218–24.

92. Pacchierotti F, Eichenlaub-Ritter U. Environmental hazard in the aetiology of somatic and germ cell aneuploidy. Cytogenet Genome Res 2011;133(2–4):254–68.

93. Hunt PA, Koehler KE, Susiarjo M, et al. Bisphenol A exposure causes meiotic aneuploidy in the female mouse. Curr Biol 2003;13(7):546–53.

94. George O, Bryant BK, Chinnasamy R, et al. Bisphenol A directly targets tubulin to disrupt spindle organization in embryonic and somatic cells. ACS Chem Biol 2008; 3(3):167–79.

95. Dolinoy DC, Huang D, Jirtle RL. Maternal nutrient supplementation counteracts bisphenol A-induced DNA hypomethylation in early development. Proc Natl Acad Sci USA 2007;104(32):13056–61.

96. Avissar-Whiting M, Veiga KR, Uhl KM, et al. Bisphenol A exposure leads to specific microRNA alterations in placental cells. Reprod Toxicol 2010;29(4):401–6.

97. Herrera LA, Prada D, Andonegui MA, et al. The epigenetic origin of aneuploidy. Curr Genomics 2008;9(1):43–50.

98. Kerkel K, Schupf N, Hatta K, et al. Altered DNA methylation in leukocytes with trisomy 21. PLoS Genet 2010;6(11):e1001212.

99. Pangalos C, Avramopoulos D, Blouin JL, et al. Understanding the mechanism(s) of mosaic trisomy 21 by using DNA polymorphism analysis. Am J Hum Genet 1994; 54(3):473–81.

100. Niikawa N, Kajii T. The origin of mosaic Down syndrome: four cases with chromosome markers. Am J Hum Genet 1984;36(1):123–30.

101. Jacobs PA, Court Brown WM, Doll R. Distribution of human chromosome counts in relation to age. Nature 1961;191:1178–80.

102. Jacobs PA, Brunton M, Court Brown WM, et al. Change of human chromosome count distribution with age: evidence for a sex differences. Nature 1963;197: 1080–1.

103. Fitzgerald PH, McEwan CM. Total aneuploidy and age-related sex chromosome aneuploidy in cultured lymphocytes of normal men and women. Hum Genet 1977; 39(3):329–37.

104. Galloway SM, Buckton KE. Aneuploidy and ageing: chromosome studies on a random sample of the population using G-banding. Cytogenet Cell Genet 1978; 20(1–6):78–95.

105. Brown T, Fox DP, Robertson FW, et al. Non-random chromosome loss in PHA-stimulated lymphocytes from normal individuals. Mutat Res 1983;122(3-4):403–6.

106. Ford JH, Russell JA. Differences in the error mechanisms affecting sex and auto-somal chromosomes in women of different ages within the reproductive age group. Am J Hum Genet 1985;37(5):973–83.

107. Martin JM, Kellett JM, Kahn J. Aneuploidy in cultured human lymphocytes: I. Age and sex differences. Age Ageing 1980;9(3):147–53.

108. Nowinski GP, Van Dyke DL, Tilley BC, et al. The frequency of aneuploidy in cultured lymphocytes is correlated with age and gender but not with reproductive history. Am J Hum Genet 1990;46(6):1101–11.

109. Catalan J, Autio K, Wessman M, et al. Age-associated micronuclei containing centromeres and the X chromosome in lymphocytes of women. Cytogenet Cell Genet 1995;68(1-2):11–6.

110. Mukherjee AB, Alejandro J, Payne S, et al. Age-related aneuploidy analysis of human blood cells in vivo by fluorescence in situ hybridization (FISH). Mech Ageing Dev 1996;90(2):145–56.

111. Guttenbach M, Koschorz B, Bernthaler U, et al. Sex chromosome loss and aging: in situ hybridization studies on human interphase nuclei. Am J Hum Genet 1995;57(5): 1143–50.

112. Richard F, Aurias A, Couturier J, et al. Aneuploidy in human lymphocytes: an extensive study of eight individuals of various ages. Mutat Res 1993;295(2): 71–80.

113. Ford JH, Lester P. Factors affecting the displacement of human chromosomes from the metaphase plate. Cytogenet Cell Genet 1982;33(4):327–32.

114. Neurath P, DeRemer K, Bell B, et al. Chromosome loss compared with chromosome size, age and sex of subjects. Nature 1970;225(5229):281–2.

115. Wenger SL, Golden WL, Dennis SP, et al. Are the occasional aneuploid cells in peripheral blood cultures significant? Am J Med Genet 1984;19(4):715–9.

116. Mukherjee AB, Thomas S. A longitudinal study of human age-related chromosomal analysis in skin fibroblasts. Exp Cell Res 1997;235(1):161–9.

117. Ford JH. A model for the mechanism of aneuploidy involving chromosome displace-ment. In: Dellarco VL, Voytek PE, Hollaender A, editors. Aneuploidy: etiology and mechanisms. New York: Plenum Press; 1985. p. 291–5.

118. Wojda A, Zietkiewicz E, Mossakowska M, et al. Correlation between the level of cytogenetic aberrations in cultured human lymphocytes and the age and gender of donors. J Gerontol A Biol Sci Med Sci 2006;61(8):763–72.

119. Aboalela N. The Effects of Age and Heterochromatin on Frequencies of Acquired Chromosomal Aneuploidy in Uncultured Human Leukocytes. Richmond: Virginia Commonwealth University; 2001.

120. Fauth E, Scherthan H, Zankl H. Frequencies of occurrence of all human chromo-somes in micronuclei from normal and 5-azacytidine-treated lymphocytes as re-vealed by chromosome painting. Mutagenesis 1998;13(3):235–41.

121. Leach NT, Rehder C, Jensen K, et al. Human chromosomes with shorter telomeres and large heterochromatin regions have a higher frequency of acquired somatic cell aneuploidy. Mech Ageing Dev 2004;125(8):563–73.

122. Maurer B, GM, Schmid M. Chromosomal instability in normative aging. In: Hisama FM, Weissman SM, Martin G, editors. Chromosomal instability and aging. New York: Marcel Dekker; 2003. p. 125–47

123. Fenech M, Morley AA. The effect of donor age on spontaneous and induced micronuclei. Mutat Res 1985;148(1-2):99–105.

124. Ford JH, Schultz CJ, Correll AT. Chromosome elimination in micronuclei: a common cause of hypoploidy. Am J Hum Genet 1988;43(5):733–40.

125. Hando JC, Nath J, Tucker JD. Sex chromosomes, micronuclei and aging in women. Chromosoma 1994;103(3):186–92.
126. Guttenbach M, Schakowski R, Schmid M. Aneuploidy and ageing: sex chromosome exclusion into micronuclei. Hum Genet 1994;94(3):295–8.
127. Nath J, Tucker JD, Hando JC. Y chromosome aneuploidy, micronuclei, kinetochores and aging in men. Chromosoma 1995;103(10):725–31.
128. Zijno A, Leopardi P, Marcon F, et al. Analysis of chromosome segregation by means of fluorescence in situ hybridization: application to cytokinesis-blocked human lymphocytes. Mutat Res 1996;372(2):211–9.
129. Catalan J, Autio K, Kuosma E, et al. Age-dependent inclusion of sex chromosomes in lymphocyte micronuclei of man. Am J Hum Genet 1998;63(5):1464–72.
130. Jones KH, York, TP, Juusola J, et al. Genetic and environmental factors contributing to spontaneous micronuclei frequencies in children and adults: a twin study. Mutagenesis. 2011. [Epub ahead of print].
131. Norppa H, Falck GC. What do human micronuclei contain? Mutagenesis. 2003; 18(3):221–33.
132. Leach NT, Jackson-Cook C. The application of spectral karyotyping (SKY) and fluorescent in situ hybridization (FISH) technology to determine the chromosomal content(s) of micronuclei. Mutat Res 2001;495(1-2):11–9.
133. Jones KH. Age-related genetic and epigenetic chromosomal changes: A twin study. Richmond: Virginia Commonwealth University; 2009.
134. Hernandez R, Frady A, Zhang XY, et al. Preferential induction of chromosome 1 multibranched figures and whole-arm deletions in a human pro-B cell line treated with 5-azacytidine or 5-azadeoxycytidine. Cytogenet Cell Genet 1997;76(3-4): 196–201.
135. Rodriguez MJ, Lopez MA, Garcia-Orad A, et al. Sequence of centromere separation: effect of 5-azacytidine-induced epigenetic alteration. Mutagenesis 2001;16(2):109–14.
136. Stacey M, Bennett MS, Hulten M. FISH analysis on spontaneously arising micronuclei in the ICF syndrome. J Med Genet 1995;32(7):502–8.
137. Schmid M, Grunert D, Haaf T, et al. A direct demonstration of somatically paired heterochromatin of human chromosomes. Cytogenet Cell Genet 1983;36(3): 554–61.
138. Iourov IY, Liehr T, Vorsanova SG, et al. Visualization of interphase chromosomes in postmitotic cells of the human brain by multicolour banding (MCB). Chromosome Res 2006;14(3):223–9.
139. Martens UM, Zijlmans JM, Poon SS, et al. Short telomeres on human chromosome 17p. Nat Genet 1998;18(1):76–80.
140. Ye JZ, de Lange T. TIN2 is a tankyrase 1 PARP modulator in the TRF1 telomere length control complex. Nat Genet 2004;36(6):618–23.
141. Dynek JN, Smith S. Resolution of sister telomere association is required for progression through mitosis. Science 2004;304(5667):97–100.
142. Azzalin CM, Lingner J. Cell biology. Telomere wedding ends in divorce. Science 2004;304(5667):60–2.
143. Pampalona J, Soler D, Genesca A, et al. Whole chromosome loss is promoted by telomere dysfunction in primary cells. Genes Chromosomes Cancer 2010;49(4): 368–78.
144. Zou Y, Gryaznov SM, Shay JW, et al. Asynchronous replication timing of telomeres at opposite arms of mammalian chromosomes. Proc Natl Acad Sci USA 2004; 101(35):12928–33.

145. Samassekou O, Gadji M, Drouin R, et al. Sizing the ends: normal length of human telomeres. Ann Anat 2010;192(5):284–91.

146. Graakjaer J, Der-Sarkissian H, Schmitz A, et al. Allele-specific relative telomere lengths are inherited. Hum Genet 2006;119(3):344–50.

147. Andrew T, Aviv A, Falchi M, et al. Mapping genetic loci that determine leukocyte telomere length in a large sample of unselected female sibling pairs. Am J Hum Genet 2006;78(3):480–6.

148. Epel ES. Psychological and metabolic stress: a recipe for accelerated cellular aging? Hormones (Athens) 2009;8(1):7–22.

149. Norppa H, Renzi L, Lindholm C. Detection of whole chromosomes in micronuclei of cytokinesis-blocked human lymphocytes by antikinetochore staining and in situ hybridization. Mutagenesis 1993;8(6):519–25.

150. Scarpato R, Landini E, Migliore L. Acrocentric chromosome frequency in spontaneous human lymphocyte micronuclei, evaluated by dual-colour hybridization, is neither sex- nor age-related. Mutat Res 1996;372(2):195–204.

151. Beetstra S, Thomas P, Salisbury C, et al. Folic acid deficiency increases chromosomal instability, chromosome 21 aneuploidy and sensitivity to radiation-induced micronuclei. Mutat Res 2005;578(1-2):317–26.

152. Ni J, Lu L, Fenech M, et al. Folate deficiency in human peripheral blood lymphocytes induces chromosome 8 aneuploidy but this effect is not modified by riboflavin. Environ Mol Mutagen 2010;51(1):15–22.

153. Wang X, Thomas P, Xue J, et al. Folate deficiency induces aneuploidy in human lymphocytes in vitro-evidence using cytokinesis-blocked cells and probes specific for chromosomes 17 and 21. Mutat Res 2004;551(1-2):167–80.

154. Stopper H, Schmitt E, Gregor C, et al. Increased cell proliferation is associated with genomic instability: elevated micronuclei frequencies in estradiol-treated human ovarian cancer cells. Mutagenesis 2003;18(3):243–7.

155. Fisk HA, Mattison CP, Winey M. Human Mps1 protein kinase is required for centrosome duplication and normal mitotic progression. Proc Natl Acad Sci USA 2003;100(25):14875–80.

156. Ganem NJ, Godinho SA, Pellman D. A mechanism linking extra centrosomes to chromosomal instability. Nature 2009;460(7252):278–82.

157. Acilan C, Saunders WS. A tale of too many centrosomes. Cell 2008;134(4):572–5.

158. Smith L, Liu SJ, Goodrich L, et al. Duplication of ATR inhibits MyoD, induces aneuploidy and eliminates radiation-induced G1 arrest. Nat Genet 1998;19(1):39–46.

159. Bassing CH, Suh H, Ferguson DO, et al. Histone H2AX: a dosage-dependent suppressor of oncogenic translocations and tumors. Cell 2003;114(3):359–70.

160. Weaver Z, Montagna C, Xu X, et al. Mammary tumors in mice conditionally mutant for Brca1 exhibit gross genomic instability and centrosome amplification yet display a recurring distribution of genomic imbalances that is similar to human breast cancer. Oncogene 2002;21(33):5097–107.

161. Cleveland DW, Mao Y, Sullivan KF. Centromeres and kinetochores: from epigenetics to mitotic checkpoint signaling. Cell 2003;112(4):407–21.

162. Babu JR, Jeganathan KB, Baker DJ, et al. Rae1 is an essential mitotic checkpoint regulator that cooperates with Bub3 to prevent chromosome missegregation. J Cell Biol 2003;160(3):341–53.

163. Diaz-Martinez LA, Clarke DJ. Chromosome cohesion and the spindle checkpoint. Cell Cycle 2009;8(17):2733–40.

164. Gurvich N, Perna F, Farina A, et al. L3MBTL1 polycomb protein, a candidate tumor suppressor in del(20q12) myeloid disorders, is essential for genome stability. Proc Natl Acad Sci USA 2010;107(52):22552–7.

165. Thompson SL, Bakhoum SF, Compton DA. Mechanisms of chromosomal instability. Curr Biol 2010;20(6):R285–95.

166. Matos I, Maiato H. Prevention and correction mechanisms behind anaphase synchrony: implications for the genesis of aneuploidy. Cytogenet Genome Res 2011; 133(2–4):243–53.

167. Melcher M, Schmid M, Aagaard L, et al. Structure-function analysis of SUV39H1 reveals a dominant role in heterochromatin organization, chromosome segregation, and mitotic progression. Mol Cell Biol 2000;20(10):3728–41.

168. Folco HD, Pidoux AL, Urano T, et al. Heterochromatin and RNAi are required to establish CENP-A chromatin at centromeres. Science 2008;319(5859):94–7.

169. Wojda A, Witt M. Manifestations of ageing at the cytogenetic level. J Appl Genet 2003;44(3):383–99.

170. Aviv A, Aviv H. Telomeres, hidden mosaicism, loss of heterozygosity, and complex genetic traits. Hum Genet 1998;103(1):2–4.

171. Available at: www.goodreads.com/quotes/2476.Noam_Chomsky. Accessed August 15, 2011.

Chromosomal Structural Rearrangements: Detection and Elucidation of Mechanisms Using Cytogenomic Technologies

Sarah T. South, PhD,[a,b,*]

KEYWORDS
- Genomic microarray • Insertions • Low copy repeats
- Translocations • Fluorescence in situ hybridization
- Karyotype

With whole genome analyses, various chromosome rearrangements are observed. The higher the resolution of the analysis, the more likely one may observe unexpected complexity. As this complexity is explored, we may better understand the various mechanisms leading to chromosome rearrangements and discover new mechanisms. This requires technologies that can both look at the copy number changes associated with rearrangements, the genomic architecture surrounding the copy number alteration, and the location of rearranged material. This requires well-established technologies, such as analysis of chromosome banding patterns (traditional karyotypes), sequence analysis by polymerase chain reaction and fluorescence in situ hybridization (FISH), as well as newer technologies such as high-resolution genomic microarray.

GENOMIC MICROARRAY CAN HELP TO FURTHER CHARACTERIZE A CHROMOSOME ABNORMALITY
Unexpected Loss or Gain at de Novo Breakpoints

The finding of a de novo balanced rearrangement increases the risk for a serious congenital anomaly to approximately 6.7%.[1] This increased risk is often attributed to disruption of genes or regulatory elements. Using this logic, numerous studies focused on breakpoint mapping of de novo balanced rearrangements in an individual

The author has nothing to disclose.

[a] Cytogenetics, Genomic Microarray, Genetic Processing at ARUP Laboratories, 500 Chipeta Way, Salt Lake City, UT 84108, USA
[b] Department of Pediatrics and Pathology, University of Utah, Salt Lake City, UT 84108, USA
* Cytogenetics, Genomic Microarray, Genetic Processing at ARUP Laboratories, 500 Chipeta Way, Salt Lake City, UT 84108.
E-mail address: sarah.south@aruplab.com

Clin Lab Med 31 (2011) 513–524
doi:10.1016/j.cll.2011.08.010
0272-2712/11/$ – see front matter © 2011 Elsevier Inc. All rights reserved.

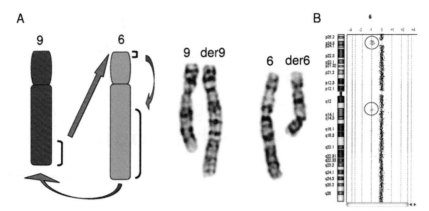

Fig. 1. (A) Complex rearrangement between chromosomes 6 and 9 that by banding seems to be balanced with a translocation of 9q32-qter to 6p, a translocation of 6pter-p24.2 to 6q13, and a translocation of 6q13-qter to 9q. (B) Genomic microarray of the same case shows a 4.9-Mb deletion at 6p25.1-24.1 and a 2.1-Mb deletion at 6q13-q14.1, consistent with deletions at 2 of the breakpoints of this rearrangement.

with phenotypic abnormalities have identified genes involved in important developmental pathways.[2]

In addition, numerous studies have also shown that de novo apparently balanced translocations associated with an abnormal phenotype often have a cryptic imbalance at or near 1 of the translocation breakpoints (**Fig. 1**), or have cryptic imbalances elsewhere in the genome. These cryptic imbalances certainly are associated in some cases with the increased risk of the rearrangement resulting in a clinical consequence and justify the further characterization of an apparently balanced cytogenetic rearrangement with high-resolution copy number analysis via genomic microarray.[3–9]

The Unbalanced Chromosome Banding Pattern May Mimic a Normal Pattern

Not only is genomic microarray preferable for the detection of small copy number changes, it is also preferable for the detection of many large copy number changes. The standard resolution of a chromosome analysis is between 5 and 10 megabases. However, the detection of a chromosomal rearrangement depends on the disruption of normal banding patterns, and there can be many large rearrangements that do not alter the normal banding pattern. For example, an unbalanced translocation results in a terminal deletion of 1 chromosome end and a duplication of another chromosome end, with the duplicated material residing in the genomic location of the deleted material (**Fig. 2A**). Because the majority of unbalanced translocations arise from balanced translocations in a carrier parent (see **Fig. 2B**), recognition of the imbalance is both critical for detection of the etiology of the abnormal phenotype, and critical for recurrence risk assessment. However, if the duplication and deletion are of similarly sized and similarly banded chromosome regions, this rearrangement will not be detected by a chromosome analysis (see **Fig. 2E**), even if the alteration results in greater than 10 megabases of DNA undergoing gains and losses; however, this imbalance is easily detected by genomic microarray (see **Fig. 2C, D**).

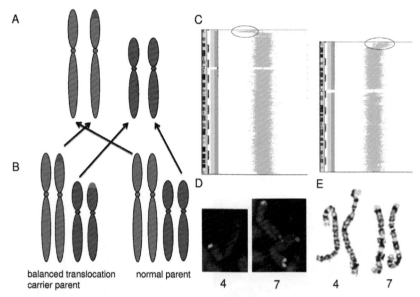

Fig. 2. (*A*) An unbalanced translocation consists of a terminal deletion (in example, p-arm of blue chromosome) with terminal duplication of other chromosome (in example, p-arm of red chromosome) with the duplicated material in the location of deleted material. (*B*) Unbalanced translocations can be de novo, but often arise from the segregation of balanced parental chromosomes. (*C*) Genomic microarray clearly shows a 4-Mb terminal deletion of 4p and a 7-Mb terminal duplication of 7p. (*D*) FISH with the 7p subtelomere probe in green (7q subtelomere probe in red) shows the additional copy of 7p on 4p, consistent with an unbalanced translocation. (*E*) Because the banding pattern of the tip of 4p is similar to the banding pattern of the tip of 7p, chromosome banding patterns for these 2 chromosomes seems to be normal.

Abnormal Banding Pattern May Not Show All Relevant Imbalances

It is also possible for multiple chromosome alterations to exist in 1 individual. The cytogenetic recognition of 1 alteration may satisfy the inquiry for the etiology of the patient's phenotype; however, a higher resolution analysis may reveal an unexpected additional alteration that has clinical significance. Examples include the initial interpretation of a pure terminal deletion, which then by genomic microarray shows both the terminal deletion and an unsuspected terminal duplication of a different chromosome end, leading to the reclassification of the rearrangement as an unbalanced translocation. As an example, an analysis of 4p deletions associated with Wolf–Hirschhorn syndrome showed a higher frequency of unbalanced translocations than predicted by chromosome analysis alone.[10] It is also possible for the multiple chromosome alterations to be independent, and yet both contributory to the clinical phenotype.

These concepts of loss of genomic material at translocation breakpoints, large but cytogenetically cryptic rearrangements, and multiple likely independent rearrangements is demonstrated by a recent case in our laboratory. Cytogenetic analysis showed an apparently balanced translocation between 2q and 18q (**Fig. 3A**), subsequent genomic microarray showed a loss of 18q material at the cytogenetic location of the 18q breakpoint. In addition, the genomic microarray also showed a terminal deletion of 9p and terminal duplication of 18p of similar sizes and banding

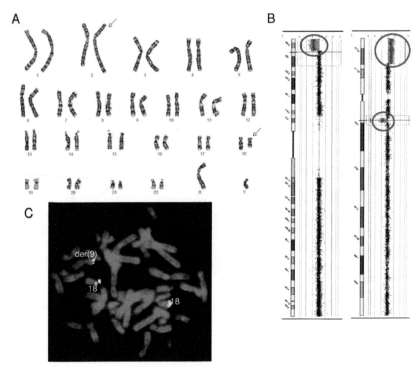

Fig. 3. (*A*) Chromosome banding shows a translocation between 2q and 18q. (*B*) Genomic microarray shows a 1.2-Mb interstitial deletion at the 18q breakpoint (right), but also a 5.9-Mb terminal deletion of 9p (left) and a 6.0-Mb terminal duplication of 18p (right). (*C*) FISH with the 18p subtelomere probe (fusion signal) shows additional signal is on 9p, consistent with an unbalanced translocation not detected in chromosome analysis owing to similar a banding pattern and size of affected 9p and 18p regions.

patterns (see **Fig. 3**B). FISH with the 18p subtelomere probe confirmed an unbalanced translocation between 9p and 18p (see **Fig. 3**C).

Inherited Identical Banding Patterns May Not Represent the Same Genomic Alteration

The utility of genomic microarray for further characterization of a chromosome rearrangement is not limited to de novo alterations. Identical banding patterns in family members are generally assumed to represent the same genomic architecture. However, it is possible for balanced and unbalanced rearrangements to have identical banding patterns, and the unbalanced rearrangements may originate from the segregation of a balanced parental rearrangement. Two independent published cases from our laboratory showed an identical banding pattern between the unaffected balanced parent and the affected unbalanced child. In 1 case, the parent carried a balanced double intrachromosomal insertion that underwent recombination to produce both an interstitial deletion and duplication. In the other case, the carrier parent had a double interchromosomal insertion with unbalanced segregation of the derivative chromosomes in the affected child.[11] Therefore, if phenotypic differences exist in the individuals showing the same chromosome banding patterns, a higher resolution copy number analysis is recommended for further characterization of the imbalances that may be associated with the banding patterns.

Deletion Size May Change Between Generations

Phenotypic differences between a parent and child with a deletion may rarely be explained by changes in the size of the inherited deletion. Two studies have reported the identification of a small, cytogenetically cryptic, subtelomeric deletion in a phenotypically mildly abnormal or normal mother that expanded into a clinically consequential and cytogenetically visible deletion in their affected child[12,13] (**Fig. 4**). Because only 2 reports currently exist, the frequency of deletion size expansion is not certain, and may be rare. Still, these reports illustrate the need for more comprehensive analyses of parental chromosome structure when characterizing an abnormality in a child.

CHROMOSOME ANALYSIS OR FISH CAN FURTHER CHARACTERIZE AN IMBALANCE OBSERVED BY GENOMIC MICROARRAY
Identification of Unbalanced Translocation or Unbalanced Recombinant

Genomic microarray can identify copy number changes, but it does not always show the structural rearrangement of the genomic material associated with the imbalance. In some cases, that structural rearrangement may be the unbalanced segregation of a balanced rearrangement in either parent, and as such there is a significant risk for the carrier parent to produce unbalanced gametes that may result in either miscarriage or another liveborn child with an unbalanced chromosome complement.

For some genomic imbalances, the pattern of gain and loss is highly suggestive of a particular structural rearrangement. As discussed, the pattern of a terminal deletion of 1 chromosome coupled with the terminal duplication of a different chromosome is highly suggestive of an unbalanced translocation, and this can be confirmed by either FISH with a probe in the duplicated region or in some cases a standard chromosome analysis. Terminal deletion of 1 end of a chromosome with duplication of the other end would be highly suggestive of a recombinant from a pericentric inversion (**Fig. 5**). Again, FISH can confirm this with a probe in the duplicated interval, which would show the additional copy is located at the deleted end. With this additional information of the structural rearrangement, appropriate parental follow-up studies can be performed to rule out the potential parental balanced rearrangements. However, not all copy number changes identified by genomic microarray have a pattern clearly suggestive of a concerning structural rearrangement. The pattern of trisomy 21 owing to nondisjunction versus a Robertsonian translocation is indistinguishable using current genomic microarray platforms. However, the recurrence risk is significantly different for the 2 mechanisms, because an unbalanced Robertsonian carrier likely has a parent with a balanced Robertsonian translocation. In contrast, the recurrence risk for nondisjunction is very low. Genomic microarray technology has not been amenable to evaluation of the structural rearrangements associated with the short arm of the acrocentrics owing to the highly repetitive sequence of the acrocentric short arms. As such, terminal deletions and duplications of the p-arms of the acrocentric chromosomes are not recognized with this technology. This copy number change of repetitive sequence is not itself clinically pathogenic; however, it precludes the recognition of the genomic microarray pattern that would suggest an unbalanced translocation or recombinant from a pericentric inversion. For these types of rearrangements involving the p-arms of the acrocentrics, only a deletion or only a duplication of the other partner of this structural rearrangement would be seen by the genomic microarray analysis. Translocations involving the acrocentric short arms are

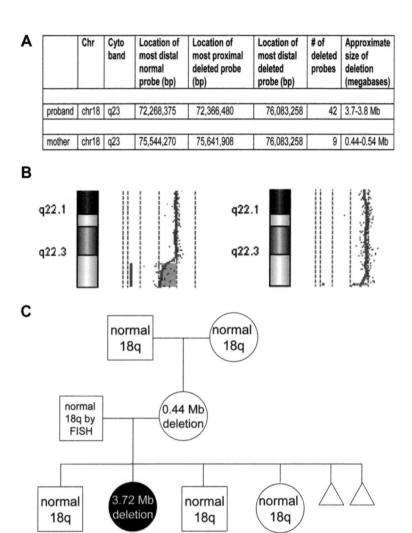

Fig. 4. (A) Table and (B) images of high-resolution genomic microarray results showing a terminal deletion involving 42 probes with an estimated deletion size of 3.7 to 3.8 Mb in the proband (image on left) and a terminal deletion involving 9 probes with an estimated deletion size of 0.44 to 0.54 Mb in her mother (image on right) within chromosome band 18q23. (C) High-resolution genomic microarray of maternal grandparents and siblings of proband showed a normal pattern for chromosome 18.

not rare events; indeed, a study by Ravnan and colleagues[14] looking at the rate of cryptic chromosome imbalances using a subtelomeric FISH analysis, found that of 145 unbalanced translocations identified, 17 (11.7%) involved a duplication of a non-acrocentric subtelomeric region onto an acrocentric short arm. Because the subtelomere assay could only detect a duplication on an acrocentric short arm and not the reciprocal alteration (a duplication of an acrocentric short arm on another chromosome), and both would be predicted to occur at equal frequencies, it is reasonable to conclude the frequency of unbalanced translocations involving an acrocentric short arm is twice that found in the study, around 23%. This is similar to

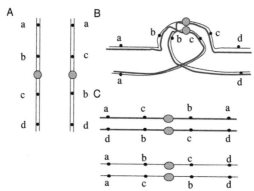

Fig. 5. (*A*) Pericentric inversion involving loci b and c around the centromere. (*B*) To allow pairing of homologous regions, the inverted region of 1 chromosome forms a loop. A recombination event may occur within this loop between 1 of each of the sister chromatids. (*C*) The final 4 versions of this chromosome that segregate into the four gametes include 2 recombinant chromosomes which each have a partial monosomy of 1 end and a partial trisomy of the other end, with the additional copy in the location of the deleted copy. Because there were also sister chromatids not involved in the recombination event, the parental chromosomes segregate into the other 2 gametes.

the 20% frequency for acrocentric p-arm involvement found in a smaller study focusing on unbalanced translocations of 4p.[10]

DISRUPTION OF A GENE OWING TO A COPY NUMBER GAIN

Duplications detected by genomic microarray present unique considerations, such as location, orientation, and breakpoints of the additional copy of genomic material. When the breakpoints do not seem to disrupt coding or regulatory sequences within the duplicated material, it is likely that the clinical consequence of the duplication will be primarily due to the consequence of an additional copy of any genes within that duplicated interval. However, the location of the additional material may itself require consideration. A tandem duplication is the most common scenario and likely does not require additional considerations. However, if the additional copy is inserted elsewhere in the genome, it is possible the insertion event could disrupt genes or regulatory elements. This disruption may not be accompanied by any genomic copy number changes at the site of insertion and, therefore, may not be detected by the genomic microarray. A recent report of such a scenario involved a 126-kb duplicated region from 19p13.3 inserted into MECP2 at Xq28 in a patient with symptoms of Rett syndrome.[15] FISH with a probe in the duplicated region can often show the genomic location of the additional material, and support either a tandem duplication or insertion event. For insertion events, it may be prudent to consider any strong candidates for the patient's phenotype at the site of the insertion.

An additional consideration for insertions is the increased likelihood of a balanced carrier parent. Furthermore, a parent carrying a balanced insertion is at risk of producing gametes with both deletions alone and duplications alone of the inserted region, or both deletions and duplications dependent on the orientation and location of the inserted material.[16,17]

When the breakpoints of the duplicated segment fall within the coding sequence and the duplication is tandem, the orientation of the duplicated material bears

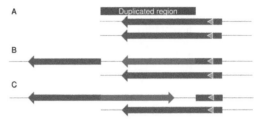

Fig. 6. (*A*) Duplication with a breakpoint in the coding sequence of 1 copy of a haploin-sufficient gene. (*B*) Direct orientation of the duplicated copy can leave 2 intact copies of the gene. (*C*) Inverted orientation of the duplicated copy can leave only 1 intact copy of the gene.

consideration, although with current techniques in the clinical laboratory, it is often outside the capabilities of the laboratory to determine the orientation. If the duplicated material is in direct orientation to the original copy, there are likely still 2 intact open reading frames for the affected gene, with a third disrupted open reading frame (**Fig. 6A, B**). This is less likely to result in a clinical consequence. However, if the duplicated material is inverted, there may be only 1 intact open reading frame, increasing the likelihood of a clinical consequence owing to haploinsufficiency of the disrupted gene (see **Fig. 6C**). This simplified model does not take into consideration any additional complexities at the breakpoints that may occur as part of DNA repair processes that may insert or delete genomic material at the breakpoints. Therefore, because it is difficult in the clinical setting to determine the true consequence to the coding sequence when a duplication breakpoint is within a gene, it is prudent to consider alternative approaches, such as familial studies or functional assays when available.

Considerations of the Sequence Flanking Imbalances

The genomic architecture associated with the imbalance may also be identified by evaluation of the sequence flanking the imbalance. If the flanking sequence consists of low-copy repeats (LCRs), which are stretches of duplicated DNA that are between 10 and 500 kb in size with sequence homologies greater than 95%, then the likely mechanism for the observed deletion or duplication is non-allelic homologous recombination.[18] As such, it is very unlikely that the deletion or duplication is related to a balanced parental insertion, and the recurrence risk within the family is most associated with the likelihood of a parent carrying the same deletion or duplication, which will be a consideration of the penetrance, expressivity, and potential imprinting of the imbalance as well as a careful evaluation of the phenotype of each parent.

Another pattern observed in genomic microarray studies involves a terminal deletion with an adjacent duplication. Three mechanisms are commonly proposed to explain the origin of an inverted duplication with terminal deletion, and sequence analysis between the duplicated and deleted region can distinguish between these 3. All 3 mechanisms involve the formation of a dicentric chromosome that subsequently breaks during meiosis to form a monocentric duplicated and deleted chromosome. However, the means by which the dicentric chromosome is created differs among the 3 mechanisms.

The first mechanism involves the presence of a paracentric inversion in one of the parents.[19] During meiosis, the chromosome carrying the paracentric inversion pairs with its normal homologue by forming an inversion loop (**Fig. 7A**). Crossing over within the loop creates a dicentric chromosome and an acentric fragment. A subsequent

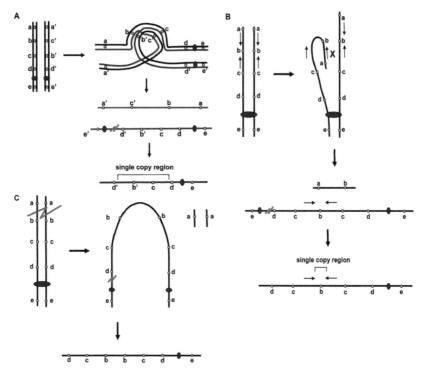

Fig. 7. Three models commonly used to explain formation of a terminal deletion with inverted duplication. (*A*) A paracentric inversion in a parental chromosome results in a 1-chromosome forming a loop to allow homologous pairing during prophase I of meiosis. A recombination event within the loop then results in 2 recombinant chromosomes, 1 acentric and the other dicentric with each having a terminal deletion of 1 end and a duplication of the other end on the opposite chromosome arm. Prezygotic breakage of the dicentric outside the inverted region leads to a monocentric chromosome with a terminal deletion of the "a" locus and an inverted duplication of the "d" locus with a single copy region for the "b" and "c" loci. (*B*) The presence of inverted LCRs within the same arm on 1 parental chromosome results in a folding of this chromosome with pairing and recombination between the repeats on sister chromatids within 1 chromosome. This results in a dicentric chromosome having a terminal deletion of 1 end and a duplication of the other end on the opposite chromosome arm. Prezygotic breakage of the dicentric outside the inverted repeats leads to a monocentric chromosome with a terminal deletion of the "a" locus and an inverted duplication of the "c" and "d" loci with a single copy region for the "b" locus, which is flanked by the inverted repeats. (*C*) A double-strand break of 1 chromosome is repaired by fusion of the 2 sister chromatids (U-type exchange), which results in a dicentric chromosome having a terminal deletion of 1 end and a duplication of the other end on the opposite chromosome arm. Prezygotic breakage of the dicentric outside the fusion region leads to a monocentric chromosome with a terminal deletion of the "a" locus and an inverted duplication of the "b," "c," and "d" loci with no single copy region between the duplication.

prezygotic breakage of the dicentric outside the inverted region leads to a monocentric chromosome with a terminal deletion and an inverted duplication with a single copy region between the 2 duplicated segments. This single copy represents the region inverted in the parent. Although paracentric inversions occur in approximately 0.1% to 0.5% of the population,[20] there is believed to be a negligible risk for producing viable offspring because the resulting acentric and dicentric chromosomes are unstable. However, there are individual reports of viable monocentric chromosomes owing to breakage of the dicentric prezygotically.[16,21]

The second commonly proposed mechanism involves the presence of LCRs. A possible consequence of inverted LCRs in the same chromosome arm is partial folding of 1 homologue onto itself with a recombination event between the inverted repeats (see **Fig. 7**B).[22] This could also occur between inverted repeats on homologous chromosomes. The recombination results in a dicentric chromosome and an acentric fragment. As with the first mechanism, prezygotic breakage of the dicentric outside the inverted repeats leads to a monocentric chromosome with a terminal deletion and an inverted duplication with a single copy region between the duplication that is flanked by the inverted repeats.

The third mechanism suggests that the inverted duplication with terminal deletion arises from an initial double-strand break of the 2 sister chromatids (see **Fig. 7**C).[23] Fusion of the broken ends results in a symmetric U-type reunion between the sister chromatids producing a dicentric chromosome. The broken chromosome may also inappropriately recombine with the unbroken homologous chromosome in a U-type exchange mechanism to heal the broken end. The resulting dicentric chromosome then undergoes random breakage distal to the fusion site. Prezygotic breakage of the dicentric outside the fusion region leads to a monocentric chromosome with a terminal deletion and an inverted duplication with no single copy region between the duplication. However, a number of such cases have been sequenced across the breakpoints and small single copy regions exist on the order of tens to hundreds of base pairs, with microhomology flanking the single copy region, suggesting the U-type reunion involves microhomology-mediated mechanisms.[24]

SUMMARY

By identifying both the imbalance and the genomic architecture associated with the imbalance, the mechanism leading to the imbalance can often be identified. Understanding the mechanism leads to a more accurate recurrence risk assessment. Common mechanisms that lead to imbalances include loss or gain at translocation breakpoints, unbalanced translocations, recombination within a pericentric or paracentic inversion, intra- and interchromosomal insertions leading to deletions and duplications or gene disruption, instability of size of a deletion between generations, deletions and duplications mediated by non-allelic homologous recombination of LCRs and U-type exchange that may be mediated by microhomology. A combination of technologies is required for both the identification of the imbalance and characterization of the genomic architecture. As our technologies improve and increase in resolution, it is likely that our understanding of genomic rearrangement mechanisms will also change and we will continue to be impressed by the dynamic nature of chromosome structure and its relationship to human disease.

ACKNOWLEDGEMENTS

The authors thank Allen Lamb and Hutton Kearney for discussions of data presented in **Figs. 3 and 6**.

REFERENCES

1. Warburton D. De novo balanced chromosome rearrangements and extra marker chromosomes identified at prenatal diagnosis: clinical significance and distribution of breakpoints. Am J Hum Genet 1991;49:995–1013.

2. Tommerup N. Mendelian cytogenetics. Chromosome rearrangements associated with mendelian disorders. J Med Genet 1993;30:713–27.
3. Patsalis PC, Evangelidou P, Charalambous S, et al. Fluorescence in situ hybridization characterization of apparently balanced translocation reveals cryptic complex chromosomal rearrangements with unexpected level of complexity. Eur J Hum Genet 2004;12:647–53.
4. Gribble SM, Prigmore E, Burford DC, et al. The complex nature of constitutional de novo apparently balanced translocations in patients presenting with abnormal phenotypes. J Med Genet 2005;42:8–16.
5. Astbury C, Christ LA, Aughton DJ, et al. Detection of deletions in de novo "balanced" chromosome rearrangements: further evidence for their role in phenotypic abnormalities. Genet Med 2004;6:81–9.
6. De Gregori M, Ciccone R, Magini P, et al. Cryptic deletions are a common finding in "balanced" reciprocal and complex chromosome rearrangements: a study of 59 patients. J Med Genet 2007;44:750–62.
7. Higgins AW, Alkuraya FS, Bosco AF, et al. Characterization of apparently balanced chromosomal rearrangements from the developmental genome anatomy project. Am J Hum Genet 2008;82:712–22.
8. Baptista J, Mercer C, Prigmore E, et al. Breakpoint mapping and array CGH in translocations: comparison of a phenotypically normal and an abnormal cohort. Am J Hum Genet 2008;82:927–36.
9. Schluth-Bolard C, Delobel B, Sanlaville D, et al. Cryptic genomic imbalances in de novo and inherited apparently balanced chromosomal rearrangements: array CGH study of 47 unrelated cases. Eur J Med Genet 2009;52:291–6.
10. South ST, Whitby H, Battaglia A, et al. Comprehensive analysis of Wolf-Hirschhorn syndrome using array CGH indicates a high prevalence of translocations. Eur J Hum Genet 2008;16:45–52.
11. South ST, Rector L, Aston E, et al. Large clinically consequential imbalances detected at the breakpoints of apparently balanced and inherited chromosome rearrangements. J Mol Diagn 2010;12:725–9.
12. Faravelli F, Murdolo M, Marangi G, et al. Mother to son amplification of a small subtelomeric deletion: a new mechanism of familial recurrence in microdeletion syndromes. Am J Med Genet A 2007;143A:1169–73.
13. South ST, Rope AF, Lamb AN, et al. Expansion in size of a terminal deletion: a paradigm shift for parental follow-up studies. J Med Genet 2008;45:391–5.
14. Ravnan JB, Tepperberg JH, Papenhausen P, et al. Subtelomere FISH analysis of 11 688 cases: an evaluation of the frequency and pattern of subtelomere rearrangements in individuals with developmental disabilities. J Med Genet 2006;43:478–89.
15. Neill NJ, Ballif BC, Lamb AN, et al. Recurrence, submicroscopic complexity, and potential clinical relevance of copy gains detected by array CGH that are shown to be unbalanced insertions by FISH. Genome Res 2011;21:535–44.
16. Madan K, Nieuwint AW. Reproductive risks for paracentric inversion heterozygotes: Inversion or insertion? That is the question. Am J Med Genet 2002;107:340–3.
17. Gardner R, Sutherland G. Chromosome abnormalities and genetic counseling. 3rd edition. New York: Oxford University Press; 2004.
18. Shaffer LG, Lupski JR. Molecular mechanisms for constitutional chromosomal rearrangements in humans. Annu Rev Genet 2000;34:297–329.
19. Gorinati M, Caufin D, Minelli A, et al. Inv dup (p21.1----22.1): further case report and a new hypothesis on the origin of the chromosome abnormality. Clin Genet 1991;39: 55–9.

20. Pettenati MJ, Rao PN, Phelan MC, et al. Paracentric inversions in humans: a review of 446 paracentric inversions with presentation of 120 new cases. Am J Med Genet 1995;55:171–87.

21. South ST, Swensen JJ, Maxwell T, et al. A new genomic mechanism leading to cri-du-chat syndrome. Am J Med Genet A 2006;140:2714–20.

22. Giglio S, Broman KW, Matsumoto N, et al. Olfactory receptor-gene clusters, genomic-inversion polymorphisms, and common chromosome rearrangements. Am J Hum Genet 2001;68:874–83.

23. Weleber RG, Verma RS, Kimberling WJ, et al. Duplication-deficiency of the short arm of chromosome 8 following artificial insemination. Ann Genet 1976;19:241–7.

24. Rudd K, Rosenfeld JA, Ballif B, et al. Large inverted duplications are separated by disomic spacers: Implications for CNV formation. Paper presented at: 2011 ACMG Annual Clinical Genetics Meeting. March 16–20, Vancouver, British Columbia, Canada, 2011.

Fluorescence In Situ Hybridization

Karen D. Tsuchiya, MD[a,b,]*

KEYWORDS

- Fluorescence in situ hybridization • FISH • Interphase FISH
- Metaphase FISH

Fluorescence in situ hybridization (FISH) is a versatile technique that allows visualization of nucleic acid sequences in their native context at the single cell level. FISH can be performed on a variety of targets, including RNA within cells, DNA in metaphase chromosome preparations obtained from mitotic cells, or DNA in interphase nuclei from cells in the non-mitotic phases of the cell cycle. Interphase nuclei can be obtained from cultured or uncultured cells, sorted cells, or paraffin-embedded tissue. FISH has been widely used for research applications, including physical mapping; studies of biological processes such as DNA replication, RNA processing, and gene expression; and studies of chromosome evolution, including conservation of sequences and chromosome rearrangements between species. In the clinical laboratory, FISH has become not only an indispensible adjunct to banded chromosome analysis, but also a stand-alone method for the detection and characterization of both constitutional and acquired chromosomal abnormalities.

The basic elements of the FISH procedure include selection of probe(s) for sequence that is complementary to the target of interest, probe labeling, slide preparation, slide pretreatment, denaturation of probe and target, hybridization, washing, analysis, and interpretation. For genomic DNA analysis, FISH probes can target unique DNA sequences, repetitive DNA sequences, entire chromosome arms, or whole chromosomes. Unique sequence probes are useful for identifying gains and losses of specific genes or genomic regions, as well as genomic rearrangements, such as translocations. Repetitive sequence probes are primarily used for interrogating centromeric or pericentromeric regions. Probes that hybridize along the length of entire chromosome arms or whole chromosomes, also known as chromosome paints, can be used to confirm or further characterize chromosomal rearrangements identified by banded chromosome analysis (**Fig. 1**). Most FISH probes used for detecting unique sequences are currently made from bacterial artificial chromosomes that contain genomic inserts on the order of 100 to 300 Kb. Propagation and extraction of

[a] Department of Laboratory Medicine, University of Washington School of Medicine, 1959 NE Pacific Street, Box 357110, Seattle, WA 98195, USA
[b] Department of Laboratories, Seattle Children's Hospital, Seattle, 4800 Sand Point Way NE, A-6901, PO Box 5371, WA 98105-0371, USA
* Seattle Children's Hospital, 4800 Sand Point Way NE, A-6901, PO Box 5371, Seattle, WA 98105-0371.
E-mail address: karen.tsuchiya@seattlechildrens.org

Clin Lab Med 31 (2011) 525–542
doi:10.1016/j.cll.2011.08.011   labmed.theclinics.com
0272-2712/11/$ – see front matter © 2011 Elsevier Inc. All rights reserved.

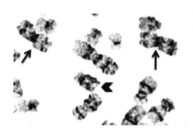 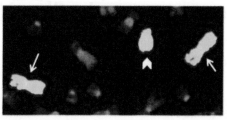

Fig. 1. Partial G-banded metaphase cell (*left*) and FISH image of a chromosome 3 whole chromosome paint probe (*right*). A low percentage of G-banded cells from a patient with multiple congenital anomalies showed a supernumerary marker chromosome (*arrowhead*) whose chromosome of origin, by definition, could not be identified without additional characterization. By array CGH, there was a suggestion of very low level gain of part of the long arm of chromosome 3 (not shown). A chromosome 3 whole chromosome paint probe confirmed that the marker chromosome was derived from chromosome 3 (*arrowhead*). The two normal chromosomes 3 in both images are designated with arrows.

DNA from bacterial artificial chromosomes is relatively straightforward, and the size of the insert produces signal that can be easily visualized. Probes can also be made from vectors containing smaller inserts, such as fosmids or even plasmids, particularly if the target consists of repetitive DNA that will result in a larger signal. FISH using oligonucleotide probes was originally limited to repetitive targets; however, recent advances in the synthesis of long oligonucleotides promises to provide a source of probes that can be used to visualize nonrepetitive targets at a much greater resolution than can be achieved using large insert clones.[1]

FISH probes can be labeled either by incorporation of biotin or digoxigenin-conjugated nucleotides into the probe with subsequent detection using a fluorescently labeled antibody (indirect method), or by incorporation of fluorophore-conjugated nucleotides (direct method). Probes used in clinical laboratories are currently labeled using the direct method because fewer steps and less time are involved in performing tests using these probes. Indirect labeling may also produce more background from nonspecific antibody binding. However, indirect labeling allows for more flexibility, because different fluorophores can be attached to the detection antibody for the same indirectly labeled probe, and multiple rounds of detection with antibody can be performed for signal amplification. Probes made from cloned genomic DNA typically require suppression of repetitive sequence within the probe to avoid cross-hybridization with other regions of the genome. A significant advantage of oligonucleotide probes is that they can be selected in silico for unique sequence, resulting in high signal to noise without the need for suppression of repetitive elements.

Slide preparation, pretreatment, and other aspects of the FISH procedure vary depending on specific applications, and some of the relevant variables are discussed within the specific techniques or applications that follow. There are also unique issues related to signal analysis and interpretation depending on the specific FISH application, although recommendations that apply to many situations encountered in clinical laboratories are available.[2] With the exception of FISH tests that are approved by the US Food and Drug Administration (FDA), clinical laboratories must validate FISH probes prior to use. For the detection of nonmosaic abnormalities, steps involved in this validation process include confirmation of correct probe localization, and assessment of probe sensitivity and specificity. For mosaic conditions or minimal residual disease detection, additional validation is required. Details on performing these validation steps are published elsewhere.[2]

FISH TECHNIQUES
Comparative Genomic Hybridization

Comparative genomic hybridization (CGH) is a method for detecting genomic gains and losses (copy number changes) that can be performed on either metaphase chromosome preparations or arrays. For metaphase-based CGH, a test DNA is labeled in one fluorophore, a reference DNA is labeled in another fluorophore, and equal amounts of labeled test and reference DNA are hybridized to metaphase chromosome preparations from a normal specimen. The ratio of fluorescence intensity of the hybridized test and reference DNA is measured along the length of the chromosomes using digital image analysis. Regions of loss in the test DNA result in a decreased ratio of test to reference DNA over those chromosome regions, whereas gains in the test DNA result in an increased ratio. Metaphase-based CGH requires only DNA from the test specimen, because the hybridization is performed on metaphase cells from a normal specimen. Thus, this technique was useful in the past for detection of copy number alterations in neoplastic specimens that were highly complex and not readily amenable to G-banded chromosome analysis, or from paraffin-embedded tissue and other specimens for which metaphase chromosomes could not be obtained.[3–5] Limitations of CGH include the inability to detect balanced genomic rearrangements, and a limit of resolution of 3 to 5 Mb at best.[6] Because of its vastly superior resolution, array-based CGH has essentially replaced metaphase-based CGH.

Multicolor FISH

In the mid 1990s, techniques using multicolor whole chromosome paint probes that allowed simultaneous visualization of the 24 different human chromosomes in one hybridization experiment were introduced. The two main techniques, known as spectral karyotyping and multicolor FISH, involve combinatorial labeling of flow sorted chromosomes using different combinations of five fluorochromes.[7,8] Spectral karyotyping utilizes spectral imaging and spectroscopy for image acquisition, whereas multicolor FISH utilizes a series of filters with defined emission spectra. These techniques have been helpful for the identification of marker chromosomes, although marker chromosomes are now often identified, and their content more precisely characterized, using array-based copy number assessment. Spectral karyotyping/multicolor FISH may still be useful for characterizing balanced interchromosomal rearrangements, particularly in neoplastic specimens that have poor banded morphology and complex rearrangements (**Fig. 2**); however, the limit of resolution is approximately 1 to 2 Mb for the detection of reciprocal terminal translocations.[9] The use of these techniques in clinical laboratories is also limited by their expense and the time involved in performing the experiments and analysis.

Fiber FISH

The linear nature of metaphase chromosomes allows mapping of the position and orientation of sequences with respect to each other by FISH, but resolution is limited to probes that are at least 1 to 3 Mb apart.[10] Interphase FISH provides much better resolution than metaphase FISH, but the DNA in this less condensed state is arranged in a random, nonlinear fashion. FISH on extended chromatin or DNA combines the qualities of both metaphase and interphase FISH in that it allows for high-resolution mapping on linear stretches of chromatin or DNA. This technique has been referred to by a variety of names, including FISH on free chromatin or DNA, FISH on extended or elongated chromatin or DNA fibers, FISH on DNA halos, and FISH on single or

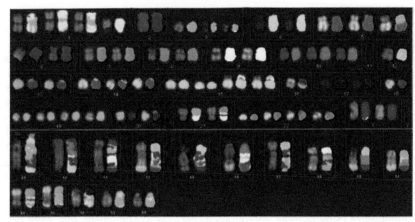

Fig. 2. Spectral karyotype of a cell from an osteosarcoma. For each chromosome, the raw spectral color image is on the left and the classified image with an assigned color is on the right. The chromosomes in the last two rows show complex structural rearrangements, with each chromosome consisting of portions of two or more chromosomes. This spectral karyotype is typical of the genomic complexity seen in osteosarcoma, which often precludes karyotyping by G-banded analysis.

individual stretched DNA molecules, but the term "fiber FISH" has been used to encompass all of these variations.[11] Fiber FISH mapping can distinguish probes separated by as little as 1 Kb on a DNA fiber.

Different methods have been developed for releasing extended chromatin or DNA from the nucleus, but subsequent FISH is similar to that performed on more conventional preparations.[10] Methods for release include alkaline lysis or detergents, which is sometimes followed by mechanical stretching of the released fibers. DNA fibers can also be released from previously fixed cells, and molecular combing is a method that can be used to generate extended DNA from isolated DNA instead of lysed cells. Fiber FISH is not well-suited for use in the clinical laboratory owing to a number of factors, such as the time involved in preparing slides and nonstandard slide preparation; however, it has been used for a number of research applications that require high-resolution mapping. Some of these applications include determination of the size and structure of viral DNA integrated into a host genome; determination of the size, number, and orientation of amplicons within amplified regions of DNA; determination of the relationship and orientation of repetitive DNA elements (satellite sequences, arrays of alpha-satellites, etc); recognition of length differences in telomeres; and the study of the spatial and temporal distribution of DNA replication sites.

Flow FISH for the Determination of Telomere Length

Alteration of telomere length has been studied in the context of aging, cancer, and other disorders. A number of different techniques have been developed to measure telomere length.[12] Analysis of terminal restriction fragment length by Southern blotting is reproducible but time consuming, requires a relatively large amount of DNA, and can overestimate the average telomere length by many Kb because of the distance between terminal restriction sites and the telomeric repeats. Polymerase chain reaction-based methods have also been used to determine telomere length, and these have their advantages and disadvantages as well. A quantitative FISH technique for measurement of telomere length on individual metaphase chromosomes has been developed that uses peptide nucleic acid probes that are complementary to single-stranded TTAGGG target sequences. Quantitative hybridization to telomere repeats is achieved by using conditions that allow peptide nucleic acid probes to hybridize to only the telomere repeat target sequences. This technique originally used image analysis, but was subsequently adapted for analysis of cells in suspension by flow cytometry (flow FISH). Additional modifications to the technique have included partial automation, inclusion of control cells with known telomere length, and the capability of limited immunophenotyping to analyze telomere length in subpopulations of leukocytes.

Although flow FISH is time consuming and technically demanding, it has been used in many research studies.[12] Flow FISH is also being used as a diagnostic tool in patients who are suspected to have dyskeratosis congenita (DC), an inherited bone marrow failure syndrome that is characterized by short telomeres. Germline mutations in genes in the telomerase maintenance pathway are known to cause DC and other related disorders with short telomeres; however, mutations have only been identified in approximately half of the patients to date who meet clinical criteria for DC.[13] Very short telomeres, defined as telomere length below the first percentile compared with healthy controls, have been found by flow FISH in leukocytes from individuals with DC.[13,14] The finding of very short telomeres seems to have a high diagnostic sensitivity for DC, but the specificity for distinguishing DC from other bone marrow failure disorders differed between two studies.[13,14] It is not known at present if this difference in specificity is real or owing to technical differences.

Oligonucleotide-Based High-Resolution FISH

FISH with oligonucleotide probes was originally limited to repetitive DNA targets, but recent advances in the de novo synthesis of long oligonucleotides (>150 mers) allow visualization of unique sequence targets at a resolution that has not been possible with probes generated from cloned DNA. Careful in silico selection of oligonucleotides for non-repetitive, unique genomic sequence generates high signal to noise without the need for suppression of repetitive DNA sequence. With selected, tiled oligonucleotide probes, Yamada and colleagues[1] were able to visualize regions as small as 6.7 Kb by FISH using conventional cytogenetic preparations and standard FISH protocols. These investigators were also able to determine the genomic structure of the same 479-Kb duplication in 15q13.3 in two different individuals using a 2-color oligonucleotide probe set. The duplication was visualized as a direct duplication in one individual, whereas in the second individual the signal pattern was consistent with an inverted duplication. Thus, oligonucleotide FISH may provide an easier alternative to fiber FISH for high-resolution mapping of genomic structure in some situations. Oligonucleotide FISH would also be useful in the clinical laboratory for visualizing deletions and duplications detected by microarray that are below the level of resolution of FISH using bacterial artificial chromosome probes.

APPLICATIONS OF INTERPHASE FISH
Technical Considerations

A significant advantage of interphase FISH over metaphase FISH is that actively dividing cells are not necessary; therefore, interphase FISH can be performed on a wider range of specimens. A much larger number of nuclei can also be scored very quickly by interphase FISH, allowing for the detection of low level mosaicism and minimal residual disease. For interphase FISH analysis, probe design or strategy for the identification of chromosomal abnormalities depends on the specific alteration to

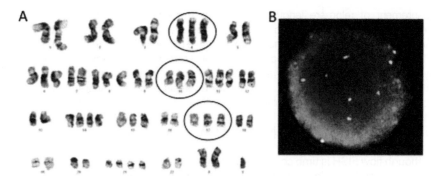

Fig. 3. Karyotype and interphase FISH image from the bone marrow of a patient with precursor B-cell acute lymphoblastic leukemia. (A) The karyotype shows trisomies for chromosomes 4, 10, and 17 (circled), among other abnormalities. (B) The interphase nucleus, hybridized with a probe set consisting of centromere probes for chromosomes 4 (red), 10 (green), and 17 (aqua), has three signals for each probe, reflecting trisomies for all three chromosomes.

be detected. Enumeration probes consist of either centromeric/pericentromeric probes for detecting aneusomies, or unique sequence probes for detecting aneusomies, deletions, duplications, or amplification (**Figs. 3** and **4**). Fusion probe strategies are used for identifying specific translocations or inversions, and consist of probes from the two targets involved in the rearrangement that are labeled in two different colors (eg, red probe for *PML* at 15q24.1 and green for *RARA* at 17q21.2). In the normal state, the two probes are separated; however, the presence of the relevant rearrangement results in juxtaposition of the probes to give a fusion signal. First-generation fusion probes gave single fusion signals that can result in false-positive

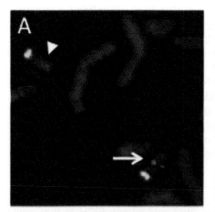

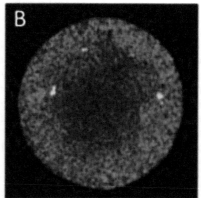

Fig. 4. Partial metaphase (A) and interphase (B) FISH images from a patient with the 22q11.2 (DiGeorge/Velocardiofacial) deletion syndrome. The probe set includes a locus specific probe containing the *HIRA* gene from 22q11.2 (red) and a control probe from 22q13 .3 (green). The non-deleted (*arrow*) and the deleted (*arrowhead*) chromosomes 22 from a metaphase cell are shown. The nucleus demonstrates the same signal pattern, with 2 green signals from the control probe, but only a single red signal from the 22q11.2 region.

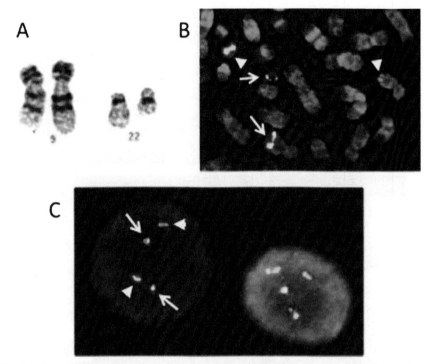

Fig. 5. G-banded chromosomes, and metaphase and interphase FISH images demonstrating a *BCR/ABL1* gene rearrangement due to the t(9;22)(q34;q11.2). (*A*) G-banded pairs of chromosomes 9 and 22 show the reciprocal t(9;22), with the homologues involved in the translocation on the right of each chromosome pair. (*B*) Metaphase cell hybridized with a dual fusion BCR/ABL1 probe, with the ABL1 probe in red and the BCR probe in green. The translocation breakpoints fall within the ABL1 and BCR probes, resulting in juxtaposition (fusion) of the red and green signals on both derivative chromosomes involved in the translocation (*arrows*). The BCR and ABL1 probe signals from the non-translocated chromosomes 9 and 22 are also present (*arrowheads*). (*C*) Interphase nuclei with the same dual fusion signal pattern. When following patients with a *BCR/ABL1* gene rearrangement for minimal residual disease, hundreds of interphase nuclei, which are much more abundant than metaphase cells, can be scored for this dual fusion signal pattern relatively quickly.

results in some proportion of interphase nuclei owing to coincidental overlap of probes. Dual-fusion probe designs circumvent this problem by creating two fusion signals, thereby essentially eliminating the possibility of false-positive signals owing to chance probe overlap (**Fig. 5**). Translocations and inversions can also be identified using a break-apart probe strategy, in which different color probes that flank the breakpoints of the rearrangement are utilized. In the normal state, the break-apart probe gives two fusion signals, whereas a rearrangement results in separation of the fused signal to give a red signal and green signal (**Fig. 6**). For informative schematic diagrams illustrating the dual fusion and break-apart probe strategies, refer to the review by Ventura and colleagues.[15]

The choice of a fusion probe versus a break-apart probe usually depends on the variability of fusion partners that can be involved in a rearrangement. Rearrangements with consistent partners (eg, *BCR/ABL1* gene rearrangements) lend themselves well to a dual-fusion probe strategy that allows for optimal probe specificity and sensitivity.

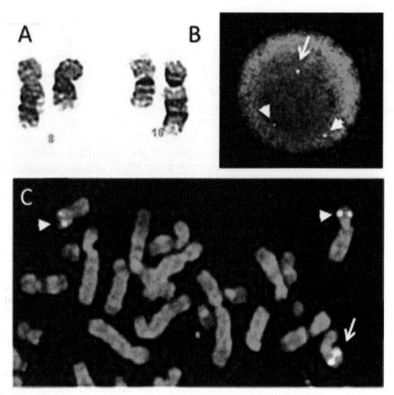

Fig. 6. G-banded chromosomes, and metaphase and interphase FISH images, demonstrating a *CBFB* gene rearrangement owing to a complex rearrangement between chromosomes 8 and 16. (*A*) G-banded pairs of chromosomes 8 and 16, with the homologues involved in the rearrangement on the right of each pair. Interphase nucleus (*B*) and metaphase cell (*C*) hybridized with a CBFB break-apart probe. The normal state for this probe is a fusion signal (*arrow*) at 16q22.1, which is the location of the *CBFB* gene. When a rearrangement of the *CBFB* gene occurs owing to an inversion or translocation, the red and green probe become separated (*arrowheads*). In this example, the green signal is located on the derivative chromosome 8 involved in a translocation with chromosome 16, and the red signal is located on the short arm of the derivative chromosome 16 owing to an inversion in addition to the translocation. Although the complex structure of this rearrangement cannot be appreciated in interphase nuclei, the relevant abnormality, which is rearrangement of the *CBFB* gene, is evident from the split red and green signals, allowing subsequent detection of minimal residual disease without the need for metaphase cells or G-banded chromosome analysis.

Break-apart probes are more suitable for rearrangements in which one of the translocation partners is highly variable, such as those involving the *MLL* gene. Thus, a break-apart probe can recognize a rearrangement involving *MLL* regardless of the translocation partner, although the specific partner cannot be identified with this type of probe, and sensitivity for detecting a low proportion of nuclei with the rearrangement is inferior to a dual-fusion probe strategy.

FISH for Prenatal Detection of Aneuploidies and Preimplantation Genetic Diagnosis

Conventional karyotyping is a reliable method for prenatal detection of aneuploidies and structural rearrangements, with an accuracy of more than 99.5%.[16] The main drawback of standard G-banded chromosome analysis in this setting is the time needed for culturing of fetal cells, which can cause anxiety for patients and providers. Aneuploidies for chromosomes 13, 18, 21, X, and Y account for more than 60% of all chromosomal abnormalities detected at amniocentesis and for 85% to 95% of those that are responsible for live-born birth defects.[17,18] In the early 1990s, studies were performed that established the potential for rapid detection of aneuploidies for these chromosomes in uncultured amniocytes using interphase FISH.[17,18] In 1997, an assay utilizing two multicolor probe sets, one consisting of locus-specific probes for chromosomes 13 and 21 and the other consisting of centromere probes for chromosomes 18, X, and Y, was approved by the FDA for the enumeration of these chromosomes in amniocytes (AneuVysion, Abbott Molecular Inc, Des Plaines, IL, USA). This FDA-approved assay allows for prenatal detection of aneuploidies of the targeted chromosomes within 24 hours. The assay does not detect other chromosomal abnormalities such as aneuploidies for other chromosomes or structural rearrangements.

After FDA approval, many laboratories worldwide adopted the AneuVysion assay. Results from almost 30,000 cases confirmed the reliability and accuracy of the assay for the detection of aneuploidies for chromosomes 13, 18, 21, X, and Y in uncultured amniocytes.[16] Rare false-positive and false-negative results have been attributed to technical factors, or rare polymorphisms that result in probe cross-hybridization or significant decrease in probe signal. Although very infrequent, there is no tolerance for false-positive results that lead to termination of an unaffected fetus; therefore, it is recommended that clinical decision making be based on two of three of the following: Positive FISH result, routine chromosome analysis, or clinical information.[19] Although FDA approval is only for amniocytes, studies suggest that interphase FISH for the common aneuploidies may have comparable accuracy for uncultured chorionic villus cells.[20,21]

Interphase FISH also plays a role in preimplantation genetic diagnosis (PGD), where it can be used if a parent is known to carry a structural chromosome abnormality, or for the detection of aneuploidies. FISH for PGD involves single-cell analysis. Cells for PGD can be obtained from polar body biopsy, blastomere biopsy, or trophectoderm biopsy from the blastocyst, depending on the center performing the procedure and the specific question. Polar bodies cannot be used to assess paternally derived chromosomal abnormalities. For reciprocal translocations, PGD FISH strategies involving probes that span translocation breakpoints or probes that flank breakpoints have been employed.[22] Flanking probes are most commonly used because of the commercial availability of subtelomeric probes that are specific for each chromosome arm. For aneuploidies, 70% to 80% can be detected using probes for eight to twelve different chromosomes, with combinations of probes hybridized in two to three sequential rounds of FISH.[23] Whole-genome screening for chromosomal imbalances in PGD has also been attempted using whole-genome amplification and metaphase-based CGH, and more recently using array-based methods.[22,23]

FISH and Bladder Cancer

FISH has been increasingly used in the clinical laboratory for monitoring patients previously diagnosed with bladder cancer for recurrence, and for diagnosing bladder cancer. Bladder cancer is characterized by a number of recurrent genomic imbalances that are detectable by FISH. Homozygous deletions of 9p21 that include the *CDKN2A* (*p16*) gene tend to occur early in the development of bladder cancer. As tumors progress, chromosomal instability and the acquisition of aneuploidy for multiple chromosomes is common.[24] In 2000, Sokolova and colleagues[25] determined that the combination of FISH probes that had the highest sensitivity for detecting bladder cancer consisted of a locus specific probe for the 9p21, *CDKN2A* gene region, and centromere probes for chromosomes 3, 7, and 17. This probe set (UroVysion, Abbott Molecular Inc) received FDA approval in 2001 for detection of recurrence in voided urine from patients with a history of bladder cancer, and subsequently received approval in 2005 for diagnosing bladder cancer in patients with hematuria. Although FDA approval is only for voided urine specimens, laboratories have also used other specimen types, including bladder washings, urine obtained by catheterization, and stomal urine specimens. A few recent studies also suggest that this assay may be useful for detecting urothelial carcinoma that arises in the upper urinary tract (ureters and renal pelvis), and biliary tract malignancies.[26]

Multiple studies have demonstrated that compared with urine cytology, which has traditionally been used to detect bladder cancer in urine specimens, the sensitivity of FISH is higher for all stages and grades of bladder cancer.[26] The specificity for FISH is only slightly lower than cytology. Cases that are positive by FISH can be polysomic (greater than or equal to two of the four probes show gains), tetrasomic, trisomic, or have homozygous loss of 9p21. Polysomy is typically found in high-grade tumors, and constitutes the majority of positive cases.[26]

FISH on Paraffin-Embedded Tissue

Most pathology laboratories receive surgical biopsies already fixed in formalin; therefore, the ability to perform interphase FISH on formalin-fixed, paraffin-embedded material has utility in many situations. FISH on paraffin-embedded tissue is used as an aid in the classification of many neoplasms, including soft tissue tumors, gliomas, and lymphomas.[15,27–29] This technique is also used as a predictor of prognosis or response to specific therapies in breast carcinoma and gastric carcinoma (*HER2* amplification), neuroblastoma (*MYCN* amplification), and non-small cell lung cancer (*ALK* rearrangement).[30–33] FISH on paraffin-embedded tissue can also be used to look for constitutional aneuploidies in autopsy tissue if material was not cultured for routine cytogenetic analysis at the time of demise. FISH of paraffin-embedded tissue is most frequently performed on sections, typically 3 to 6 microns in thickness, but it can also be performed on nuclei extracted from thicker sections or from cores of paraffin blocks.[34] FISH performed on tissue sections preserves specimen architecture and allows correlation of FISH results with specific cells, but sectioning causes nuclear truncation, which results in signal loss in some nuclei. The latter is more of a problem with enumeration probes for the assessment of aneuploidy or deletions than for other probe types, such as those that utilize a dual-fusion strategy. The nuclear extraction technique leaves nuclei intact, but specimen architecture is not maintained; therefore, extracted nuclei are not suitable for certain applications. For example, FISH for *HER2* (*ERBB2*) amplification status in breast cancer should be performed on tissue sections to ensure that the invasive component of the tumor can be distinguished from benign tissue and in situ tumor.

There are a number of aspects of slide preparation and signal scoring that are specific to paraffin-embedded FISH assays. The quality of paraffin-embedded FISH and brightfield ISH (BRISH) results has been demonstrated to depend on the type of fixative, length of time from excision to fixation, and time of fixation.[35,36] The quality of BRISH results has also been determined to be influenced by the age of paraffin blocks, use of decalcifying solutions, and section thickness, and these variables most likely apply to FISH as well.[35] FISH on paraffin-embedded material requires deparaffinization, pretreatment, and protease treatment of the tissue before hybridization.[15,37] Fixation results in cross-linking of nucleic acids and proteins; therefore, heat or chemical pretreatment and protease treatment are necessary to increase probe accessibility and reduce background. Analysis of FISH signals also requires special considerations owing to nuclear truncation, possible suboptimal hybridization efficiency, tissue autofluorescence, and the need for correlation with histology. Cutoffs for distinguishing a positive (abnormal) from a negative (within normal limits) result for some assays that assess gene amplification status, such as *HER2* amplification in breast cancer and *MYCN* amplification in neuroblastoma, are based on published literature. For other paraffin-embedded FISH tests, each laboratory needs to establish their own cutoff values. Published guidelines for determining cutoffs are provided elsewhere, but it should be noted that cutoffs that have been established for interphase FISH from cultured cells should not be used for interphase FISH from paraffin-embedded material.[2]

One of the most common applications of FISH performed on paraffin-embedded sections is the assessment of *HER2* amplification in breast cancer. Overexpression of the HER2 protein, usually caused by gene amplification, occurs in 10% to 30% of invasive breast cancers. HER2 overexpression/gene amplification are prognostic markers for aggressive disease and predict response to several systemic therapies, including trastuzumab and lapatinib in adjuvant, neoadjuvant, and metastatic disease.[33,38] Immunohistochemistry and FISH are currently the two predominant assays for assessing either protein overexpression or gene amplification, respectively, in invasive breast cancer. Both methods have advantages and disadvantages, and the choice of which one to use is dependent on resources, expertise, and preference at a given institution.[33,39] Recommendations to help ensure optimal assay performance, interpretation, and reporting, regardless of which technique is employed, have been published.[38,40] Commercially available FISH tests consist of either a single probe to assess absolute *HER2* copy number, or a dual probe assay that includes a chromosome 17 control probe, with results given as a *HER2*/chromosome 17 centromere ratio. The purpose of the control probe is to distinguish true *HER2* amplification from polysomy for chromosome 17, because the clinical significance of the latter is unclear. Based on the 2007 American Society of Clinical Oncology/College of American Pathologists guidelines,[38] a result is considered non-amplified if there is an average of fewer than 4.0 *HER2* copies per nucleus using the single probe assay or if the ratio is below 1.8 using the dual probe assay (**Fig. 7**A). An average of greater than 6.0 *HER2* copies per nucleus or a ratio of greater than 2.2 are considered amplified (see **Fig. 7**B). Equivocal results fall in between the non-amplified and amplified values. A recent study found that benefit from trastuzumab therapy seemed to be independent of chromosome 17 copy number, raising the question of whether or not the ratio should be used to determine amplification status.[41,42]

Determination of *MYCN* amplification status in neuroblastoma is another application of paraffin-embedded FISH. *MYCN* amplification is strongly associated with rapid tumor progression and poor prognosis in patients of all ages with any stage of disease, and the International Neuroblastoma Risk Group Biology Committee recommends that *MYCN* status should be evaluated in every resected neuroblastoma.[30] Different definitions for *MYCN* amplification have been published, with the Children's Oncology Group defining amplification as ten or more copies of *MYCN* per nucleus and the International Neuroblastoma Risk Group Biology Committee defining amplification as a ratio of *MYCN* to chromosome 2 control signal of greater than 4.0.[30,43] In contrast with *HER2* amplification in breast cancer, *MYCN* amplification in many cases is high level, with *MYCN* signals that are too numerous to accurately count (**Fig. 8**). It is important to be able to differentiate this type of true amplification from diffuse, nonspecific background. When present, *MYCN* amplification is usually present in all

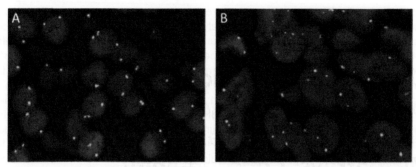

Fig. 7. FISH results demonstrating *HER2* non-amplified and amplified breast cancers. FISH was performed on paraffin-embedded tissue using a probe containing the *HER2* gene (red signals) and a chromosome 17 centromere probe (green signals). (*A*) The non-amplified case shows two *HER2* and 2 chromosome 17 centromere signals in the majority of nuclei, resulting in a ratio of less than 1.8. (*B*) The amplified case shows multiple *HER2* signals and two or three chromosome 17 centromere signals, resulting in a ratio of greater than 2.2. Note the overlap of some nuclei, which can make it difficult to determine which signals belong to a given nucleus. Also note that not all signals within a given nucleus can be captured within a single plane of focus, requiring focusing through the thickness of the nucleus to enumerate all signals. (*Courtesy of* Dr Diane Persons, University of Kansas Medical Center.)

tumor cells, but occasionally there is heterogeneity with a mixture of amplified and non-amplified tumor cells, or amplification in a minority of tumor cells. Heterogenous amplification should be distinguished from the presence of normal cells. There are also rare cases that have gain of *MYCN* that is not considered amplification. Heterogeneous amplification or *MYCN* gain without amplification should be noted in reports, because the clinical significance of these findings has not yet been determined.[30]

Although the topic is beyond the scope of this article, BRISH has been gaining in popularity as an alternative to paraffin-embedded FISH, particularly for assessing

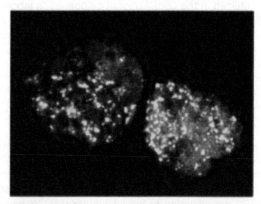

Fig. 8. FISH showing *MYCN* amplification in nuclei from a neuroblastoma. Green signals are from a probe containing the *MYCN* gene and red signals are from a chromosome 2 centromere probe. The nuclei have two red signals representing two copies of chromosome 2, and innumerable green signals representing amplification of the *MYCN* gene.

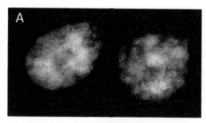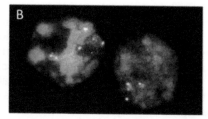

Fig. 9. FISH on touch preparation slides without and with protease digestion. (*A*) Without protease treatment, nuclei show diffuse green background and lack of probe signals. (*B*) A slide made from the same tumor treated with protease has significantly less background and visible probe signals.

HER2 status in breast cancer.[44–46] BRISH techniques include chromogenic in situ hybridization and silver in situ hybridization. A significant advantage of BRISH is that tissue architecture and morphology are much easier to interpret compared with FISH. Thus, with BRISH it is easier to ensure that the appropriate area of the tissue (invasive tumor, tumor versus normal, etc) is analyzed. Other advantages of BRISH include the use of bright field as opposed to fluorescence microscopy and the ability to archive the hybridized slides for a longer period of time.

FISH on Nuclei From Touch Preparations

Touch preparations may provide an alternative to paraffin-embedded FISH if fresh or frozen tissue is available. Touch preparations are made by touching unfixed tissue to the slide that will be used for FISH, followed by fixation of the cells on the slide. It can be difficult to control the density of cells deposited on the slide. A friable tumor may result in clumps of cells that are difficult to analyze, whereas a tumor with a large amount of fibrous stroma may yield few cells. This technique is also not suitable if specific nuclei need to be analyzed within a heterogeneous mixture, but if a sample is relatively homogeneous, it can yield intact nuclei that do not require as much manipulation as that required for FISH of paraffin-embedded sections. Protease digestion may be required for some specimens to increase probe accessibility and decrease background (**Fig. 9**). The main drawback of this technique is that the slides need to be made before tissue fixation.

FISH on Targeted Cell Populations

There are a number of techniques for performing FISH on targeted cells within a heterogeneous population. Some of these techniques, such as flow cytometry or immunomagnetic cell selection, involve purification of cells of interest before FISH, whereas others entail prior or simultaneous identification of specific cells with conventional or immunochemical stains in conjunction with FISH. FISH on targeted cells has become increasingly important in clinical cytogenetics laboratories for the evaluation of multiple myeloma and other plasma cell disorders. Cytogenetic aberrations in plasma cell disorders have important prognostic implications (see the article on Multiple Myeloma). Because of the low proliferative activity of plasma cells and patchy bone marrow involvement, conventional cytogenetics and even interphase FISH on cultured specimens can fail to detect abnormalities that are present. Multiple studies have shown significantly increased FISH detection rates of prognostically important alterations when some form of plasma cell identification or purification is used.[47–49] One method of targeting plasma cells for analysis involves cytoplasmic immunostaining with antibodies against immunoglobulin kappa or lambda in combination with FISH, for simultaneous identification of plasma cells and visualization of FISH signals.[50,51] The most widely used method entails purification of plasma cells before FISH using immunomagnetic cell selection and anti-CD138–specific antibodies.[52] Cutoffs for determination of abnormal FISH results using these techniques vary depending on the study, and the biologic significance of chosen cutoffs still needs to be analyzed in a large cohort of patients.[47]

In addition to plasma cell neoplasms, combined immunostaining and FISH has been used to evaluate other forms of neoplasia.[53,54] Combined immunostaining and FISH is not just limited to cellular phenotyping, but has also been utilized for studying DNA–protein interactions in various other basic and translational research applications. Simultaneous DNA–protein detection has been used in studies that investigate the structure and function of meiotic chromosomes, genome organization, and correlation of changes in protein and DNA localization within the nucleus with changes in gene expression.[55]

AUTOMATION OF FISH ANALYSIS

Interphase FISH scoring is a time-consuming process that requires a high level of skill and subjective interpretation of signal patterns. As the volume of FISH testing in clinical laboratories has increased, so has interest in automated scoring of FISH signals to increase efficiency, and reduce inter- and intra-individual variation. Theodosiou and colleagues[56] have written an in-depth review on several methods of FISH image analysis on various tissue types from a number of research groups. The two main aspects involved in automated analysis of FISH images are spot (signal) detection and segmentation of nuclei. In tissue sections, it is difficult to correctly segment nuclei because of nuclear overlap. Different software analysis methods have been developed to overcome this limitation by defining small regions of interest for automated analysis, including tile sampling and grid sampling.[57,58] For fusion probe sets, the optimal distance between red and green signals for defining fusion events needs to be determined for each unique probe set.[57] Before automated analysis can be put into clinical use, each probe or probe set needs to be validated against manual scoring in each laboratory. After implementation, manual review of captured images or manual rescoring is still necessary in some cases, for example, if an equivocal result is obtained for *HER2* amplification in breast cancer.[58] Studies have compared automated against manual analysis for many different FISH assays, including aneuploidy detection in amniocytes, *HER2* amplification status in breast cancer, dual-fusion and break-apart probes in paraffin-embedded tissue sections, and FISH for bladder cancer.[57–60] All of these studies showed good correlation between automated and manual FISH interpretations.

SUMMARY

This article presents many applications of FISH technology, including recent advances in areas such as high-resolution oligonucleotide FISH, flow FISH, and automated analysis. Despite dramatic changes in the field of cytogenetics owing to the implementation of array technology, FISH remains useful in both the research and clinical laboratory because of its unique ability to visualize nucleic acid sequences in their native context within individual cells. Although array-based copy number detection allows discovery of gains and losses at a very high level of resolution, the structure of gains is not evident and detection of mosaicism is limited. Thus, FISH will continue to be useful in conjunction with arrays and G-banded chromosome analysis for further characterization of the structure of chromosome alterations, and also as a stand alone technique for detection of minimal residual disease in patients with neoplasia.

ACKNOWLEDGMENTS

The author thanks Billy Davis for assistance with many of the FISH images.

REFERENCES

1. Yamada NA, Rector LS, Tsang P, et al. Visualization of fine-scale genomic structure by oligonucleotide-based high-resolution FISH. Cytogenet Genome Res 2010;132:248.
2. Mascarello JT, Hirsch B, Kearney HM, et al. Section E9 of the ACMG technical standards and guidelines: Fluorescence in Situ Hybridization (FISH). Genet Med 2011;13:667–75.
3. Hermsen MA, Meijer GA, Baak JP, et al. Comparative genomic hybridization: a new tool in cancer pathology. Hum Pathol 1996;27:342.
4. Kallioniemi A, Kallioniemi OP, Sudar D, et al. Comparative genomic hybridization for molecular cytogenetic analysis of solid tumors. Science 1992;258:818.
5. Levy B, Dunn TM, Kaffe S, et al. Clinical applications of comparative genomic hybridization. Genet Med 1998;1:4.
6. Kirchhoff M, Rose H, Lundsteen C. High resolution comparative genomic hybridisation in clinical cytogenetics. J Med Genet 2001;38:740.
7. Schrock E, du Manoir S, Veldman T, et al. Multicolor spectral karyotyping of human chromosomes. Science 1996;273:494.
8. Speicher MR, Gwyn Ballard S, Ward DC. Karyotyping human chromosomes by combinatorial multi-fluor FISH. Nat Genet 1996;12:368.
9. Fan YS, Siu VM, Jung JH, et al. Sensitivity of multiple color spectral karyotyping in detecting small interchromosomal rearrangements. Genet Test 2000;4:9.
10. Heng HH, Tsui LC. High resolution free chromatin/DNA fiber fluorescent in situ hybridization. J Chromatogr A 1998;806:219.
11. Raap AK, Florijn RJ, Blonden LAJ, et al. Fiber FISH as a DNA mapping tool. Methods 1996;9:67.
12. Baerlocher GM, Vulto I, de Jong G, et al. Flow cytometry and FISH to measure the average length of telomeres (flow FISH). Nat Protoc 2006;1:2365.
13. Alter BP, Baerlocher GM, Savage SA, et al. Very short telomere length by flow fluorescence in situ hybridization identifies patients with dyskeratosis congenita. Blood 2007;110:1439.
14. Du HY, Pumbo E, Ivanovich J, et al. TERC and TERT gene mutations in patients with bone marrow failure and the significance of telomere length measurements. Blood 2009;113:309.
15. Ventura RA, Martin-Subero JI, Jones M, et al. FISH analysis for the detection of lymphoma-associated chromosomal abnormalities in routine paraffin-embedded tissue. J Mol Diagn 2006;8:141.
16. Tepperberg J, Pettenati MJ, Rao PN, et al. Prenatal diagnosis using interphase fluorescence in situ hybridization (FISH): 2-year multi-center retrospective study and review of the literature. Prenat Diagn 2001;21:293.
17. Klinger K, Landes G, Shook D, et al. Rapid detection of chromosome aneuploidies in uncultured amniocytes by using fluorescence in situ hybridization (FISH). Am J Hum Genet 1992;51:55.

18. Ward BE, Gersen SL, Carelli MP, et al. Rapid prenatal diagnosis of chromosomal aneuploidies by fluorescence in situ hybridization: clinical experience with 4,500 specimens. Am J Hum Genet 1993;52:854.

19. American College of Medical Genetics, American College of Genetics. Technical and clinical assessment of fluorescence in situ hybridization: an ACMG/ASHG position statement. I. Technical considerations. Test and Technology Transfer Committee. Genet Med 2000;2:356.

20. Cai LS, Lim AS, Tan A. Rapid one-day fluorescence in situ hybridisation in prenatal diagnosis using uncultured amniocytes and chorionic villi. Ann Acad Med Singapore 1999;28:502.

21. Evans MI, Klinger KW, Isada NB, et al. Rapid prenatal diagnosis by fluorescent in situ hybridization of chorionic villi: an adjunct to long-term culture and karyotype. Am J Obstet Gynecol 1992;167:1522.

22. Fragouli E. Preimplantation genetic diagnosis: present and future. J Assist Reprod Genet 2007;24:201.

23. Simpson JL. Preimplantation genetic diagnosis at 20 years. Prenat Diagn 2010;30: 682.

24. Wolff DJ. The genetics of bladder cancer: a cytogeneticist's perspective. Cytogenet Genome Res 2007;118:177.

25. Sokolova IA, Halling KC, Jenkins RB, et al. The development of a multitarget, multicolor fluorescence in situ hybridization assay for the detection of urothelial carcinoma in urine. J Mol Diagn 2000;2:116.

26. Halling KC, Kipp BR. Fluorescence in situ hybridization in diagnostic cytology. Hum Pathol 2007;38:1137.

27. Kim YH, Nobusawa S, Mittelbronn M, et al. Molecular classification of low-grade diffuse gliomas. Am J Pathol 2010;177:2708.

28. Rodriguez FJ, Giannini C. Oligodendroglial tumors: diagnostic and molecular pathology. Semin Diagn Pathol 2010;27:136.

29. Tanas MR, Goldblum JR. Fluorescence in situ hybridization in the diagnosis of soft tissue neoplasms: a review. Adv Anat Pathol 2009;16:383.

30. Ambros PF, Ambros IM, Brodeur GM, et al. International consensus for neuroblastoma molecular diagnostics: report from the International Neuroblastoma Risk Group (INRG) Biology Committee. Br J Cancer 2009;100:1471.

31. Bang YJ, Van Cutsem E, Feyereislova A, et al. Trastuzumab in combination with chemotherapy versus chemotherapy alone for treatment of HER2-positive advanced gastric or gastro-oesophageal junction cancer (ToGA): a phase 3, open-label, randomised controlled trial. Lancet 2010;376:687.

32. Gerber DE, Minna JD. ALK inhibition for non-small cell lung cancer: from discovery to therapy in record time. Cancer Cell 2010;18:548.

33. Ross JS, Slodkowska EA, Symmans WF, et al. The HER-2 receptor and breast cancer: ten years of targeted anti-HER-2 therapy and personalized medicine. Oncologist 2009;14:320.

34. Paternoster SF, Brockman SR, McClure RF, et al. A new method to extract nuclei from paraffin-embedded tissue to study lymphomas using interphase fluorescence in situ hybridization. Am J Pathol 2002;160:1967.

35. Babic A, Loftin IR, Stanislaw S, et al. The impact of pre-analytical processing on staining quality for H&E, dual hapten, dual color in situ hybridization and fluorescent in situ hybridization assays. Methods 2010;52:287.

36. Khoury T, Sait S, Hwang H, et al. Delay to formalin fixation effect on breast biomarkers. Mod Pathol 2009;22:1457.

37. Summersgill B, Clark J, Shipley J. Fluorescence and chromogenic in situ hybridization to detect genetic aberrations in formalin-fixed paraffin embedded material, including tissue microarrays. Nat Protoc 2008;3:220.
38. Wolff AC, Hammond ME, Schwartz JN, et al. American Society of Clinical Oncology/College of American Pathologists guideline recommendations for human epidermal growth factor receptor 2 testing in breast cancer. Arch Pathol Lab Med 2007;131:18.
39. Laudadio J, Quigley DI, Tubbs R, et al. HER2 testing: a review of detection methodologies and their clinical performance. Expert Rev Mol Diagn 2007;7:53.
40. Vance GH, Barry TS, Bloom KJ, et al. Genetic heterogeneity in HER2 testing in breast cancer: panel summary and guidelines. Arch Pathol Lab Med 2009;133:611.
41. Perez EA, Reinholz MM, Hillman DW, et al. HER2 and chromosome 17 effect on patient outcome in the N9831 adjuvant trastuzumab trial. J Clin Oncol 2010;28:4307.
42. Ross JS. Saving lives with accurate HER2 testing. Am J Clin Pathol 2010;134:183.
43. Schneiderman J, London WB, Brodeur GM, et al. Clinical significance of MYCN amplification and ploidy in favorable-stage neuroblastoma: a report from the Children's Oncology Group. J Clin Oncol 2008;26:913.
44. Gruver AM, Peerwani Z, Tubbs RR. Out of the darkness and into the light: bright field in situ hybridisation for delineation of ERBB2 (HER2) status in breast carcinoma. J Clin Pathol 2010;63:210.
45. Lambros MB, Natrajan R, Reis-Filho JS. Chromogenic and fluorescent in situ hybridization in breast cancer. Hum Pathol 2007;38:1105.
46. Penault-Llorca F, Bilous M, Dowsett M, et al. Emerging technologies for assessing HER2 amplification. Am J Clin Pathol 2009;132:539.
47. Christensen JH, Abildgaard N, Plesner T, et al. Interphase fluorescence in situ hybridization in multiple myeloma and monoclonal gammopathy of undetermined significance without and with positive plasma cell identification: analysis of 192 cases from the region of Southern Denmark. Cancer Genet Cytogenet 2007;174:89.
48. Put N, Lemmens H, Wlodarska I, et al. Interphase fluorescence in situ hybridization on selected plasma cells is superior in the detection of cytogenetic aberrations in plasma cell dyscrasia. Genes Chromosomes Cancer 2010;49:991.
49. Slovak ML, Bedell V, Pagel K, et al. Targeting plasma cells improves detection of cytogenetic aberrations in multiple myeloma: phenotype/genotype fluorescence in situ hybridization. Cancer Genet Cytogenet 2005;158:99.
50. Ahmann GJ, Jalal SM, Juneau AL, et al. A novel three-color, clone-specific fluorescence in situ hybridization procedure for monoclonal gammopathies. Cancer Genet Cytogenet 1998;101:7.
51. Boersma-Vreugdenhil GR, Peeters T, Bast BJ, et al. Translocation of the IgH locus is nearly ubiquitous in multiple myeloma as detected by immuno-FISH. Blood 2003;101:1653.
52. Zojer N, Schuster-Kolbe J, Assmann I, et al. Chromosomal aberrations are shared by malignant plasma cells and a small fraction of circulating CD19+ cells in patients with myeloma and monoclonal gammopathy of undetermined significance. Br J Haematol 2002;117:852.
53. Martin-Subero JI, Chudoba I, Harder L, et al. Multicolor-FICTION: expanding the possibilities of combined morphologic, immunophenotypic, and genetic single cell analyses. Am J Pathol 2002;161:413.
54. Weber-Matthiesen K, Winkemann M, Muller-Hermelink A, et al. Simultaneous fluorescence immunophenotyping and interphase cytogenetics: a contribution to the characterization of tumor cells. J Histochem Cytochem 1992;40:171.
55. Ye CJ, Stevens JB, Liu G, et al. Combined multicolor-FISH and immunostaining. Cytogenet Genome Res 2006;114:227.

56. Theodosiou Z, Kasampalidis IN, Livanos G, et al. Automated analysis of FISH and immunohistochemistry images: a review. Cytometry A 2007;71:439.
57. Alpar D, Hermesz J, Poto L, et al. Automated FISH analysis using dual-fusion and break-apart probes on paraffin-embedded tissue sections. Cytometry A 2008;73:651.
58. Stevens R, Almanaseer I, Gonzalez M, et al. Analysis of HER2 gene amplification using an automated fluorescence in situ hybridization signal enumeration system. J Mol Diagn 2007;9:144.
59. Smith GD, Bentz JS. "FISHing" to detect urinary and other cancers: validation of an imaging system to aid in interpretation. Cancer Cytopathol 2010;118:56.
60. Wauters J, Assche EV, Antsaklis A, et al. Fully automated FISH examination of amniotic fluid cells. Prenat Diagn 2007;27:951.

The Evolving Picture of Microdeletion/Microduplication Syndromes in the Age of Microarray Analysis: Variable Expressivity and Genomic Complexity

Kristen L. Deak, PhD, Sarah R. Horn, PhD,
Catherine W. Rehder, PhD*

KEYWORDS

- Microdeletion • Microduplication • Syndrome • Microarray
- 1q21 • 15q13 • 15q24 • 16p13.1 • 16p11.2 • 17q21.3

Submicroscopic genomic copy number changes not visible by routine chromosome analysis are a common cause of congenital anomalies, developmental delay, and neuropsychiatric disorders. In previous decades, most recurrent genomic rearrangements were identified in a phenotype-first manner. In other words, a distinct collection of features and congenital anomalies distinguished a particular patient population, which was then interrogated for a common genetic anomaly. The clinical phenotypes of Prader-Willi and DiGeorge syndromes were described in 1956 and 1968, respectively, but the underlying genomic lesions were not described until 1981.[1,2] The advent of genomic microarray testing has ushered in a new age of discovery in which the genomic change is often identified before a clear common clinical picture has emerged.

Many of the classic microdeletion syndromes, such as DiGeorge, Prader-Willi, Angelman, and Williams syndromes, for example, as well as many more-recently described deletions and duplications, are recurrent because of the underlying architecture of the genome (**Table 1**). Approximately 5% of the human genome comprises blocks of repetitive sequences greater than 1 kilobase (kb) in size that share 90% sequence homology with other regions of the genome.[27] When these segmental duplications flank an intervening block of unique sequence, nonallelic

---

The authors have nothing to disclose.

Department of Pathology, Duke University, Durham, NC USA
* Corresponding author.
E-mail address: catherine.rehder@duke.edu

Clin Lab Med 31 (2011) 543–564
doi:10.1016/j.cll.2011.08.008
0272-2712/11/$ – see front matter © 2011 Elsevier Inc. All rights reserved.

labmed.theclinics.com

Table 1
Summary of genomic and clinical characteristics of 3 classic and 9 new syndromic disorders

	Genomic Coordinates (Mb)	Size (Mb)	Clinical Features	Reported in Unaffected Individuals	Candidate Genes	Selected References
Classic Disorders						
Williams	chr7:72.3–74.0	~1.6–1.9	MR, short stature, SVAS, hypercalcemia, hoarse voice, friendly disposition, periorbital fullness, stellate pattern of iris, full lips, long philtrum	—	ELN, LIMK1, GTF2I, STX1A, BAZ1B, CYLN2, GTF2IRD1, NCF1	Morris[3]
Prader-Willi	Class I chr15:20.4–26.2 Class II chr15:21.3–26.2	~5.8–6.0 ~5.0	Neonatal hypotonia and feeding difficulties followed by hyperphagia and obesity, cognitive impairment, hypogonadism, behavioral phenotype	—	SNURF-SNRPN, MKRN3, MAGEL2, NDN	Cassidy & Schwartz[4]
Angelman	Class I chr15:20.4–26.2 Class II chr15:21.3–26.2	~5.8–6.0 ~5.0	Severe developmental delay or intellectual disability, speech impairment, gait ataxia and/or tremulousness of limbs, inappropriate happy demeanor, microcephaly, seizures	—	UBE3A	Williams et al[5]

(continued on next page)

Table 1
(continued)

	Genomic Coordinates (Mb)	Size (Mb)	Clinical Features	Reported in Unaffected Individuals	Candidate Genes	Selected References
DiGeorge	Class I chr22:17.2–19.8	~2.5	CHD (especially conotruncal defects), learning difficulties, characteristic facial features, immune deficiency, hypocalcemia, palatal abnormalities, psychiatric illness	− (deletions)	TBX1, UFD1L CDC45L	McDonald-McGinn et al[6]
New Syndromic Loci						
TAR (1q21)	chr1:144.1–144.6	0.2–0.5	Thrombocytopenia, bilateral absence of the radii	+	LIX1L, PIAS3	Klopocki et al[7]
1q21	chr1:145.0–146.4	1.4	Microcephaly (deletions)/ macrocephaly (duplications), mild facial dysmorphisms, DD, cardiac abnormalities, FTT, joint laxity	− (deletions) + (duplications)	PRKAB2,FMO5, CHD1L, BCL9, ACP6, GJA5, GJA8, GPR89B	Mefford et al[8]; Brunetti-Pierri et al[9]
BP1-BP2(15q11.2)	chr15:20.2–20.7	0.5	Speech delay, behavioral and neuropsychiatric abnormalities (deletions and duplications)	+ (deletions) + (duplications)	TUBGCP5, NIPA1, NIPA2, CYF1P1	Doornbos et al[10]; Burnside et al[11]

(continued on next page)

Table 1
(continued)

Genomic Coordinates (Mb)	Size (Mb)	Clinical Features	Reported in Unaffected Individuals	Candidate Genes	Selected References
15q13.3 chr.15:29.0–30.5	1.5	Cognitive impairment, behavior problems (poor attention span, hyperactivity, aggressive/impulsive behaviors), learning difficulties, seizures, schizophrenia, neuropsychiatric abnormalities	+ (deletions) − (duplications)	CHRNA7	Sharp et al[12]; van Bon et al[13]; Helbig et al[14]; Miller et al[15]
15q24 chr15:72.15–73.85	1.7–3.9	Growth retardation, microcephaly, digital abnormalities, hypospadias, loose connective tissue, facial dysmorphisms	− (deletions) + (duplications)	CYP11A1, SEMA7A, CPLX3, SRTA6, ARID3B, SIN3A, CSK, P450scc	Sharp et al[16]; Klopocki et al[17]
16p13.11 chr16:14.7–16.3	1.5–1.7	Cognitive impairment with psychomotor/language delays, congenital abnormalities (such as dysmorphic facies, microcephaly, short stature, cleft lip/midline defects), and neuropsychiatric disorders	+ (duplications) + (deletions)	NDE1, NTAN1	Ullmann et al[18]; Hannes et al[19]

(continued on next page)

Table 1
(continued)

Genomic Coordinates (Mb)	Size (Mb)	Clinical Features	Reported in Unaffected Individuals	Candidate Genes	Selected References
16p11.2 (distal) chr.16:28.7–28.95	0.2	DD, behavioral problems, obesity, seizures, unusual facial morphology (prominent forehead, narrow, downslanting palpebral fissures)	+(deletions)	*SH2B1*	Bochukova et al[20]; Bachmann-Gagescu et al[21]; Barge-Schaapveld et al[22]
16p11.2 (Proximal) chr.16:29.5–30.1	0.5–0.6	Language delays, learning difficulties, intellectual disability, neuropsychological impairments (with or without a diagnosis of ASD), minor dysmorphic facies, obesity, seizures	+(duplications) +(deletions)	*MVP, CDIPT1, SEZ6L2, ASPHD1, KCTD13*	Kumar et al[23]; Marshall et al[24]; Weiss et al[25]; Miller et al[26]
17q21.3 chr17:41.0–41.4	0.4–0.6	Mild to moderate MR, seizures, hypotonia, motor and speech delay, long fingers, amiable personality, large and low-set ears, tubular/pear-shaped nose	−(deletions)	*MAPT, CRHR1*	Sharp et al[27]; Koolen et al[28]; Shaw-Smith et al[29]; Koolen et al[30]; Tan et al[31]

Abbreviations: ASD, autistic spectrum disorders; CHD, congenital heart defect; DD, developmental delay; FTT, failure to thrive; MR, mental retardation; SVAS, supravalvular aortic stenosis.

Note: Genomic coordinates are approximate and are based on Build 36 [hg 18]. Unless otherwise noted, the features listed describe individuals carrying deletion of the corresponding region.

homologous recombination (NAHR) can cause deletion, duplication, or inversion of that unique sequence. The internal structure and orientation of these repetitive blocks is polymorphic, and often a particular orientation such as an inversion facilitates NAHR. In this review, the authors focus on 9 regions of the genome that are flanked by repetitive sequences. Whereas the phenotypic consequences of aberrations in some of these regions are clear, the clinical significance of copy number changes in other regions remains to be fully elucidated. Many of the rearrangements discussed in this review and other recent reviews[32,33] are members of the "susceptibility" genre, characterized by variable expressivity and reduced penetrance. By themselves these genomic changes may not be sufficient to cause a clinically abnormal phenotype; however, when combined with other genomic and environmental insults, the cumulative or epistatic effects may result in an abnormal phenotype.[34]

1q21.1

The genomic architecture of the 1q21 region predisposes it to NAHR-mediated rearrangements due to the presence of 4 segmental duplications of very high sequence identity, termed BP1-BP4, or break point 1, 2, 3. . .[8] (**Fig. 1**). These regions of segmental duplication can serve as substrates for atypical recombination. Three deletions or duplications involving this region have been reported. The first aberration is deletion/duplication of the BP2-BP3 region that is associated with thrombocytopenia absent radius (TAR) syndrome.[7] The distal 1.35 Mb deletion of 1q21.1, involving BP3 to BP4, is typically considered to be the classic 1q21.1 microdeletion syndrome.[8] Deletions of BP2 to BP4 are often termed class II deletions and involve both the proximal TAR region as well as the 1.35 Mb distal 1q21.1 region and are approximately 2 Mb in total size.[35]

TAR Deletion/Duplication

TAR syndrome is characterized by the bilateral absence of the radius bone and a dramatically reduced platelet count or hypomegakaryocytic thrombocytopenia. The syndrome is associated with a microdeletion within 1q21.1, with a minimum deletion interval of 200 kb between BP2 and BP3 that is necessary, but not sufficient, to cause the phenotype.[7] The most frequently observed deletion is roughly 500 kb (chr.1: 144.1–144.6 Mb, hg18) and contains approximately 17 known genes. Parental analyses have shown that this deletion is de novo in only 25% of affected individuals. Therefore, it has been postulated that the phenotype develops only in the presence of additional, although still unknown, modifiers.[7] It is unclear whether reciprocal duplications of this region may have phenotypic consequences[36] or represent benign variants, because they are sometimes seen in unaffected parents (KLD and CWR unpublished observation). Within the minimum interval, 2 candidate genes seem to be the most promising contributors to the phenotype seen in these individuals. The *PIAS3* gene product has interactions with *STAT3*,[37] a transcription factor involved in hematopoietic growth factor signaling, and the *LIX1L* gene shares sequence homology to the *Lix1* gene, which is expressed during chick hind-limb development.[38]

1q21.1 Deletion

The 1q21.1 microdeletion involves minimally the material between segmental duplication blocks BP3 and BP4, which spans an approximately 1.35 Mb region (chr.1: 145.0–146.35 Mb, hg18).[8] Clinical features are variable, and unlike some copy number changes, do not seem to lead to a clinically distinguishable phenotype. Typically, individuals with aberrations of 1q21 are discovered by microarray analysis,

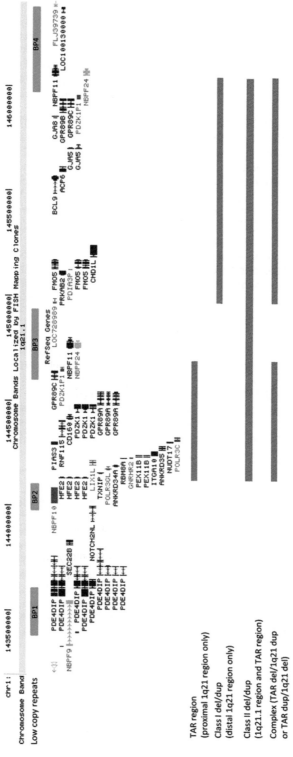

Fig. 1. The repetitive sequence blocks of 1q21 and related disorders. Based on Build 36 [hg 18].

representing a genotype-first model of diagnosis. The most common clinical findings in these individuals are microcephaly, mild intellectual disability, dysmorphic facial features, and eye abnormalities. Many other features may also be present but are typically seen in less than 25% of individuals.[8] These findings include seizures, skeletal malformations, cardiac defects, and genitourinary anomalies. Deletions of 1q21.1 are also considered to be a risk factor for psychiatric disorders such as autism spectrum disorder (ASD), attention deficit hyperactivity disorder, sleep disturbances, and schizophrenia.[39]

There are a total of 8 OMIM genes found in the 1.35 Mb region of 1q21.1: *PRKAB2*, *FMO5*, *CHD1L*, *BCL9*, *ACP6*, *GJA5*, *GJA8*, and *GPR89B*. Although no genotype-phenotype correlations have been described, 2 of these genes, *GJA5* and *GJA8*, have been suggested to contribute to some of the clinical features seen in patients with 1q21.1 deletions. Mutations and deletions of the *GJA5* gene have been identified in individuals with atrial fibrillation and structural cardiac defects.[40,41] In a study of individuals with congenital heart defects, .6% of these patients were found to have deletions involving *GJA5*.[40] Mutations in the *GJA8* gene have been detected in cases of several types of cataracts as well as cataract-microcornea syndrome.[42–46] Deletions of *GJA5* and *GJA8* are therefore hypothesized to play a role in the cardiac and eye abnormalities observed in individuals with 1q21.1 deletions.[8] The *BCL9* (B cell CLL/lymphoma 9) gene, a transcription factor in the Wnt signaling pathway, has been proposed as a candidate gene for schizophrenia because this signaling pathway influences neuroplasticity, cell survival, and neurogenesis.[47]

Class II Deletion

Larger deletions that involve both the TAR and the 1.35 Mb critical region are known as class II deletions. The clinical features of these individuals seem to be similar to those of the distal 1q21.1 deletions and can also be variable. These features include developmental delay, cardiac defects, genitourinary anomalies, and dysmorphic features.[9,35] Complex deletions and/or duplications can also occur where an individual has a deletion of the TAR region and duplication of the distal 1q21.1 region[9] or vice versa.[36]

1q21.1 Duplication

Duplications of the distal 1q21.1 region (BP2–BP3) have also been described.[8,9] Like many reciprocal duplications of microdeletion syndromes, the overall incidence seems to be lower, which is thought to be due to ascertainment bias because the duplication is associated with a less severe phenotype and therefore may not come to clinical attention. Common clinical features of 1q21.1 microduplications include dysmorphic features, developmental delay and intellectual disability, and autistic features, although the duplication has been observed in control cohorts.[8] Unlike the 1q21.1 microdeletions where microcephaly is consistently seen, macrocephaly seems to be a prominent feature of the 1q21.1 microduplications. It is thought that one or more dosage-sensitive genes, related to the size and the development of the brain, are located in this region.[9,48]

CHROMOSOME 15
15q13.3 Deletion/Duplication

The genomic architecture of chromosome 15 is complex (**Fig. 2**). Six regions of low copy repeats have been identified and are commonly referred to as break points 1 to 6 (BP1–6). Prader-Willi and Angelman syndromes are caused by deletions mediated

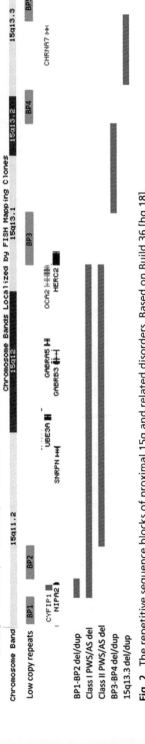

Fig. 2. The repetitive sequence blocks of proximal 15q and related disorders. Based on Build 36 [hg 18].

proximally by either BP1 or BP2 and distally by BP3. More distally, deletions between BP4 and BP5 in the 15q13.3 region have also been reported. First described in a series of 5 probands identified by a whole-genome microarray screen of patients with mental retardation and/or congenital anomalies,[12] additional studies[13-15] have widened the phenotypic spectrum. In the cohort of probands described by van Bon and colleagues[13] (N = 15), 14 displayed some degree of cognitive impairment ranging from mild learning problems to severe mental retardation. In that study, the only other features observed in over 50% of the probands were behavior problems such as poor attention span, hyperactivity, and aggressive and impulsive behavior. No common dysmorphic features were noted. When additional family members were examined to determine inheritance, 13 relatives with no cognitive deficits carrying the deletion were identified. Other carrier family members displayed abnormal phenotypes ranging from mild mental retardation to learning difficulties. Other studies have shown that deletion carriers demonstrate an increased frequency of seizures,[14] schizophrenia,[39] and other neuropsychiatric abnormalities.[15] The deletion is thought to account for .24% of cases of idiopathic mental retardation,[13] 1% of cases of idiopathic generalized epilepsy,[14] and .2% of cases of schizophrenia with only a general population frequency of less than .02%.[39] However, given the wide interfamily and intrafamily variability in the phenotype, it seems unlikely that the deletion, in isolation, is sufficient to cause an abnormal phenotype. It has been hypothesized that some individuals possess the ability to outgrow the abnormal phenotype such that they display learning disabilities at a young age but grow to become normal functioning adults.[13]

The BP4-BP5 region (chr.15: 29.0–30.5 Mb, hg18) contains 7 known genes: ARHGAP11B, MTMR15, MTMR10, TRPM1, KLF13, OTUD7A, and CHRNA7. CHRNA7 encodes the human alpha-7 neuronal nicotinic receptor subunit, which is a member of a family of ligand-gated ion channel proteins that mediate fast signal transmission at synapses. This gene is the most thoroughly investigated candidate gene in the region. Outside of microdeletion studies, polymorphisms in the gene have been linked to schizophrenia[49] and epilepsy,[50] and the knockout mouse displays an abnormal EEG,[51] making CHRNA7 a promising contender as an important causative gene.

Duplication of the BP4-BP5 region has also been reported.[13,15,52] These duplications were found in individuals being investigated because of developmental delay/mental retardation, multiple congenital anomalies, dysmorphic features, autism or autistic spectrum, or seizures (typical indications for chromosomal microarray analysis). The clinical significance of the BP4-BP5 microduplications as well as smaller duplications of the CHRNA7 gene is unclear, because many families have both affected and unaffected individuals who carry the duplication. It too may be a risk factor for neuropsychiatric disease.

BP1-BP2 Deletion/Duplication and Other Abnormalities in the Region

Because of the unique structure of chromosome 15, additional deletions and duplications have been reported that use atypical combinations of the break points. Van Bon and colleagues[13] described one family in which a BP3-BP4 deletion failed to segregate with an abnormal phenotype supporting the characterization of this deletion as a benign variant. Subsequent studies have suggested that although not sufficient to cause an abnormal phenotype, BP3-BP4 deletions could be contributory. Common features cited include failure to thrive, hypotonia, renal anomalies, and premature puberty, although variable expressivity and inheritance of the deletion from a "normal" parent were also documented.[53] Maternally derived deletions mediated by BP1 or BP2 proximally and BP4 or BP5 distally have been shown to result in a more severe Angelman phenotype, with these individuals scoring lower on assessments across all areas of mental, social, and language development.[54] In fact, some studies have reported phenotypic differences between patients with Prader-Willi syndrome depending on the proximal deletion break point, BP1 (type 1) or BP2 (type 2).[55]

Recently, two studies have reported cohorts of patients (N = 9[10] and N = 146[11]) with deletions and duplications mediated proximately by BP1 and distally by BP2. Both studies indicate that phenotypic consequences of both deletion and duplication of this region are highly variable. The abnormal features most significantly associated with deletion were behavioral/neuropsychiatric anomalies and speech delay, observed in 67% and 92% of evaluated individuals, respectively.[11] Some probands showed inheritance of the deletion or duplication from an apparently normal or mildly affected parent; however, most parents did not undergo rigorous behavioral or psychiatric evaluation. The authors of both studies acknowledge that their data could be skewed by ascertainment bias and/or small control populations, but both advocate that copy number changes in this region could contribute to an abnormal phenotype. Additional investigation including a control study in which participants undergo in-depth psychiatric testing is recommended. Four genes are contained in the region, *TUBGCP5*, *NIPA1*, *NIPA2*, *CYF1P1*. These genes are highly conserved, not imprinted, and may play roles in cognition and behavior.[10,11,55,56]

A third study that specifically examined candidate loci in a large cohort of patients with idiopathic generalized epilepsies reported BP1-BP2 deletions in 1% of their patient population (n = 1234) and in .2% of their control population.[57] Although enriched in the affected population, the deletion failed to segregate with the seizure phenotype in 3 large families, emphasizing the fact that other factors (stochastic events, environmental effects, recessive mutations on the other allele, and background genomic variation) must play a role in the phenotypic expression of this deletion.

15q24 Deletion

Sharp and colleagues[16] first described a cohort of 4 patients, all with mild to moderate developmental delay, growth retardation, hypospadias, microcephaly, digital abnormalities, and joint laxity, who were found to have microdeletions of the 15q24 region. The investigators suggested that individuals with these deletions could share enough common features to potentially represent a clinically recognizable syndrome. To date, few additional patients have been described to both clarify the clinical presentation and to delineate the smallest region of overlap (SRO) for the 15q24 microdeletion syndrome. The reported phenotypic features of individuals with deletions of 15q24 have consistently included developmental delay that is mild to moderate, growth retardation or short stature, hypotonia, digital abnormalities, skeletal deformities such as joint laxity, genital abnormalities, and characteristic facial features. [7,58–61]

NAHR has been proposed as the mechanism underlying these rearrangements because of the presence of 3 highly identical segmental duplications located within this region, and the majority of the described 15q24 deletions do have break points in these repetitive regions. The discovery of additional repetitive elements in the region has come from the analysis of alternative break points in newly described individuals.[58] The total size of the 15q24 deletions range from approximately 1.7 to 6.1 Mb, and the current SRO has been defined as an approximately 1.2 Mb region between break points termed 15q24B and 15q24C.[17,61] This region is gene-rich, and genes such as *CYP11A1*, *SEMA7A*, *CPLX3*, *SRTA6*, *ARID3B*, *SIN3A*, and *CSK* have been proposed to contribute to the phenotype.

15q24 Duplication

One patient with duplication of the 15q24 region has been described by Kiholm Lund and colleagues.[62] Although the duplication was inherited from a healthy father, features similar to that of the 15q24 microdeletion syndrome were noted, such as global developmental delay and dysmorphic features, along with digital and genital abnormalities. One additional case with 15q24 microduplication that encompasses the SRO for the reciprocal microdeletion has been documented. A male with mild mental retardation, decreased joint mobility, digital abnormalities, and characteristic facial features was described.[58] He was also described as having attention deficit hyperactivity disorder and Asperger syndrome. Cukier and colleagues[63] identified a small 10-kb duplication located within the 15q24 critical region, found to be inherited identical by descent in first cousins with autism. Because this duplication encompasses only a single gene, *UBL7*, it was suggested that these individuals effectively narrowed the critical region for susceptibility to the development of ASDs in 15q24 rearrangements.

Duplications adjacent and distal to the minimal critical region for the 15q24 deletions have also been described in 2 families. These duplications are also likely to be NAHR-mediated because of the abundance of low copy repeats located in this region. In both studies, 3 individuals are described including 2 siblings and their mother. All individuals exhibited mild developmental delay, hypotonia, digital abnormalities, and characteristic facial features.[58,64] Because of the lack of described cases, it remains unclear if 15q24 duplications, especially those outside of the SRO described in the 15q24 deletions, result in a distinct clinical phenotype.

CHROMOSOME 16

With high levels of segmentally duplicated sequence,[65,66] regions of chromosome 16 are primed for the generation of rearrangements via NAHR. The short arm in particular features clusters of segmental duplications,[65,66] and several new microdeletion and microduplication syndromes have been recently described for 16p, including those within 16p13.11 and 16p11.2 (**Fig. 3**).

16p13.11 Deletion/Duplication

Reciprocal microdeletions and microduplications of 1.5 to 1.65 Mb of 16p13.11 (chr.16: 14.7–16.3 Mb, hg18) were first discovered using array comparative genomic hybridization in individuals referred for autism and mental retardation.[18,19] Hannes and colleagues[19] concluded that deletions within this region are considered to be a risk factor for multiple congenital abnormalities and moderate to severe mental retardation.[19] Although the phenotypic findings vary, affected individuals may show cognitive impairment with psychomotor and language delays and variable congenital abnormalities such as dysmorphic facial features, microcephaly, short stature, and cleft lip/midline defects, as well as brain and ear abnormalities.[18,19,67,68]

A striking association of both deletions *and* duplications of this region with autism and other neuropsychiatric disorders like schizophrenia, idiopathic epilepsy, and behavioral problems has subsequently emerged. Specifically, deletions at 16p13.11 confer susceptibility to generalized and focal epilepsies,[49,69,70] whereas both deletions and duplications of this region confer an increased risk of schizophrenia.[71,72]

Both of the initial reports on recurrent 16p13.11 microdeletions describe individuals who carry the microdeletion but are unaffected by mental retardation[18] and/or multiple congenital abnormalities.[19] Similarly, de Kovel and colleagues[57] identified the

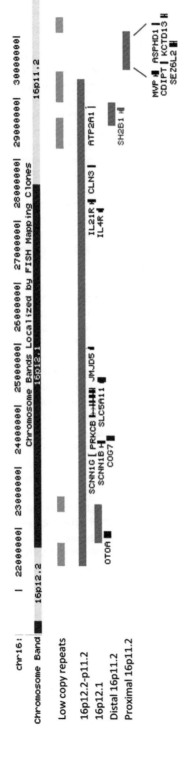

Fig. 3. Genomic schematic highlighting the repetitive sequence blocks of proximal 16p and related disorders. Based on Build 36 [hg 18].

recurrent deletion in .04% of their controls unaffected by schizophrenia, and in their study of generalized epilepsies, Ingason and colleagues[72] identified 2 unaffected parents who transmitted the microdeletion to their affected offspring.[57,72] These reports of unaffected carriers and the varied clinical spectrum of affected individuals suggest that factors such as incomplete penetrance, variable expressivity, or additional modifiers likely contribute to the phenotypes associated with 16p13 imbalance.

Although 14 to 15 protein-encoding genes and 2 microRNA-encoding genes are present within the region of imbalance on 16p13.11, two genes are cited repeatedly as possible candidates for the observed neurocognitive phenotypes: NDE1 (nudE nuclear distribution gene homolog 1) and NTAN1 (N-terminal asparagines amidase).[18,19,67] NDE1 encodes a centrosomal protein that functions in cellular proliferation-differentiation decisions important for the normal development of the cerebral cortex, as evidenced by the microcephaly and reduced cerebral cortex observed in Nde-null mice and in individuals with NDE1 mutations.[73–77] Likewise, Ntan1-/- mice also exhibited neurologic abnormalities, showing alterations in spontaneous activity, spatial memory, and a socially conditioned exploratory phenotype.[78] These gene functions do correlate with the neurocognitive features resulting from 16p13.11 imbalances, and together with other factors, these candidate genes may contribute to the phenotypic findings in a dosage-sensitive manner.

16p11.2 Deletions

In addition to the 16p13.11 microdeletion, other recurrent microdeletions within 16p have been reported, several located in the proximal region of 16p11.2. The typical, or proximal, 16p11.2 microdeletion is a deletion of 550 to 600 kb at approximately 29.5 to 30.1 Mb (chr.16: 29.5–30.1 Mb, hg18, OMIM #611913), whereas the atypical, or distal, 16p11.2 deletion is smaller (220 kb) and located at 28.7 to 29.0 Mb (chr.16: 28.74–28.95 Mb, hg18, OMIM #613444). Even more distal is the 16p12.2–p11.2 deletion syndrome, a large recurrent deletion of 7.1 to 8.7 Mb (OMIM #613604), which extends into 16p11.2 and can encompass the distal 16p11.2 deletion.[79,80] Within this large 16p12.2–p11.2 deletion there is a smaller recurrent deletion of approximately 520 kb (at 16p12.1, OMIM 136570)[35] (see **Fig. 3**). For the purposes of this review, only the distal and the proximal 16p11.2 microdeletion syndromes will be summarized further.

Distal 16p11.2 Deletion

Reports of patients with the distal 16p11.2 deletion (or the "atypical" deletion)[81] have been published by several groups.[20–22,81–83] Whereas phenotypic variability exists, commonly reported findings include developmental delay, behavioral problems, obesity, seizures, and an unusual facial morphology (prominent forehead and narrow, downslanting palpebral fissures).[22] Deletions of the distal region of 16p11.2 encompass 9 genes. Of these, the SH2B1 gene is a candidate for the severe early-onset obesity reported in almost 20% of individuals with the microdeletion.[20–22] The SH2B1 gene encodes a protein involved in leptin and insulin signaling, and disruption of the gene in mouse models results in hyperphagia, obesity, and insulin resistance.[84]

Proximal 16p11.2 Deletion/Duplication

Initially reported as a benign copy number variant,[85,86] the proximal 16p11.2 microdeletion was later described as a recurrent microdeletion in individuals with ASD by 3 groups in 2008.[23–25] Subsequently, recurrent imbalances of this region (microdeletions and microduplications) have been reported to confer susceptibility to ASD in up to 1% of all ASD patients.[23–25, 87,] Clinically, this microdeletion is characterized by language delays (with expressive language more affected than receptive language), learning difficulties and intellectual disability, neuropsychological impairments (with or without a diagnosis of ASD), minor dysmorphic features, and a propensity for obesity and seizure activity.[26] The proximal 16p11.2 microdeletion may also contribute to psychiatric diseases (such as schizophrenia, ADHD, and bipolar disorder) and minor cardiac abnormalities.[26] An association between the reciprocal 16p11.2 microduplication and an increased risk of schizophrenia has also been reported,[88] although the full clinical significance of the microduplication remains unclear.[26]

The proximal 16p11.2 microdeletion contains 25 genes or transcripts, several of which have functions known to correlate with the phenotypic findings. Based on expression data and cellular functions (including roles in neurodevelopment), a number of the potential candidate genes within this region have been indentified, such as *MAPK3*, *MAZ*, *DOC2A*, *SEZ6L2*, *HIRIP3*, *TBX6*, and *ALDOA*.[23,81,89] A report by Crepel and colleagues[90] recently narrowed the critical region for autism within the microdeletion to 5 candidate genes, *MVP*, *CDIPT1*, *SEZ6L2*, *ASPHD1* and *KCTD13*, and 2 in particular, *SEZ6L2* (seizure-related 6 homolog 2) and *MVP* (major vault protein) ranked especially high.[90]

Like many of these new microdeletion syndromes, the proximal 16p11.2 microdeletion has been reported in control individuals.[25,91] Miller and colleagues[26] suggested that both the recent nature of its description and the ascertainment bias inherent in some study designs make it difficult to calculate the exact penetrance of the proximal 16p11.2 microdeletion.[26] The distal 16p11.2 microdeletion has similarly been reported in control patients and in patients showing no particular clinical phenotype,[20,21] highlighting the need for additional research and the consideration of modifying factors in understanding the clinical effects of these microdeletions.

Although phenotypic variability is a hallmark feature of the 16p microdeletion syndromes discussed here, some degree of neuropsychological and/or cognitive impairment is commonly observed in individuals carrying either of the microdeletions of 16p11.2 (proximal or distal) and in those with a microdeletion within 16p13.11. Together, reports of recurrent microdeletions in the short arm of chromosome 16 provide growing evidence of the phenotypic impact of NAHR within this region, riddled with segmental duplications.

CHROMOSOME 17
17q21.3 Deletion/Duplication

In September of 2006, three groups published reports of multiple patients with deletions of 17q21.3, approximately 480 to 600 kb in size.[27–29] These patients all shared a common phenotype that included mild to moderate mental retardation, hypotonia, motor and speech delay, long fingers, an amiable or friendly disposition, and dysmorphic features including large and low-set ears, and a tubular, pear-shaped nose with a bulbous tip. Subsequent reports of larger collections of patients[30,31] added epilepsy/seizures, other central nervous system defects, cardiac defects, urologic anomalies, musculoskeletal defects, and abnormal hair, nails, and teeth as characteristics found in at least 50% of affected individuals in at least one of these larger studies. The estimated prevalence of the deletion is 1:16,000 and may account for up to .64% of idiopathic mental retardation. Little is known with regard to the reciprocal duplication that has only been reported in 5 patients with an abnormal neuropsychiatric phenotype and, in some cases, multiple congenital anomalies.[92,93]

Using a high-density array, the common region of deletion has been refined (chr17: 41.0–41.4 Mb, hg18).[30] The segmental duplications,[27,28] which likely mediate this recurrent copy number change, are complex. Two ancestral variants have been delineated, H1 and H2, which vary in the orientation of some of the duplication blocks.[94,95] H2, which has a frequency of 20% in the European population, is characterized by a 900-kb inversion. Analysis of parent/proband trios,[29,30] showed that in each case the de novo deletion occurred on an allele transmitted by a parent who carried at least one H2 allele. It is therefore hypothesized that NAHR may only occur in the presence of an H2 allele. This phenomenon, of an inversion polymorphism within a region of segmental duplication serving as a predisposing factor for genomic rearrangement, occurs in other regions of the genome[96,97] including the Williams syndrome region. Large percentages of the population carry these polymorphisms; however, the incidences of these genomic rearrangements including Williams syndrome and the 17q21.3 deletion are relatively rare. Therefore the inversion is likely necessary, but not sufficient, for deletion generation, and preconception carrier testing is likely of limited utility.

Six genes are found within the deletion region, C17orf69, CRHR1, IMP5, MAPT, STH, and KIAA1267,[30] with 2 genes, CRHR1 and MAPT, thought to be of particular significance. CRHR1 encodes a hormone receptor (corticotrophin-releasing factor receptor 1) involved in endocrine, behavioral, autonomic, and immune responses to stress.[98] Deficient mice show decreased anxiety, impaired stress response, and abnormal neuroendocrine development.[99] Similar to the CRHR1 gene, the MAPT gene is also highly expressed in the brain. MAPT encodes the microtubule-associated protein tau, which is found in the neurofibrillary tangles of Alzheimer disease patients. Mutations in the MAPT gene have been observed in 10% of patients with frontotemporal dementia or Pick disease. More relevant to the deletion phenotype, mice lacking tau protein show muscle weakness and behavioral and learning deficits.[100,101]

Because the MAPT gene held so much promise as the critical gene within the deletion region, Koolen and colleagues[30] performed full gene sequencing in 122 patients fitting the 17q21.3 microdeletion phenotypic profile but lacking the genomic deletion. In their study, no sequence changes of clear clinical significance were identified, leading the investigators to conclude that the phenotype associated with the 17q21.3 microdeletion is due to the combined effects of haploinsufficiency for multiple genes in the interval rather than a single gene. Recently, 2 patients have been identified with deletions only involving the MAPT gene.[102] The phenotype of both patients falls within the spectrum of those carrying the full deletion, arguing that MAPT is most likely the critical gene.

SUMMARY

Although the disorders discussed in this review are only a subset of all of the segmental aneusomy syndromes, they represent the variety and complexity of the phenotypes and penetrance levels observed in this class of disorders. As the use of microarrays as a first-line genomic screen increases, no doubt these as well as many additional imbalances will become better characterized. Several deletions and duplications that have been touted as "susceptibility" regions have also been detected in control cohorts and in unaffected relatives. Additional population-based studies that include thorough cognitive and psychiatric examinations are necessary to truly elucidate the phenotypic spectrum and penetrance associated with this new class of disorders.

REFERENCES

1. Ledbetter DH, Riccardi VM, Airhart SD, et al. Deletions of chromosome 15 as a cause of the Prader-Willi syndrome. N Engl J Med 1981;304(6):325–9.

2. de la Chapelle A, Herva R, Koivisto M, et al. A deletion in chromosome 22 can cause DiGeorge syndrome. Hum Genet 1981;57(3):253–6.
3. Morris CA. Williams syndrome. In: Pagon RA, Bird TD, Dolan CR, et al, editors. GeneReviews. Seattle (WA): NCBI Bookshelf; 2006.
4. Cassidy SB, Schwartz S. Prader-Willi syndrome. In: Pagon RA, Bird TD, Dolan CR, et al, editors. GeneReviews. Seattle (WA): NCBI Bookshelf; 2009.
5. Williams CA, Dagli AI, Driscoll DJ. Angelman syndrome. In: Pagon RA, Bird TD, Dolan CR, et al, editors. GeneReviews. Seattle (WA): NCBI Bookshelf; 2008.
6. McDonald-McGinn DM, Emanuel BS, Zackai EH. 22q11.2 deletion syndrome. In: Pagon RA, Bird TD, Dolan CR, et al, editors. GeneReviews. Seattle (WA): NCBI Bookshelf; 2005.
7. Klopocki E, Schulze H, Strauss G, et al. Complex inheritance pattern resembling autosomal recessive inheritance involving a microdeletion in thrombocytopenia-absent radius syndrome. Am J Hum Genet 2007;80(2):232–40.
8. Mefford HC, Sharp AJ, Baker C, et al. Recurrent rearrangements of chromosome 1q21.1 and variable pediatric phenotypes. N Engl J Med 2008;359(16):1685–99.
9. Brunetti-Pierri N, Berg JS, Scaglia F, et al. Recurrent reciprocal 1q21.1 deletions and duplications associated with microcephaly or macrocephaly and developmental and behavioral abnormalities. Nat Genet 2008;40(12):1466–71.
10. Doornbos M, Sikkema–Raddatz B, Ruijvenkamp CA, et al. Nine patients with a microdeletion 15q11.2 between breakpoints 1 and 2 of the Prader–Willi critical region, possibly associated with behavioural disturbances. Eur J Med Genet 2009; 52(2–3):108–15.
11. Burnside RD, Pasion R, Mikhail FM, et al. Microdeletion/microduplication of proximal 15q11.2 between BP1 and BP2: a susceptibility region for neurological dysfunction including developmental and language delay. Hum Genet 2011. [Epub ahead of print].
12. Sharp AJ, Mefford HC, Li K, et al. A recurrent 15q13.3 microdeletion syndrome associated with mental retardation and seizures. Nat Genet 2008;40(3):322–8.
13. van Bon BW, Mefford HC, Menten B, et al. Further delineation of the 15q13 microdeletion and duplication syndromes: a clinical spectrum varying from non-pathogenic to a severe outcome. J Med Genet 2009;46(8):511–23.
14. Helbig I, Mefford HC, Sharp AJ, et al. 15q13.3 microdeletions increase risk of idiopathic generalized epilepsy. Nat Genet 2009;41(2):160–2.
15. Miller DT, Shen Y, Weiss LA, et al. Microdeletion/duplication at 15q13.2q13.3 among individuals with features of autism and other neuropsychiatric disorders. J Med Genet 2009;46(4):242–8.
16. Sharp AJ, Selzer RR, Veltman JA, et al. Characterization of a recurrent 15q24 microdeletion syndrome. Hum Mol Genet 2007;16(5):567–72.
17. Klopocki E, Graul-Neumann LM, Grieben U, et al. A further case of the recurrent 15q24 microdeletion syndrome, detected by array CGH. Eur J Pediatr 2008;167(8): 903–8.
18. Ullmann R, Turner G, Kirchhoff M, et al. Array CGH identifies reciprocal 16p13.1 duplications and deletions that predispose to autism and/or mental retardation. Hum Mutat 2007;28(7):674–82.
19. Hannes FD, Sharp AJ, Mefford HC, et al. Recurrent reciprocal deletions and duplications of 16p13.11: the deletion is a risk factor for MR/MCA while the duplication may be a rare benign variant. J Med Genet 2009;46(4):223–32.
20. Bochukova EG, Huang N, Keogh J, et al. Large, rare chromosomal deletions associated with severe early-onset obesity. Nature 2010;463(7281):666–70.

21. Bachmann-Gagescu R, Mefford HC, Cowan C, et al. Recurrent 200-kb deletions of 16p11.2 that include the SH2B1 gene are associated with developmental delay and obesity. Genet Med 2010;12(10):641–7.

22. Barge-Schaapveld DQ, Maas SM, Polstra A, et al. The atypical 16p11.2 deletion: a not so atypical microdeletion syndrome? Am J Med Genet A 2011;155(5):1066–72.

23. Kumar RA, KaraMohamed S, Sudi J, et al. Recurrent 16p11.2 microdeletions in autism. Hum Mol Genet 2008;17(4):628–38.

24. Marshall CR, Noor A, Vincent JB, et al. Structural variation of chromosomes in autism spectrum disorder. Am J Hum Genet 2008;82(2):477–88.

25. Weiss LA, Shen Y, Korn JM, et al. Association between microdeletion and microduplication at 16p11.2 and autism. N Engl J Med 2008;358(7):667–75.

26. Miller DT, Nasir R, Sobeih MM, et al. 16p11.2 microdeletion. In: Pagon RA, Bird TD, Dolan CR, et al, editors. GeneReviews. Seattle (WA): NCBI Bookshelf; 2011.

27. Sharp AJ, Hansen S, Selzer RR, et al. Discovery of previously unidentified genomic disorders from the duplication architecture of the human genome. Nat Genet 2006;38(9):1038–42.

28. Koolen DA, Vissers LE, Pfundt R, et al. A new chromosome 17q21.31 microdeletion syndrome associated with a common inversion polymorphism. Nat Genet 2006; 38(9):999–1001.

29. Shaw-Smith C, Pittman AM, Willatt L, et al. Microdeletion encompassing MAPT at chromosome 17q21.3 is associated with developmental delay and learning disability. Nat Genet 2006;38(9):1032–7.

30. Koolen DA, Sharp AJ, Hurst JA, et al. Clinical and molecular delineation of the 17q21.31 microdeletion syndrome. J Med Genet 2008;45(11):710–20.

31. Tan TY, Aftimos S, Worgan L, et al. Phenotypic expansion and further characterisation of the 17q21.31 microdeletion syndrome. J Med Genet 2009;46(7):480–9.

32. Slavotinek AM. Novel microdeletion syndromes detected by chromosome microarrays. Hum Genet 2008;124(1):1–17.

33. Girirajan S, Eichler EE. Phenotypic variability and genetic susceptibility to genomic disorders. Hum Mol Genet 2010;19(R2):R176–87.

34. Girirajan S, Rosenfeld JA, Cooper GM, et al. A recurrent 16p12.1 microdeletion supports a two-hit model for severe developmental delay. Nat Genet 2010;42(3): 203–209.

35. Velinov M, Dolzhanskaya N. Clavicular pseudoarthrosis, anomalous coronary artery and extra crease of the fifth finger-previously unreported features in individuals with class II 1q21.1 microdeletions. Eur J Med Genet 2010;53(4):213–6.

36. Brunet A, Armengol L, Heine D, et al. BAC array CGH in patients with Velocardiofacial syndrome-like features reveals genomic aberrations on chromosome region 1q21.1. BMC Med Genet 2009;10:144.

37. Chung CD, Liao J, Liu B, et al. Specific inhibition of Stat3 signal transduction by PIAS3. Science 1997;278(5344):1803–5.

38. Swindell EC, Moeller C, Thaller C, et al. Cloning and expression analysis of chicken Lix1, a founding member of a novel gene family. Mech Dev 2001;109(2):405–8.

39. Stefansson H, Rujescu D, Cichon S, et al. Large recurrent microdeletions associated with schizophrenia. Nature 2008;455(7210):232–6.

40. Christiansen J, Dyck JD, Elyas BG, et al. Chromosome 1q21.1 contiguous gene deletion is associated with congenital heart disease. Circ Res 2004;94(11):1429–35.

41. Gollob MH. Cardiac connexins as candidate genes for idiopathic atrial fibrillation. Curr Opin Cardiol 2006;21(3):155–8.

42. Shiels A, Mackay D, Ionides A, et al. A missense mutation in the human connexin50 gene (GJA8) underlies autosomal dominant "zonular pulverulent" cataract, on chromosome 1q. Am J Hum Genet 1998;62(3):526–32.

43. Willoughby CE, Arab S, Gandhi R, et al. A novel GJA8 mutation in an Iranian family with progressive autosomal dominant congenital nuclear cataract. J Med Genet 2003;40(11):e124.

44. Devi RR, Vijayalakshmi P. Novel mutations in GJA8 associated with autosomal dominant congenital cataract and microcornea. Mol Vis 2006;12:190–5.

45. Arora A, Minogue PJ, Liu X, et al. A novel connexin50 mutation associated with congenital nuclear pulverulent cataracts. J Med Genet 2008;45(3):155–60.

46. Kumar M, Agarwal T, Khokhar S, et al. Mutation screening and genotype phenotype correlation of alpha-crystallin, gamma-crystallin and GJA8 gene in congenital cataract. Mol Vis 2011;17:693–707.

47. Li J, Zhou G, Ji W, et al. Common variants in the BCL9 gene conferring risk of schizophrenia. Arch Gen Psychiatry 2011;68(3):232–40.

48. Dumas L, Sikela JM. DUF1220 domains, cognitive disease, and human brain evolution. Cold Spring Harb Symp Quant Biol 2009;74:375–82.

49. Freedman R, Coon H, Myles-Worsley M, et al. Linkage of a neurophysiological deficit in schizophrenia to a chromosome 15 locus. Proc Natl Acad Sci USA 1997;94(2):587–92.

50. Elmslie FV, Rees M, Williamson MP, et al. Genetic mapping of a major susceptibility locus for juvenile myoclonic epilepsy on chromosome 15q. Hum Mol Genet 1997;6(8):1329–34.

51. Orr-Urtreger A, Goldner FM, Saeki M, et al. Mice deficient in the alpha7 neuronal nicotinic acetylcholine receptor lack alpha-bungarotoxin binding sites and hippocampal fast nicotinic currents. J Neurosci 1997;17(23):9165–71.

52. Szafranski P, Schaaf CP, Person RE, et al. Structures and molecular mechanisms for common 15q13.3 microduplications involving CHRNA7: benign or pathological? Hum Mutat 2010;31(7):840–50.

53. Rosenfeld JA, Stephens LE, Coppinger J, et al. Deletions flanked by breakpoints 3 and 4 on 15q13 may contribute to abnormal phenotypes. Eur J Hum Genet 2011;19(5):547–54.

54. Sahoo T, Bacino CA, German JR, et al. Identification of novel deletions of 15q11q13 in Angelman syndrome by array-CGH: molecular characterization and genotype-phenotype correlations. Eur J Hum Genet 2007;15(9):943–9.

55. Bittel DC, Kibiryeva N, Butler MG. Expression of 4 genes between chromosome 15 breakpoints 1 and 2 and behavioral outcomes in Prader–Willi syndrome. Pediatrics 2006;118(4):e1276–83.

56. Chai JH, Locke DP, Greally JM, et al. Identification of four highly conserved genes between breakpoint hotspots BP1 and BP2 of the Prader-Willi/Angelman syndromes deletion region that have undergone evolutionary transposition mediated by flanking duplicons. Am J Hum Genet 2003;73(4):898–925.

57. de Kovel CG, Trucks H, Helbig I, et al. Recurrent microdeletions at 15q11.2 and 16p13.11 predispose to idiopathic generalized epilepsies. Brain 2010;133(Pt 1):23–32.

58. El-Hattab AW, Smolarek TA, Walker ME, et al. Redefined genomic architecture in 15q24 directed by patient deletion/duplication breakpoint mapping. Hum Genet 2009;126(4):589–602.

59. Van Esch H, Backx L, Pijkels E, et al. Congenital diaphragmatic hernia is part of the new 15q24 microdeletion syndrome. Eur J Med Genet 2009;52(2–3):153–6.

60. Masurel-Paulet A, Callier P, Thauvin-Robinet C, et al. Multiple cysts of the corpus callosum and psychomotor delay in a patient with a 3.1 Mb 15q24.1q24.2 interstitial deletion identified by array-CGH. Am J Med Genet A 2009;149A(7):1504–10.

61. Andrieux J, Dubourg C, Rio M, et al. Genotype-phenotype correlation in four 15q24 deleted patients identified by array-CGH. Am J Med Genet A 2009;149A(12): 2813–9.

62. Kiholm Lund AB, Hove HD, Kirchhoff M. A 15q24 microduplication, reciprocal to the recently described 15q24 microdeletion, in a boy sharing clinical features with 15q24 microdeletion syndrome patients. Eur J Med Genet 2008;51(6):520–6.

63. Cukier HN, Salyakina D, Blankstein SF, et al. Microduplications in an autism multiplex family narrow the region of susceptibility for developmental disorders on 15q24 and implicate 7p21. Am J Med Genet B Neuropsychiatr Genet 2011;156(4):493–501.

64. Roetzer KM, Schwarzbraun T, Obenauf AC, et al. Further evidence for the pathogenicity of 15q24 microduplications distal to the minimal critical regions. Am J Med Genet A 2010;152A(12):3173–8.

65. Bailey JA, Gu Z, Clark RA, et al. Recent segmental duplications in the human genome. Science 2002;297(5583):1003–7.

66. Martin J, Han C, Gordon LA, et al. The sequence and analysis of duplication-rich human chromosome 16. Nature 2004;432(7020):988–94.

67. Nagamani SC, Erez A, Bader P, et al. Phenotypic manifestations of copy number variation in chromosome 16p13.11. Eur J Hum Genet 2011;19(3):280–6.

68. Balasubramanian M, Smith K, Mordekar SR, et al. Clinical report: An interstitial deletion of 16p13.11 detected by array CGH in a patient with infantile spasms. Eur J Med Genet 2011;54(3):314–8.

69. Heinzen EL, Radtke RA, Urban TJ, et al. Rare deletions at 16p13.11 predispose to a diverse spectrum of sporadic epilepsy syndromes. Am J Hum Genet 2010;86(5): 707–18.

70. Mefford HC, Muhle H, Ostertag P, et al. Genome-wide copy number variation in epilepsy: novel susceptibility loci in idiopathic generalized and focal epilepsies. PLoS Genet 2010;6(5):e1000962.

71. Kirov G, Grozeva D, Norton N, et al. Support for the involvement of large copy number variants in the pathogenesis of schizophrenia. Hum Mol Genet 2009;18(8): 1497–503.

72. Ingason A, Rujescu D, Cichon S, et al. Copy number variations of chromosome 16p13.1 region associated with schizophrenia. Mol Psychiatry 2011;16(1):17–25.

73. Feng Y, Walsh CA. Mitotic spindle regulation by Nde1 controls cerebral cortical size. Neuron 2004;44(2):279–93.

74. Pawlisz AS, Mutch C, Wynshaw-Boris A, et al. Lis1-Nde1-dependent neuronal fate control determines cerebral cortical size and lamination. Hum Mol Genet 2008; 17(16):2441–55.

75. Kim S, Zaghloul NA, Bubenshchikova E, et al. Nde1-mediated inhibition of ciliogenesis affects cell cycle re-entry. Nat Cell Biol 2011;13(4):351–60.

76. Alkuraya FS, Cai X, Emery C, et al. Human mutations in NDE1 cause extreme microcephaly with lissencephaly. Am J Hum Genet 2011;88(5):536–47.

77. Bakircioglu M, Carvalho OP, Khurshid M, et al. The essential role of centrosomal NDE1 in human cerebral cortex neurogenesis. Am J Hum Genet 2011;88(5):523–35.

78. Kwon YT, Balogh SA, Davydov IV, et al. Altered activity, social behavior, and spatial memory in mice lacking the NTAN1p amidase and the asparagine branch of the N-end rule pathway. Mol Cell Biol 2000;20(11):4135–48.

79. Ballif BC, Hornor SA, Jenkins E, et al. Discovery of a previously unrecognized microdeletion syndrome of 16p11.2-p12.2. Nat Genet 2007;39(9):1071–3.

80. Battaglia A, Novelli A, Bernardini L, et al. Further characterization of the new microdeletion syndrome of 16p11.2-p12.2. Am J Med Genet A 2009;149A(6): 1200–4.

81. Bijlsma EK, Gijsbers AC, Schuurs–Hoeijmakers JH, et al. Extending the phenotype of recurrent rearrangements of 16p11.2: deletions in mentally retarded patients without autism and in normal individuals. Eur J Med Genet 2009;52(2–3):77–87.

82. Firth HV, Richards SM, Bevan AP, et al. DECIPHER: Database of Chromosomal Imbalance and Phenotype in Humans Using Ensembl Resources. Am J Hum Genet 2009;84(4):524–33.

83. Sampson MG, Coughlin CR 2nd, Kaplan P, et al. Evidence for a recurrent microdeletion at chromosome 16p11.2 associated with congenital anomalies of the kidney and urinary tract (CAKUT) and Hirschsprung disease. Am J Med Genet A 2010; 152A(10):2618–22.

84. Ren D, Zhou Y, Morris D, et al. Neuronal SH2B1 is essential for controlling energy and glucose homeostasis. J Clin Invest 2007;117(2):397–406.

85. Sebat J, Lakshmi B, Malhotra D, et al. Strong association of de novo copy number mutations with autism. Science 2007;316(5823):445–9.

86. Ghebranious N, Giampietro PF, Wesbrook FP, et al. A novel microdeletion at 16p11.2 harbors candidate genes for aortic valve development, seizure disorder, and mild mental retardation. Am J Med Genet A 2007;143A(13):1462–71.

87. Fernandez BA, Roberts W, Chung B, et al. Phenotypic spectrum associated with de novo and inherited deletions and duplications at 16p11.2 in individuals ascertained for diagnosis of autism spectrum disorder. J Med Genet 2010;47(3):195–203.

88. McCarthy SE, Makarov V, Kirov G, et al. Microduplications of 16p11.2 are associated with schizophrenia. Nat Genet 2009;41(11):1223–7.

89. Kumar RA, Marshall CR, Badner JA, et al. Association and mutation analyses of 16p11.2 autism candidate genes. PLoS One 2009;4(2):e4582.

90. Crepel A, Steyaert J, De la Marche W, et al. Narrowing the critical deletion region for autism spectrum disorders on 16p11.2. Am J Med Genet B Neuropsychiatr Genet 2011;156(2):243–5.

91. Glessner JT, Wang K, Cai G, et al. Autism genome-wide copy number variation reveals ubiquitin and neuronal genes. Nature 2009;459(7246):569–73.

92. Grisart B, Willatt L, Destree A, et al. 17q21.31 microduplication patients are characterised by behavioural problems and poor social interaction. J Med Genet 2009; 46(8):524–30.

93. Kirchhoff M, Bisgaard AM, Duno M, et al. A 17q21.31 microduplication, reciprocal to the newly described 17q21.31 microdeletion, in a girl with severe psychomotor developmental delay and dysmorphic craniofacial features. Eur J Med Genet 2007; 50(4):256–63.

94. Stefansson H, Helgason A, Thorleifsson G, et al. A common inversion under selection in Europeans. Nat Genet 2005;37(2):129–37.

95. Rao PN, Li W, Vissers LE, et al. Recurrent inversion events at 17q21.31 microdeletion locus are linked to the MAPT H2 haplotype. Cytogenet Genome Res 2010; 129(4):275–9.

96. Shimokawa O, Kurosawa K, Ida T, et al. Molecular characterization of inv dup del(8p): analysis of five cases. Am J Med Genet A 2004;128A(2):133–7.

97. Bayes M, Magano LF, Rivera N, et al. Mutational mechanisms of Williams-Beuren syndrome deletions. Am J Hum Genet 2003;73(1):131–51.

98. De Souza EB. Corticotropin-releasing factor receptors: physiology, pharmacology, biochemistry and role in central nervous system and immune disorders. Psychoneuroendocrinology 1995;20(8):789–819.

99. Smith GW, Aubry JM, Dellu F, et al. Corticotropin releasing factor receptor 1-deficient mice display decreased anxiety, impaired stress response, and aberrant neuroendocrine development. Neuron 1998;20(6):1093–102.

100. Ikegami S, Harada A, Hirokawa N. Muscle weakness, hyperactivity, and impairment in fear conditioning in tau-deficient mice. Neurosci Lett 2000;279(3):129–32.

101. Takei Y, Teng J, Harada A, et al. Defects in axonal elongation and neuronal migration in mice with disrupted tau and map1b genes. J Cell Biol 2000;150(5):989–1000.

102. Cooper GM, Coe BP, Girirajan S, et al. A copy number variation morbidity map of developmental delay. Nat Genet 2011;43(9):838–46.

Interpretation of Copy Number Alterations Identified Through Clinical Microarray-Comparative Genomic Hybridization

Robert E. Pyatt, PhD[a,b,*], Caroline Astbury, PhD[a,b]

KEYWORDS
- Oligonucleotide microarray • Copy number alteration
- Variant of unknown significance • Deletion • Duplication

Array-comparative genomic hybridization (array-CGH) has become the first-tier technology for the clinical assessment of copy number alterations (CNAs) associated with features such as developmental delay, congenital malformations, autism, or dysmorphic features. It is a near certainty that at least 1 CNA will be identified in each array-CGH assay and the challenge then becomes differentiating between benign CNA and those copy number changes that are dosage sensitive and relate to the abnormal phenotype in question. With advances in array-CGH platform coverage, it is no longer a question of CNA identification, but rather of CNA interpretation. However, there is no single methodology employed by laboratories to conduct this process, and unfortunately all too often the end results provide no clear answer to the ordering physician or their patients. Recent approaches for interpretation of CNA have advanced to suggesting the use of first-generation computational models based on structural and functional genomic features to predict a pathologic or benign value for array-CGH findings.[1] Although such estimation procedures can be helpful, they are currently limited to a single phenotype (mental retardation) and can at best only provide an educated guess as to the true clinical significance of these alterations.

The authors have nothing to disclose.

[a] Cytogenetics and Molecular Genetics Laboratory, Department of Pathology and Laboratory Medicine, Nationwide Children's Hospital, 700 Children's Drive, Columbus, OH 43205, USA
[b] Department of Pathology, The Ohio State University College of Medicine, 129 Hamilton Hall, 1645 Neil Avenue, Columbus, OH 43210, USA
* Corresponding author. Cytogenetics and Molecular Genetics Laboratory, Department of Pathology and Laboratory Medicine, Nationwide Children's Hospital, 700 Children's Drive, Columbus, OH 43205.
E-mail address: Robert.Pyatt@nationwidechildrens.org

Clin Lab Med 31 (2011) 565–580
doi:10.1016/j.cll.2011.08.007
0272-2712/11/$ – see front matter © 2011 Elsevier Inc. All rights reserved.

CLASSIFICATION STRATEGY

A majority of clinical laboratories employ a 3-tiered system for the classification and reporting of array-CGH CNA: Likely pathogenic/abnormal, likely benign (LB), and variant of unknown significance (VUS).[2–4] For a given CNA, this process typically involves assessing the size, content, associations with benign CNA and abnormal phenotypes, and mode of inheritance, if possible. In general, larger abnormalities are thought to be more significant than smaller ones, and duplications are thought to be better tolerated than deletions. Greater significance is placed on alterations in gene-rich regions; however, this interpretation is tempered by correlation with regions of reportedly benign CNA. Large population studies documenting the instances of CNA in normal populations such as those collected within the Database of Genomic Variants[5] are extremely important to consult when beginning to identify CNA with benign features. Additionally, many laboratories maintain their own databases of benign CNA as another level of internal assessment. Connections of CNA to pathogenic features can be examined through online databases such as DECIPHER,[6] which collects information on submicroscopic chromosome imbalances, the Online Mendelian Inheritance in Man (OMIM),[7] which collects information on human genes, function, and related disorders, and, most important, through the published literature of related cases. Finally, assessing the mode of inheritance for a CNA can suggest a more benign character if the abnormality was inherited from a normal parent or a more potentially significant one if it has occurred de novo.

As recently as 3 years ago, a majority of laboratories were not typically including reportedly benign CNA along with likely pathogenic/abnormal, LB, and VUS findings on their clinical reports because there was thought to be no connection between these genomic alterations and abnormal phenotypes.[8] Many laboratories have reconsidered this practice as information has arisen suggesting that some CNA previously thought to be benign may instead have pathogenic implications. For example, microdeletions at chromosome 15q11.2 involving 4 genes, *TUBGCP5*, *NIPA2*, *NIPA1*, and *CYFIP1*, were initially thought to be benign but recently have been shown to segregate in families with features including learning delay, delayed development, and behavior issues.[9] The inclusion of all identified benign CNA in a clinical report could serve as a record of all noted array-CGH abnormalities in case such re-interpretation is ever needed in the future, but would also present a considerable burden for those responsible for writing the report.

LB findings are typically alterations in which a benign character has been suggested, but not firmly established owing to a lack of extensive evidence. Such regions frequently include gene deserts or genomic segments containing genes that do not seem to demonstrate dosage sensitivity. Correlation with limited regions of reportedly benign CNA is also frequently seen. Likely pathogenic CNA are those with concrete evidence linking the abnormality with a defined pathogenic phenotype. Variable expressivity and incomplete penetrance can further complicate a clear pathogenic connection for a CNA. VUS then are essentially everything else. Frequently, VUS are regions containing 1 or more genes with poorly defined functions, expression profiles, and/or regulatory elements. There has been some concern among clinical laboratories that the term "variant of unknown significance" can be misinterpreted to imply a more benign character than intended. Consequently, it has been suggested that this category could be split into 2 groups to better differentiate between findings with some suggestive clinical significance and those with truly unknown pathogenic potential.

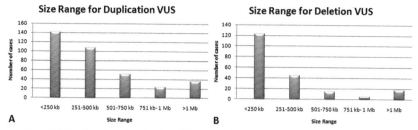

Fig. 1. Size distribution for duplication (*A*) and deletion (*B*) VUS from a consecutive series of 1998 clinical array-CGH cases.

Many laboratories utilize a size threshold, from 50 to 500 kb for deletions and 150 to 500 kb for duplications, to define what array-CGH abnormalities will or will not be clinically reported.[2] This approach can help to reduce the number of CNA of unknown significance requiring investigation, but additionally can erroneously exclude clinically significant CNA of small size. As an alternative approach to size exclusion, laboratories can utilize an approach based on the number of oligonucleotide probes altered and the significance of the shift from copy number neutral value. Although there is currently no consensus regarding the use of size cutoffs, the American College of Medical Genetics recommendations[10] for the clinical use of array-CGH may provide some guidance.

VUS

Regardless of the interpretation strategy used, VUS are a large portion of array-CGH findings and require a significant amount of time to investigate. From a consecutive series of 1998 cases submitted to our laboratory for clinical array-CGH analysis using a custom, 105,000 oligonucleotide array platform, 563 abnormalities were interpreted as a VUS from 490 patients (24.5% of cases). The 358 duplication VUS from this series ranged in size from 33 kb to 2.9 Mb with a majority being 500 kb or less (**Fig. 1**A). The 205 deletion VUS ranged in size from 24 kb to 1.54 Mb and were significantly smaller, with the majority being 250 kb or less (see **Fig. 1**B). Duplications in this series were more frequent than deletions as losses of genetic material are thought to be less well-tolerated than gains.[11] These values are similar to previously published frequencies of copy number variants in phenotypically normal individuals (65%–80% 100–500 kb; 5%–10% >500 kb; 1% >1 Mb[12]), which suggests a majority of these findings may be similarly benign.

Parental samples should always be requested for VUS to help define the significance of the abnormality. In a practice adopted from conventional cytogenetics, copy number changes that are found to be de novo are thought to be more likely pathogenic. However, in these cases, false paternity must be considered when counseling the significance of such a finding. The demonstration of CNA inheritance from a phenotypically normal parent suggests a more benign character to the alteration. However, if the normal phenotype in the parent is in question or cannot be firmly established, additional pedigree analysis may be warranted to track the occurrence of the phenotype and inheritance of the CNA within the family. Of the 285 cases from our laboratory in which the mode of inheritance for the VUS could be determined, a majority of both duplication and deletion VUS were maternally inherited (**Fig. 2**A, B). Of 167 duplication VUS, 91 (54.5%) were maternally inherited, 59 (35.3%) were paternal, and 17 (10.2%) were determined to be de novo in origin (see **Fig. 2**A).

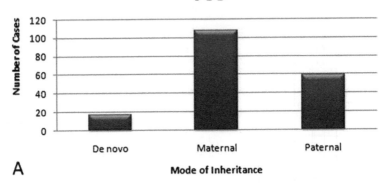

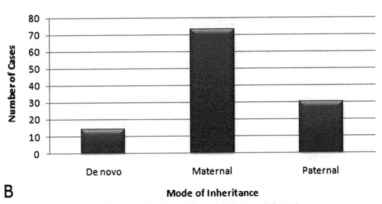

Fig. 2. Mode of inheritance for duplication (*A*) and deletion (*B*) VUS.

Similar proportions were observed for deletion VUS with 74 (62.7%) maternal, 30 (25.4%) paternal, and 124 (11.9%) de novo (see **Fig. 2**B). The size distribution for both maternally and paternally inherited VUS were similar to the entire respective series of duplication or deletion VUS with a majority of inherited duplication VUS being 500 kb or less and inherited deletion VUS being less than 250 kb (**Fig. 3**). No such trend was observed for de novo VUS, with sizes of 500 kb or greater being more common for both deletions and duplications (**Fig. 4**). Based on these results, parental analysis of VUS in our laboratory is conducted in a sequential manner starting with maternal samples, because this method will identify the inheritance in more than half of the cases while requiring the analysis of only a single parental sample.

In approximately 60% of cases in this series, the deletion or duplication VUS was the sole abnormality identified. In 34 cases, deletion or duplication VUS were co-identified along with a pathogenic finding. These instances can provide additional insight into the significance of variants because they represent either the inheritance of 2 pathogenic alterations in the same individual, the co-inheritance of a modifying factor for the pathogenic alteration, or the incidental inheritance of a benign variant

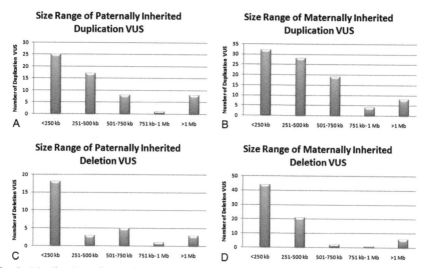

Fig. 3. Distribution of sizes for paternally inherited duplication (*A*) and deletion (*C*), and maternally inherited duplication (*B*) and deletion (*D*) VUS.

with the pathogenic one. **Fig. 5** shows one such VUS. This approximately 411kb gain at chromosome 12p11.23 includes the coding regions of 2 genes (*STK38L* and *ARNTL2*), 2 open reading frames (*C12orf71* and *C12orf70*), and a portion of a third gene (*PPFIBP1*). This duplication has been observed as the sole finding in 2 cases, both times being paternally inherited, and twice in conjunction with other variants of unknown significance. In 2 additional cases, this VUS was co-identified with a pathogenic finding including a 1.24Mb terminal loss from 22q13.33 and a 5.9Mb de novo gain at 9q21.2 through 9q13.32. In this latter case, the 12p11.23 variant was determined to have been inherited from a reportedly phenotypically normal mother. Although modifying effects cannot be excluded, the patient's phenotype seems most likely attributed to the large, de novo duplication on chromosome 9, suggesting benign consequences for the 12p11.23 gain.

Far too often, assigning array-CGH CNA to one of these categories is not a straightforward task. Interpretation frequently involves examining the size and content of a region, correlating regions of reportedly benign CNA, and associating regions, genes, or specific transcripts with abnormal phenotypes using multiple resources, including online databases, genome browsers, and the published literature. The

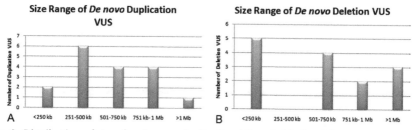

Fig. 4. Distribution of sizes for *de novo* duplication (*A*) and deletion (*B*) VUS.

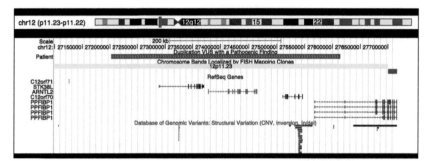

Fig. 5. Approximately 411kb gain VUS at chromosome 12p11.23 *(red bar)* co-identified with a pathogenic de novo gain at 9q21.2 through 9q13.32. The occurrence of this CNA with a pathogenic finding suggested the CNA contributes only subtly, if at all, to the patient's phenotype. [Available at: http://genome.ucsc.edu. Accessed March, 2006 (NCBI36/hg18).[31]]

following sections describe some of the specific issues our laboratory has encountered in this endeavor.

Alteration Size Versus Content

Segmental aneuploidy is often thought to be clinically significant, especially in cases involving alterations which are cytogenetically visible. **Fig. 6** shows an 18.55-Mb deletion at chromosome 13q21.31 through 13q31.1 identified in our laboratory. The large size of this loss suggests it is a pathogenic alteration; however, the region is gene poor, containing only 31 genes and 4 microRNAs. Alterations on the long arm of chromosome 13 are typically terminal losses, which are more distal to the region

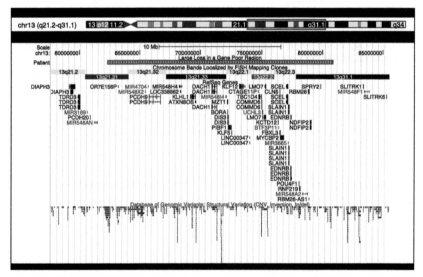

Fig. 6. Approximately18.55-Mb deletion in a gene-poor region of chromosome 13q21.31 through 13q31.1 *(red bar)*. Additional evidence suggests this is a benign variant despite its large size. [Available at: http://genome.ucsc.edu. Accessed March, 2006 NCBI36/hg18).[31]]

deleted here, and are associated with features including mental/growth retardation, dysmorphic features, malformations, holoprosencephaly, Dandy–Walker malformation, and digit abnormalities.[13–16] The literature contains 2 reports of comparable alterations at this interstitial 13q region and the associated features paint a different picture. These include a 11.2-Mb duplication at 13q12, which overlaps the proximal portion of the deleted region in **Fig. 6**, including 2 genes (*OR7E1569* and *PCDH9*) in a boy with autism[17] and a 14.5-Mb deletion identified prenatally in a male child who presented with hypotonia at birth and later with some pigmentation anomalies and slightly delayed motor development. This deletion was show to have been inherited from the child's mother and maternal grandfather, both of whom were phenotypically normal.[18] Finally, a 29.8-Mb deletion at 13q21.31 through 13q31.3 was reported in a 16-month-old girl who demonstrated micrognathia, tapering fingers, mild dysmorphic features, hypotonia, short stature, microcephaly, and moderate mental retardation.[19] Using a series of cases in addition to that one, the authors assembled a genotype–phenotype map for deletions on the long arm of chromosome 13 with micrognathia being the only feature associated with losses in the 13q21.32 through 13q31.1 region. Features such as Dandy–Walker malformations, microcephaly, and limb abnormalities were associated with more distal critical segments on 13q.[19] Based on these findings, including a lack of association with major features, demonstration of stable, multigenerational inheritance from normal individuals, and the gene-poor content of this region, alterations in this region have been proposed as benign variants.[17,18] However, additional studies are needed to firmly establish the benign nature of these variants on chromosome 13 and the 18.55-Mb deletion observed in our laboratory was consequently reported as a VUS.

MicroRNAs

The interpretation of small duplications or deletions typically relies on how well characterized functions and established pathogenic mechanisms are for genes within those regions. Unfortunately, such detailed information is only available for a small percentage of the coding regions in the human genome, leaving alterations involving coding regions, non-coding RNAs, hypothetical genes, and open reading frames to be somewhat of a mystery. **Fig. 7** shows an 836-kb gain at chromosome 13q31.3 that contains only the microRNA, MIR 622. MicroRNAs in their mature form are single stranded molecules of 20 to 23 nucleotides, which have been shown to function in controlling gene expression. Four hundred forty-five microRNAs have been identified

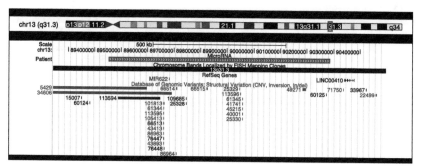

Fig. 7. Approximately 836-kb gain at chromosome 13q31.3, which contains only the microRNA MIR 622 *(red bar)*. MicroRNAs currently have no known role in congenital disorders. [Available at: http://genome.ucsc.edu. Accessed March, 2006 (NCBI36/hg18).[31]]

in the human genome with 222 of those located within protein coding genes.[20] Although they have been shown to contribute to the pathogenesis of many disorders, including cancer[21] and type II diabetes,[22] the function of microRNAs in congenital genetic syndromes remains unknown. The duplicated region shown in **Fig. 7** contains small segments of reportedly benign CNA, including both genomic losses and gains. However, there is only a single report of 2 individuals out of 1190 Canadian controls in the Database of Genomic Variants with benign CNA, including MIR 662, both of which are genomic losses.[23] Were it not for the presence of the microRNA, this gene-poor region with noted benign CNA would be considered LB. However, the presence of poorly characterized genomic elements such as a microRNA suggests a more conservative interpretation.

Incidental Carrier Identification

The clinical application of array-CGH technology primarily focuses on the identification of regions of dosage sensitivity and the correlation of those copy number changes with abnormal phenotypes. In addition to identifying single copy changes directly associated with abnormal phenotypes, single CNAs in genes associated with disorders demonstrating autosomal recessive inheritance can also be identified. **Fig. 8A** shows a 721-kb loss at chromosome 7q31.2 through 7q31.31 that contains 4 genes, including the *CFTR* gene. Cystic fibrosis is most frequently associated with homozygous mutations in *CTFR*, but exonic and whole gene deletions have also been described.[24] This case is further complicated by the loss of the 3 genes neighboring *CFTR*. Additionally, **Fig. 8B** shows a 305-kb loss at 13q12.11, including the *CRYL1* gene and a majority of the *GJB6* gene. Homozygous deletions of approximately 309 kb in the *GJB6* gene or digenic inheritance of 1 deleted *GJB6* allele and 1 mutated *GJB2* allele are associated with non-syndromic deafness *DFNB1*.[25] In both of these cases, interpretation of these CNA can be guided based on the patient's phenotype.

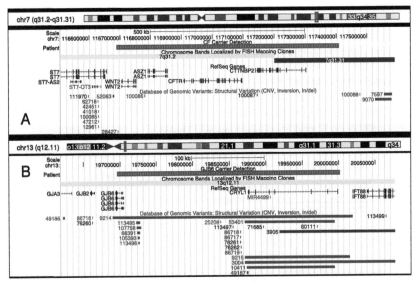

Fig. 8. Incidental carrier detection of cystic fibrosis (*A*) and congenital deafness (*B*) (*red bars*) in 2 individuals referred for clinical array-CGH analysis presenting with nonspecific indications. [Available at: http://genome.ucsc.edu. Accessed March, 2006 (NCBI36/hg18).[31]]

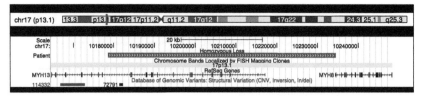

Fig. 9. Homozygous loss of an approximately 56-kb region within the *MYH13* gene (*red bar*). Although single copy alterations may be benign, homozygous deletions can unmask previously unrecognized autosomal recessive conditions. [Available at: http://genome.ucsc.edu. Accessed March, 2006 (NCBI36/hg18).[31]]

In cases where individuals are manifesting features of a suspected recessive disorder, molecular analysis of the second allele should be recommended for a comprehensive understanding of the mutation status. If no features are present, this suggests the individual is more likely to be a benign carrier, rather than manifesting the condition.

Unmasking of Recessive Conditions

Although most CNA display single copy losses or gains, rare, 2-copy deletions or duplications can also be identified. **Fig. 9** shows a 56-kb loss at chromosome 17p13.1 observed in a male referred for array-CGH analysis owing to intrauterine growth retardation and respiratory distress syndrome, which demonstrated the pattern and significance of a homozygous loss. The deleted region contains the 5' portion of the *MYH13* gene including exons 1 through 18 and the region contains limited reports of benign CNA. The *MYH13* gene encodes for a myosin heavy chain and is part of a myosin gene cluster at 17p13.1, which shows strong evolutionary conservation of gene order, transcriptional orientation, and intergenic distance between humans and mice.[26] Microarray analysis demonstrated the presence of the deletion in a heterozygous state in both parents who were subsequently determined to be related. Although fluorescence in situ hybridization (FISH) could have confirmed the homozygous loss in the child, the deletion seen here is well below the detection limit of this technique. Most resources cataloging the benign nature of CNA focus on the single-copy state of deletions or duplications. Homozygous alterations are not as well-characterized and can uncover abnormal phenotypes. This is additionally complicated when the genes in question are poorly understood.

Partial Gene Duplications

Fig. 10 shows a 53-kb duplication at 10q23.2 through 10q23.31 that includes a portion of the non-coding pseudogene *CFLP1*, the entire coding region of the *KILLIN* gene, and exon 1 of the *PTEN* gene. KILLIN seems to function as an inhibitor of DNA synthesis under the regulation of p53.[27] Mutations in the *PTEN* gene are associated with PTEN hamartoma tumor syndrome, including Cowden syndrome (OMIM: 158350), Bannayan–Riley–Ruvalcaba syndrome (OMIM: 153480), Proteus syndrome and Proteus-like syndrome (OMIM: 176920), and macrocephaly/autism syndrome (OMIM: 605309). Approximately 10% of those individuals with Bannayan–Riley–Ruvalcaba syndrome have exonic or whole gene deletions[28]; rare instances of deletions in Cowden syndrome have also been reported.[29] However, duplications in the *PTEN* gene have not. Because of the limitations of array-CGH technology, it is not possible to determine whether the duplication is in a direct or inverted orientation or if this alteration is sufficient to disrupt gene transcription/expression. Although a

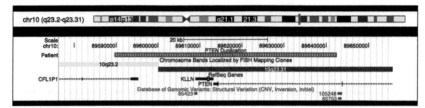

Fig. 10. Partial duplication of the *PTEN* gene as a result of an approximately 53-kb duplication at 10q23.2 through 10q23.31 (*red bar*). Although mutations in the *PTEN* gene have been well-described as pathogenic, intragenic duplications have not been previously reported. [Available at: http://genome.ucsc.edu. Accessed March, 2006 (NCBI36/hg18).[31]]

tandem duplication within the *PTEN* gene could potentially result in disrupted transcription with pathogenic consequences, these results would need to be confirmed by additional molecular testing.

Alteration in One or More Gene Transcripts

Although humans are now thought to have between 22,000 and 25,000 protein-coding genes, our understanding of the human transcriptome continues to grow as more of those genes are found to encode for multiple transcripts. **Fig. 11** shows a 186-kb gain at chromosome Xq13.1 in a male, which was determined to be maternally inherited from an apparently phenotypically normal parent. The duplicated region contains the entire coding region of the *UPRT* gene and exons 5 through 12 of the *ZDHHC15* gene. There is a single report of benign CNA in this region, including a single duplication and a single deletion from 39 Hapmap individuals.[30] Of the 3 *ZDHHC15* transcripts annotated from the March 2006 build of the human genome, the duplicated region includes coding material from the 2 long isoforms but none of the short isoform (UCSC March 2006, NCBI 36/hg18).[31] There is a single report in the literature of a woman with a balanced (X;15) translocation in which the breakpoints were mapped close to the *ZDHHC15* gene.[32] The woman reportedly presented with profound mental retardation, seizures, and normal stature. Additional testing showed the normal X chromosome to be inactive owing to 100% skewed inactivation and a complete lack of *ZDHHC15* transcripts by reverse transcriptase polymerase chain reaction compared with control lymphocytes. Consequently, the authors proposed

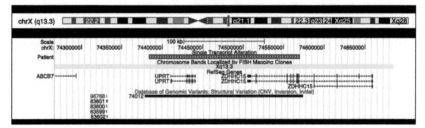

Fig. 11. Duplication of approximately 186-kb at chromosome Xq133.3 involving coding regions from 2 of 3 transcript isoforms of the *ZDHHC15* gene (*red bar*). Disruptions of all transcript isoforms have been previously suggested to have pathogenic potential. [Available at: http://genome.ucsc.edu. Accessed March, 2006 (NCBI36/hg18).[31]]

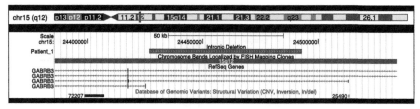

Fig. 12. Deletion localized to an intronic region of the *GABRB3* gene (*red bar*), which is associated with susceptibility to Childhood Absence Epilepsy (OMIM 612269). [Available at: http://genome.ucsc.edu. Accessed March, 2006 (NCBI36/hg18).[31]]

the *ZDHHC15* gene as a candidate for X-linked mental retardation. Although these results suggest that the complete loss of *ZDHHC15* transcripts may have pathogenic implications, the effects of a partial gene duplication disrupting only a portion of certain *ZDHHC15* transcript isoforms is unknown.

Intragenic Deletions

Fig. 12 shows a 71kb deletion within the *GABRB3* gene with no copy number variation reported for that region in the Database of Genomic Variants. The gene contains 10 exons, including 2 alternative first exons. There are rare reports of heterozygous mutations in the alternative exon 1 resulting in a hyperglycosylated protein and associated with susceptibility to childhood absence epilepsy 5 (OMIM: 612269).[33] Incomplete penetrance has also been noted. There are 4 transcripts associated with the *GABRB3* gene in the UCSC March 2006 (NCBI 36/hg18) display. The 71kb deletion contains none of the genomic material associated with the short isoform, and only intronic material associated with the 3 longer isoforms. Although it may be tempting to classify this loss as a benign variant because no coding material is disrupted, the presence of intronic regulatory elements within the alteration cannot be ruled out. Intronic deletions in the *DMD* gene have recently been reported to lead to altered splicing and the inclusion of a pseudoexon within the dystrophin transcript.[34] A comprehensive understanding of CNA must begin to include an understanding of the regulatory elements in addition to the coding material within the region. This is especially complicated because some regulatory elements have been shown to function long distances from their associated coding regions.

Array-CGH Probe Gaps

Although the probe coverage of array-CGH platforms has greatly improved, gap regions between probes can still be problematic in determining the exact size and content of alterations. Our laboratory has recently published a series of clinical array-CGH cases presenting with indications such as developmental delay, dysmorphic features, or hypotonia in which alterations in the *DMD* gene were identified.[35] Deletions and duplications causing disruption of the *DMD* gene are associated with the dystrophinopathies (OMIM: 300377), a group of disorders including Duchenne muscular dystrophy (OMIM: 310200), Becker muscular dystrophy (OMIM: 300376), and DMD-associated dilated cardiomyopathy (OMIM: 302045). The dystrophinopathies constitute a spectrum of muscle disease ranging from asymptomatic hyperCKemia to muscle cramps with myoglobinuria, and isolated quadriceps myopathy to progressive muscle diseases involving the skeletal and/or heart muscles. Learning difficulties have also been reported in some males affected with Duchenne muscular dystrophy. A

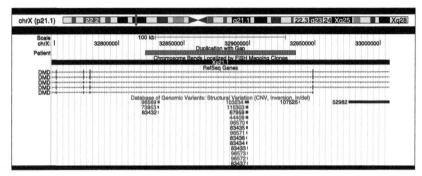

Fig. 13. Duplication within an intronic portion of the *DMD* gene (*red bar*). Exon 2 lies within the distal gap region between probes on this oligonucleotide array-CGH platform. [Available at: http://genome.ucsc.edu. Accessed March, 2006 (NCBI36/hg18).[31]]

115-kb duplication was recently identified by our laboratory in a teenage male referred for clinical testing with similar, nonspecific indications (**Fig. 13**). The duplicated region contains an intronic portion of the *DMD* gene, but exon 2 lies within the distal 18.18-kb gap on our custom oligonucleotide platform. For this case, molecular analysis of the *DMD* gene was recommended to clarify the involvement of coding material within this duplication.

Insertional Translocations

Interpretation of duplications can be further complicated by the translocation of these regions within the genome. Even if the duplicated region is benign, the significance of the finding may lie specifically in the consequences defined by the region of insertion. Complex chromosome rearrangements such as insertional translocations are rare with the frequency for microscopically visible events estimated at 1:80,000 live births[36] and submicroscopic events may be more common (~1:500).[37] Insertional translocations require at least 3 strand breaks and can be intrachromosomal or interchromosomal, resulting in a partial trisomy for the inserted region in either case. **Fig. 14**A shows a 1.78-Mb duplicated region containing the *NAALADL2* gene and some reportedly benign CNA. FISH analysis demonstrated the duplication and translocation of this region to chromosome 12q13.13 (see **Fig. 14**B). Alterations such as this can result in altered gene expression through increased expression of the duplicated genes, disruption of the genes at the insertional site, and through the creation of fusion gene products at the insertion site. Although rare, our laboratory has observed insertional translocations involving regions as small as 380 kb. This case also demonstrates the clinical utility of FISH confirmation of all duplications to exclude complex rearrangements such as this. Until there are specific molecular techniques to identify the exact site of insertion on a clinical basis, the exact genomic implications of such a finding will remain unknown.

Lineage-Specific Alterations

Bacterial artificial chromosome–based array-CGH has been demonstrated to detect mosaic cell lines as low as 10%.[37] Although the adoption of oligonucleotide based array-CGH platforms by clinical laboratories has resulted in improved probe coverage and resolution over bacterial artificial chromosomes, the sensitivity to low-level mosaicism has been markedly diminished.[38,39] A 39-Mb duplication was observed in

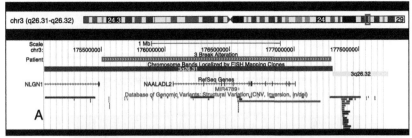

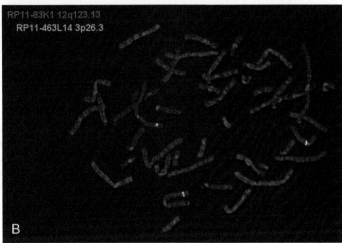

Fig. 14. Duplication of approximately 1.78 Mb at 3q26.31 (*red bar*) containing the coding region of 1 gene (*A*). FISH analysis demonstrated the insertion of the duplicated region into 12q13.13 with unknown phenotypic consequences (*B*). [Available at: http://genome.ucsc.edu. Accessed March, 2006 (NCBI36/hg18).[31]]

2 separate analyses using an oligonucleotide array-CGH platform (**Fig. 15**). Both analyses were strongly suggestive of a duplication, but the statistical significance did not reach that of a typical gain. Findings such as this, which demonstrate a consistent pattern but do not reach a level of significance, may be suggestive of mosaicism for an underlying abnormal cell line. Because of the enhanced sensitivity to low-level mosaicism, the analysis was repeated using a bacterial artificial chromosome array platform that demonstrated a clear duplication of chromosome 10q23.33 to 10q26.3. No such alteration had been observed in routine phytohemagglutinin (PHA)-stimulated peripheral blood chromosome analysis, and FISH analyses performed on both metaphase and interphase PHA-stimulated cells (primarily T lymphocytes) were inconclusive. The DNA isolation procedure used in our laboratory for array-CGH is applied nonselectively to a complete sample of peripheral blood, whereas FISH and chromosome analyses are performed on PHA-stimulated cells, which primarily selects for T lymphocytes. Consequently, these results are suggestive for a lineage specific alteration associated with a cell fraction other than T lymphocytes. FISH analyses using identical probes were performed on paraffin-embedded tissue from lung, brain, and skin with 3 signals for the 10q region identified in 10% (5/50) of lung cells and 6% (3/47) of skin cells, although no additional signal was observed in cells analyzed from the brain.

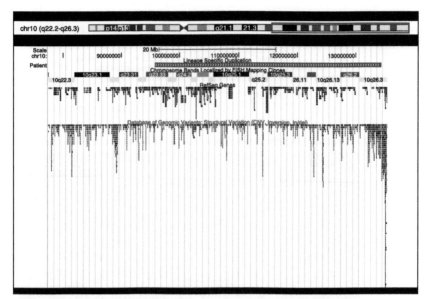

Fig. 15. Approximately 39-Mb duplication at 10q23.33 through 10qter (*red bar*). FISH analysis was only able to confirm this finding in a subset of unstimulated peripheral blood cells which suggests that this finding is a lineage restricted alteration. [Available at: http://genome.ucsc.edu. Accessed March, 2006 (NCBI36/hg18).[31]]

SUMMARY

It seems likely that many of the CNA currently interpreted as VUS will ultimately be determined to be benign. However, the classification of these VUS requires a much more extensive characterization of the human genome than exists today. Currently, there is no definitive set of rules or level of evidence required to define a CNA as benign. Evidence of the CNA in normal populations is key, but what frequency is necessary? How many times should stable inheritance of the CNA be observed? What level of phenotype information is needed to demonstrate that the parent transmitting the CNA is "normal"? Given the knowledge of variable expressivity and incomplete penetrance for many conditions, there are no consensus answers to these questions applicable to every CNA. The information needed to accurately assess the pathogenic impact of CNA is beginning to be assembled through groups such as The International Standards for Cytogenetic Arrays Consortium including their database maintained through the NCBI, which contains copy number data and phenotype information from clinical microarray cases.[40] Although the lack of understanding of the human genome can make clinical array-CGH interpretation frustrating, it is precisely why clinical human genetics is an exciting arena in which to work.

ACKNOWLEDGMENTS

The authors thank Fadel S. Alyaqoub, PhD, for his assistance in preparing this manuscript.

REFERENCES

1. Leung TY, Pooh RK, Wang CC, et al. Classification of pathogenic or benign status of CNVs detected by microarray analysis. Expert Rev Mol Diagn 2010;10:717–21.

2. Tsuchiya KD, Shaffer LG, Aradhya S, et al. Variability in interpreting and reporting copy number changes detected by array-based technology in clinical laboratories. Genet Med 2009;11:866–73.

3. Lee C, Iafrate AJ, and Brothman AR. Copy number variations and clinical cytogenetic diagnosis of constitutional disorders. Nat Genet 2007;39:S48–S54.

4. Rodriguez-Revenga L, Mila M, Rosenberg C, et al. Structural variation in the human genome: The impact of copy number variants on clinical diagnosis. Genet Med 2007; 9:600–6.

5. Available at: http://projects.tcag.ca/variation/. Accessed August 10, 2011.

6. DECIPHER. Available at: http://decipher.sanger.ac.uk/. Accessed August 15, 2011.

7. Online Mendelian Inheritance in Man. Available at: http://www.ncbi.nlm.nih.gov/omim. Accessed August 15, 2011.

8. CAP Cytogenetics Resources Committee. Comparative genomic hybridization microarray participant summary report. Survey CYCGH-B 2008. Northfield (IL): College of American Pathologists; 2008.

9. von der Lippe C, Rustad C, Heimdal K, et al. 15q11.2 microdeletion: seven new patients with delayed development and/or behavioral problems. Eur J Med Genet 2011;54:357–60.

10. Kearney HM, South ST, Wolff DJ, et al. American College of Medical Genetics recommendations for the design and performance expectations for clinical genomic copy number microarrays intended for use in the postnatal setting for detection of constitutional abnormalities. Genet Med 2011;13(7):676–9.

11. Brewer C, Holloway S, Zawalnyski P, et al. A chromosomal duplication mal of malformations: regions of suspected haplo—and triplolethality—and tolerance of segmental aneuploidy. Am J Hum Genet 1999;64:1702–8.

12. Itsara A, Cooper GM, Baker C, et al. Population analysis of large copy number variants and hotspots of human genetic disease. Am J Hum Genet 2009;84:148–61.

13. Schinzel A. Catalogue of unbalanced aberrations in man. 2nd edition. Berlin: De Gruyter; 2001. p. 552–3.

14. Brown S, Gersen S, Anyane-Yeboa K, et al. Preliminary definition of a 'critical region' of chromosome 13 in q32: report of 14 cases with 13q deletions and review of the literature. Am J Med Genet 1993;45:52–9.

15. Alanay Y, Aktas D, Utine E, et al. Is Dandy-Walker malformation associated with "distal 13q deletion syndrome"? Findings in a fetus supporting previous observations. Am J Med Genet Part A 2005;136A:265–8.

16. Gutierrez J, Sepulveda W, Saez R, et al. Prenatal diagnosis of 13q-syndrome in a fetus with holoprosencephaly and thumb agenesis. Ultrasound Obstet Gynecol 2001;2: 166–8.

17. Daniel A, Darmanian A, Peters G, et al. An innocuous duplication of 11.2 Mb at 13q21 is gene poor: sub-bands of gene paucity and pervasive CNV characterize the chromosome anomalies. Am J Med Genet Part A 2007;143A:2452–9.

18. Filges I, Rothlisberger B, Noppen C, et al. Familial 14.5 Mb interstitial deletion 13q21.1–13q21.33: clinical and array-CGH study of a benign phenotype in a three-generation family. Am J Med Genet 2009;149A: 237–41.

19. Kirchhoff M, Bisgaard AM, Stoeva R, et al. Phenotype and 244k Array-CGH Characterization of chromosome 13q deletions: an update of the phenotypic map of 13q21.1-qter. Am J Med Genet A 2009;149A:894–905.

20. Scherer S. A short guide to the human genome. New York; Cold Spring Harbor Laboratory Press; 2008. p. 57.

21. Farazi T, Spitzer J, Morozov P, et al. miRNAs in human cancer. J Pathol 2011;223: 102–15.

22. Ferland-McCollough D, Ozanne SE, Siddle K, et al. The involvement of microRNAs in type 2 diabetes. Biochem Soc Trans 2010;38:1565–70.
23. Zogopoulos G, Ha KC, Naqib F, et al. Germ-line DNA copy number variation frequencies in a large North American population. Hum Genet 2007;122:345–53.
24. Saillour Y, Cossée M, Leturcq F, et al. Detection of exonic copy-number changes using a highly efficient oligonucleotide-based comparative genomic hybridization-array method. Hum Mutat 2008;29:1083–90.
25. Pandya A, Arnos KS, Xia XJ, et al. Frequency and distribution of GJB2 (connexin 26) and GJB6 (connexin 30) mutations in a large North American repository of deaf probands. Genet Med 2003;5:295–303.
26. Weiss A, McDonough D, Wertman B, et al. Organization of human and mouse skeletal myosin heavy chain gene clusters is highly conserved. Proc Natl Acad Sci U S A 199;96:2958–63.
27. Cho YJ, Liang P. KILLIN is a p53-regulated nuclear inhibitor of DNA synthesis. Proc Natl Acad Sci U S A 2008;105:5396–401.
28. PTEN hamartoma tumor syndrome. Available at: http://www.ncbi.nlm.nih.gov/books/NBK1488/. Accessed August 15, 2011.
29. Orloff MS, Eng C. Genetic and phenotypic heterogeneity in the PTEN hamartoma tumour syndrome. Oncogene 2008;27:5387–97.
30. Conrad DF, Pinto D, Redon R, et al. Origins and functional impact of copy number variation in the human genome. Nature 2010;464:704–12.
31. Fujita PA, Rhead B, Zweig AS, et al. The UCSC Genome Browser database: update 2011. Nucleic Acids Res 2011;39:D876–82.
32. Mansouri MR, Marklund L, Gustavsson P, et al. Loss of ZDHHC15 expression in a woman with a balanced translocation t(X;15)(q13.3;cen) and severe mental retardation. Eur J Hum Genet 2005;13:970–7.
33. Tanaka M, Olsen RW, Medina MT, et al. Hyperglycosylation and reduced GABA currents of mutated GABRB3 polypeptide in remitting childhood absence epilepsy. Am J Hum Genet 2008;82:1249–61.
34. Khelifi MM, Ishmukhametova A, Van Kein PK, et al. Pure intronic rearrangements leading to aberrant pseudoexon inclusion in dystrophinopathy: a new class of mutations? Hum Mutat 2011;32:467–75.
35. Cottrell CE, Prior TW, Pyatt R, et al. Unexpected detection of dystrophin gene deletions by array comparative genomic hybridization. Am J Med Genet A 2010;152A:2301–7.
36. Van Hemel JO, Eussen HJ. Interchromosomal insertions. Identification of five cases and a review. Hum Genet 200;107:415–32.
37. Kang SH, Shaw C, Ou Z, et al. Insertional translocation detected using FISH confirmation of array-comparative genomic hybridization (aCGH) results. Am J Med Genet A 2010;152A:1111–26.
38. Ballif BC, Rorem EA, Sundin K, et al. Detection of low level mosaicism by array CGH in routine diagnostic specimens. Am J Med Genet A 2006;140:2757–67.
39. Scott SA, Cohen N, Brandt T, et al. Detection of low level mosaicism and placental mosaicism by oligonucleotide array comparative genomic hybridization. Genet Med 2010;12:85–92.
40. The International Standards for Cytogenomic Arrays Consortium. Available at: http://www.iscaconsortium.org/. Accessed August 15, 2011.

Clinical Utility of Single Nucleotide Polymorphism Arrays

Stuart Schwartz, PhD, FACMG

KEYWORDS
- Single nucleotide polymorphism microarray
- Prenatal arrays • Oncology arrays • Uniparental disomy
- Runs of homozygosity • Consanguinity

Since Tjio and Levan[1] first eloquently demonstrated in 1956 that the true chromosome number in humans was 46, cytogeneticists have striven to optimize resolution used in the analysis of chromosomes and detection of chromosomal analysis. Initial resolution of unbanded chromosomes was limited, and only abnormalities involving genomic material greater than about 20 to 25 megabase (Mb) could be detected. The resolution improved to about 10 Mb with the advent of banding and the routine analysis of chromosomes at the 500 to 550 band level. In 1976, Yunis[2] initially introduced methodology for the examination of prophase/prometaphase chromosomes (at higher resolution), where abnormalities as small as 3 to 5 Mb could be detected. However, the greatest breakthrough came over 2 decades ago in 1988, when it was demonstrated that fluorescence in situ hybridization (FISH) could be used to detect small abnormalities.[3] FISH can routinely detect changes as small as 150 kilobase (kb) in size; however, it is a directed analysis. An abnormality must first be suspected so that the appropriate probe(s) may be used to see if there is an alteration within the region of question. Initial FISH studies involved commercially developed probes and were limited in scope; however, with the sequencing of the human genome, probes are now available for any region. The combination of FISH technology, comparative genomic hybridization (CGH) involving chromosomes, and the Human Genome Project led to the development of array technology and to the detection of 50 to 150 kb alterations anywhere in the genome. Array technology allows a combination of the routine banding (which gives a whole-genome perspective) together with FISH (giving a resolution of 50–150 kb).

SINGLE NUCLEOTIDE POLYMORPHISM METHODOLOGY

Array technology is essentially the placement of a series of DNA/RNA probes on a glass slide or silicon wafer and hybridization with genomic material from a patient of

Cytogenetics Laboratory, Laboratory Corporation of America, 1904 Alexander Drive, Research Triangle Park, NC 27709, USA
E-mail address: schwas1@labcorp.com

Clin Lab Med 31 (2011) 581–594
doi:10.1016/j.cll.2011.09.002
0272-2712/11/$ – see front matter © 2011 Published by Elsevier Inc.

interest. There are several different types of arrays including (1) expression arrays, which are RNA-based, look for the expression of a series of genes, and are often used in cancer profiling; (2) molecular probe inversion arrays, which can be used to look for mutations in a series of genes of interest; and (3) genomic arrays, which look for larger changes (loss or gain) in a patient's DNA.

There are several different types of genomic arrays using different DNA probes, including bacterial artificial chromosome (BAC), oligonucleotide and single nucleotide polymorphism (SNP) arrays. Both BAC and oligonucleotide arrays are CGH arrays.[4] These arrays combine high throughput technology with genomic studies, using sequence data produced during the Human Genome Project. CGH arrays use a two-color system, in which the patient DNA is labeled in one color (eg, green), and normal control DNA is labeled using a second color (eg, red). Both patient and control DNA are hybridized together onto the probes spotted onto a glass slide, and the alterations can be detected based on the fluorescence of the probes (ie, color; yellow: normal, red: deletion, green: duplication). BAC probes are approximately 150 kb in size and in comparison with oligonucleotide probes are less sensitive and provide less coverage. Oligonucleotide probes are 60 mer in size, providing more sensitivity than BAC technology. The coverage from oligonucleotide probes is much greater than BACs and can range from 44 K (44,000 probes) to 400 K (400,000 probes), allowing for much greater resolution. Companies that initially started with and provided oligonucleotide-only arrays have recently begun to add SNPs to their array for the detection of uniparental disomy (UPD) and consanguinity (see later discussion).[5]

SNP array analysis is similar to oligonucleotide arrays in that they both combine high throughput technology with genomic studies and have become feasible because of the data produced during the Human Genome Project. In addition to detecting copy number changes, this SNP array technology will also allow detection of copy neutral changes (UPD and identity by descent or consanguinity).

As with the oligonucleotide arrays, there are numerous types of SNP arrays, all containing different numbers of probes. These arrays consist of two types of probes: nonpolymorphic copy number probes (CNP), used only for assessing copy number changes, and SNP probes, used for assessing both genotype and copy number changes. A SNP has a single base pair substitution (A, T, C, or G) of one nucleotide for another; however, this substitution is not considered a mutation.[6] To be considered a SNP, the substitution must be found in the population at a frequency of greater than 1.0%, although the closer the frequency to 50% the more useful the SNP is in this analysis. SNPs may occur within the coding sequence of a gene, the noncoding regions of genes, or the intergenic regions between genes. The alleles corresponding to the nucleotide base changes are arbitrarily given the designation allele A and allele B. Both the SNP and nonpolymorphic probes (CNP) are approximately 25 base pairs. Two high-resolution SNP arrays are the Affymetrix 6.0 array and the Illumina HumanOmni 2.5 array.

The Affymetrix SNP array CytoScan HD contains approximately 2.697 million markers across the entire human genome. There are approximately 743,304 SNPs and 1,953,246 structural CNPs. Within genes, on average there are approximately 880 base pairs between each marker. The Illumina HumanOmni 2.5 BeadChip contains approximately 2.4 million markers across the entire human genome. There are approximately 1,231,382 SNPs and 1,148,472 structural CNPs. On average there is approximately 1.19 kb between each marker.

The SNP array analysis can be used to detect both copy number changes as well as copy neutral changes. This analysis is not a CGH technique, and a concurrent control DNA sample is not used. Patient DNA is labeled with a fluorochrome, and the

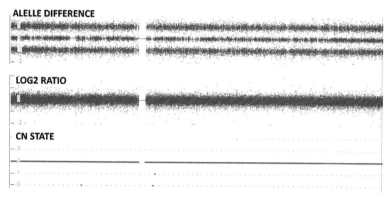

Fig. 1. Use of the Genotyping ConsoleTM (GTC) software tool with an Affymetrix 6.0 SNP array demonstrating normal copy number findings. The CN state is equal to two; the log2 ratio is equal to zero, and there are three allele difference tracts (AA, AB, and BB).

intensity is compared with a set of reference DNA in silico to derive the intensity ratio of each SNP and CNP in the patient DNA, which will provide a relative copy number, the log2 ratio (**Fig. 1**). This ratio can be determined for both the CNPs and SNPs. Determination of this ratio will indicate if there is a gain or loss of genetic material.

A second way to determine if there is a gain or loss of genetic material is by examining the genotype of the alleles of each SNP. See **Fig. 1** showing the copy number state (CN state = 2), log2 ratio (= 0) and allele difference (showing the AA, AB and BB allele tracts for the three normal genotypes). This result indicates that this sample has a normal copy number. In contrast, **Fig. 2** shows these same graphs for a deletion. All of the probes in the log2 ratio are centered on the −0.45 line indicating a deletion in this region, while at the same time the allele difference only shows two tracts instead of three. These two tracts are at 0.5 and −0.5, indicating the presence of a single A or B allele, again confirming the presence of a deletion of this region. **Fig. 3** shows these same graphs for a duplication. All of the probes in the log2 ratio are centered on the 0.3 line, indicating a duplication in this region, while at the same

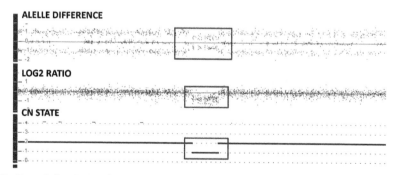

Fig. 2. Use of the GTC software tool with an Affymetrix 6.0 SNP array demonstrating a deletion (designated within the highlighted box). Within the highlighted area, the CN state is equal to one; the log2 ratio is equal to −0.45, and there are only two allele difference tracts (A and B).

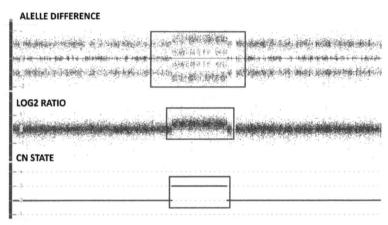

Fig. 3. Use of the GTC software tool with an Affymetrix 6.0 SNP array demonstrating a duplication (designated within the highlighted box). Within the highlighted area, the CN state is equal to three; the log2 ratio is equal to 0.3 and there are only four allele difference tracts (AAA, ABB, ABB, and BBB).

time the allele difference shows four tracts instead of three. These four tracts are at 1.5, 0.5, −0.5, and −1.5, indicating the presence of an AAA, AAB, BBA, and BBB tract, again confirming the presence of a duplication of this region.

The genotyping will also allow detection of copy neutral changes. **Fig. 4** shows normal findings with respect to the CN state and allele difference. In addition, this figure has a tract showing runs of homozygosity (ROH). These stretches can be

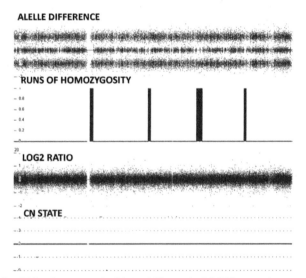

Fig. 4. Use of the GTC software tool with an Affymetrix 6.0 SNP array demonstrating normal copy number findings as well as copy neutral findings. The CN state is equal to two; the log2 ratio is equal to zero, and there are three allele difference tracts (AA, AB, and BB). Additionally, an ROH tract is also included showing only four normal small ROH.

detected when there is homozygosity of the SNPs in a 1 Mb stretch or greater of DNA. Based on examination of over 25,000 patients it is estimated that a normal individual will have between 20 and 150 Mb of homozygosity involving between 1 and 5 Mb of DNA in any stretch (data not shown). Based on a recent paper by Papenhausen and colleagues,[7] these stretches become concerning when they are greater than 10 Mb in length. UPD is associated with one long contiguous stretch of homozygosity (LCSH) when greater than 8 Mb if telomeric and greater than 15 Mb if interstitial.[7] Individuals from consanguineous unions have increased blocks of LCSH greater than 8 Mb. The more regions and chromosomes involved, the greater the consanguinity. The greater the consanguinity detected in the union, the greater the risk of recessive disease and birth defects.[8] In addition, when parental and child specimens are run on the SNP array, the genotype generated will also allow for the detection of nonpaternity and parent of origin.

Using the above parameters, SNP array studies have been used over the past 3 years to study both constitutional abnormalities and somatic changes for the elucidation of both copy number changes and copy neutral changes. Studies from a number of clinical tissue types are discussed and illustrated in detail in this article, including postnatal constitutional blood samples, prenatal diagnostic studies, preimplantation studies, products of conception analysis, and a variety of cancers.

CLINICAL APPLICATIONS AND OVERALL FINDINGS OF THE SNP ARRAY ANALYSIS
Constitutional Studies—Peripheral Blood, Copy Number Variation

The vast majority of array studies have involved an examination of constitutional postnatal bloods, looking in particular to determine the effectiveness of delineating gain or loss of material not detectable by standard cytogenetic methodology. This tendency is true for both CGH arrays as well as SNP arrays. Although the majority of studies for the detection of copy number variation have used oligonucleotide probes and CGH array, some SNP studies have been undertaken. McMullan and colleagues[9] initiated a study to validate the Affymetrix 500K SNP array for routine diagnostic use in the evaluation of patients with mental retardation. This study consisted of two separate parts. First they performed a validation study on 38 patients previously shown to have submicroscopic copy number variations (CNVs). They then prospectively studied 120 patients with unexplained mental retardation. They were able to detect all 44 CNVs previously detected in the 38 patients and the study of trios (parents and affected proband) in the retrospective study. In the 120 prospective patients, both de novo and inherited CNVs were detected. The investigators concluded that their study validated the use of the Affymetrix 500K array for the detection of de novo CNVs of greater than 100 kb in patients with unexplained mental retardation.

Gijsbers and colleagues[10] used several different commercially available SNP platforms (Affymetrix 262K Nspl, Affymetrix 238K Styl, Illumina HumanHap300, and the Illumina HumanCNV370 BeadChip) to study CNVs in 318 patients with unexplained mental retardation and/or multiple congenital anomalies. They found abnormalities in 22.6% of patients, including CNVs (14 patients with pathogenic syndromes and 63 with potentially pathogenic alterations), large segments of homozygosity (4 patients), and mosaic trisomies for an entire chromosome (2 patients). With these studies they demonstrated that the high-density SNP array analysis has the ability to detect not only CNVs but also mosaicism, uniparental disomies, and loss of heterozygosity, all in the same experiment. Based on the findings from their study they proposed that all mental retardation/multiple congenital anomaly patients be initially analyzed by SNP array analysis rather than by conventional karyotyping, which will ultimately lead to an improvement in medical care and genetic counseling.

Bruno and colleagues[11] studied 117 patients with unexplained mental retardation and/or multiple congenital anomalies using an Affymetrix 250K Nspl array. The goal of their study was to replace locus-specific testing for specific microdeletion/duplication syndromes with microarray analysis. They were able to identify 18 pathogenic and 9 "potentially pathogenic" abnormalities with the array technology. Almost all of the pathogenic CNVs were larger than 500 kb. The investigators additionally found ROH larger than 5 Mb in 5 patients. They concluded from these studies that microarray analysis has improved diagnostic success; in addition, they were able to detect newly discovered syndromes and suggested that these changes were more common than previously suspected.

Friedman and colleagues,[12] in order to study the effectiveness of the 500K Affymetrix GeneChip, analyzed 154 children with idiopathic intellectual disabilities and their parents (trios). Fifty-four of these patients were previously studied by a 100K array, and 100 of the patients were analyzed for the first time by the 500K array analysis. In the previously studied patient group, all CNVs diagnosed by the 100K were confirmed; however, at least one additional pathogenic abnormality was delineated. Pathogenic abnormalities were found in 11 of the 100 newly studied patients. As with those previously studied, these findings continue to highlight the effectiveness of SNP array analysis and indicate how array analysis is being established as the primary clinical tool in the recognition of genomic imbalance that causes intellectual disabilities and other birth defects.

More recently, Bernardini and colleagues[13] used the Affymetrix 6.0 SNP array to study 70 patients with mental retardation with/without dysmorphic features who had been previously studied on lower density arrays. The investigators demonstrated that this platform increased the ability to detect small CNVs and that they were able to detect 6 additional changes not seen in the Agilent 44K analysis. Of these 6 CNV changes detected, 3 were thought to be pathogenic.

Constitutional Studies-Peripheral Blood, Copy Neutral Changes

Although SNP array analysis can be used to detect both copy number and copy neutral changes, most of the discussion to date has focused only on copy number changes. More recently it has been established that the detection of copy neutral changes is important in the delineation of the pathology of mental retardation.

In the largest study to date, Papenhausen and colleagues[7] examined 13,000 patients with mental retardation referred for SNP analysis. Of these, 92 had a segment of homozygosity (LCSH >13.5 Mb) that suggested that UPD might be present. Of the 46 patients who had parental follow-up, 29 were confirmed as UPD. This study showed that these UPD cases could be ascertained as mixed heterodisomy/isodisomy UPD cases, complete isodisomy, or segmental UPD. The phenotypic risks for these UPD cases is obvious for imprinted chromosomes but are also important in all chromosomes because of the unmasking of recessive disorders, as well as for the developmental effects of occult trisomy. **Fig. 5** shows a case of low-level trisomy 9 mosaicism (~20%) in which UPD can also be seen. In all cases in which telomeric UPD of less than 10 Mb and interstitial UPD of greater than 20 Mb were observed, the investigators suggested that follow-up molecular testing should be done to confirm the presence of UPD. An example of the importance of detection of recessive diseases associated with UPD was recently published by Cottrell and colleagues.[14] Using SNP array technology they demonstrated segmental isodisomy at 4q12 in a child who inherited two identical *SGCB* (beta-sarcoglycan) alleles, both of which

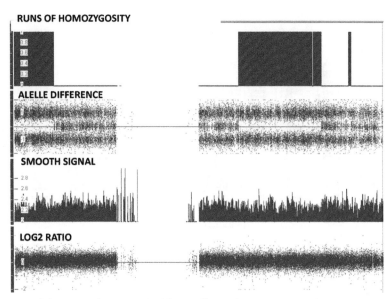

RUNS OF HOMOZYGOSITY

ALLELE DIFFERENCE

SMOOTH SIGNAL

LOG2 RATIO

Fig. 5. Use of the GTC software tool with an Affymetrix 6.0 SNP array demonstrating mosaic trisomy for chromosome 9. The CN state is slightly greater than 1.0, and the smooth signal is at about 2.3 (equivalent to about 30% mosaicism). Additionally, both the allele difference tract and the ROH tract demonstrate two large ROH, indicative of UPD for chromosome 9.

carried a missense mutation, which resulted in limb-girdle muscular dystrophy. In this case the mother was a carrier of the missense mutation and the child received two copies of the mutation because of maternal UPD 4. Conlin and colleagues[15] used SNP arrays to study mosaicism, chimerism, and UPD. The investigators were able to show that 16 cases of mosaic aneuploidy originated mitotically. However, this technology also showed that 5 trisomies originated meiotically and that 3 of the 5 had UPD in the disomic cells, confirming the increased risk for the effects of UPD in cases of meiotic nondisjunction.

One ROH is associated with UPD; however, the presence of more than one ROH (of 10 Mb or greater) detected by SNP array analysis is indicative of "identity by descent" (see also the discussion by Kearney and colleagues elsewhere in this issue). **Fig. 6** is an example of multiple stretches of ROH, which are associated with a first cousin relationship. In a report of 2,000 cases studied by Affymetrix SNP array analysis, Papenhausen and colleagues[16] demonstrated differences in ROH (LCSH) seen in first-, second-, third-, fourth-, and fifth-degree relationships (consanguinity). Theoretically, it is estimated that third-degree relatives (first cousins) would have 12.5% of their genomes in common, whereas first-degree relatives (siblings, for example) would have 50% of their genes in common. The degree of homozygosity in the child will provide insight into the genes that are in common, and the greater the degree of relationship the more ROHs that can be detected and the greater the risk for a recessive disorder. Schaaf and colleagues[17] have also recently demonstrated the effectiveness of SNP arrays in detecting incestuous parental relationships and highlighted the need to create practice guidelines dealing with the legal and ethical issues that these findings bring. Papić and colleagues[18] showed the value of homozygous mapping using a SNP-based array in a study of 2 affected siblings from a consanguineous family with limb girdle muscular dystrophy. Both of the siblings

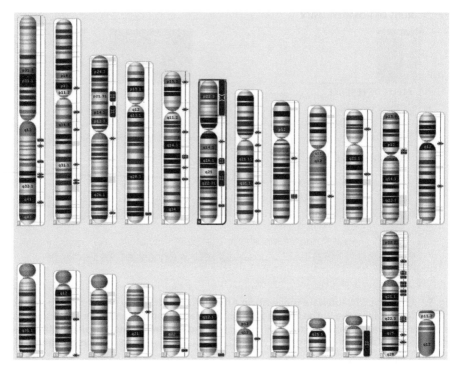

Fig. 6. Use of the Chromosome Analysis Suite (ChAS) software tool with an Affymetrix 6.0 SNP array demonstrating several large ROH regions (*in purple* on the side of several chromosomes in the ideogram). This number of ROH stretches is equivalent to an offspring of a first cousin relationship.

showed a homozygous block on chromosome 15 corresponding to the LGMD2A locus. The investigators also demonstrated that using a SNP microarray for whole-genome homozygous mapping is a low cost when helping to identify disease-causing mutations in consanguineous families.

Constitutional Studies—Prenatal

All array technology has had a tremendous impact on constitutional postnatal studies, but its impact on prenatal studies is still in its infancy (see also the discussion by Lamb elsewhere in this issue). Faas and colleagues[19] in 2010 examined the feasibility of using a 250K Affymetrix array prenatally. They detected 17 abnormalities in 38 fetuses; 6 of these were previously shown to have a chromosomal abnormality, whereas 11 abnormalities were identified in fetuses with a normal or balanced karyotype. Of these 11 abnormalities, 5 were de novo and seemed to be clinically relevant, and 2 of these involved UPD. The investigators were able to detect an abnormality in 16% of fetuses with ultrasound anomalies and a normal karyotype. This result illustrates the importance of the use of microarray technology, but the study also indicates that it must be carefully implemented.

Srebniak and colleagues[20] studied 64 prenatal samples with the Illumina Human-CytoSNP–12 array to validate its use for prenatal diagnostic studies. No false-positive or false-negatives were identified as part of the validation study. Additionally the investigators prospectively studied 61 fetuses with an abnormal ultrasound and a normal karyotype. In 4 of the 61 fetuses they found a clinically relevant abnormality, again illustrating the effectiveness of this technology.

Another prenatal diagnostic area in which this technology is beginning to be used is in preimplantation diagnosis.[21] Previous studies with FISH for preimplantation genetic diagnosis have shown that whereas FISH can diagnose abnormalities, it has not increased the successful delivery rates of fetuses. This result has been thought to be because not all of the chromosomes are studied with FISH, only those considered most clinically relevant. Array technology will allow for the analysis of all of the chromosomes, and whereas both array CGH (aCGH) and SNP arrays can determine the number of chromosomes, SNP-based arrays can also be used to haplotype the sample. Vanneste and colleagues[22] have used SNP array technology to reveal that chromosome instability is common during embryogenesis.

Another area of SNP array studies illustrating the strength of the use of SNPs in microarray analysis is the study of products of conception (POCs).[23] Four specific areas in which SNP array analysis has been beneficial for the study of POCs include (1) the detection of copy number change when chromosomal analyses have failed, (2) the detection of triploidy, (3) the detection of molar pregnancies, and (4) the detection of maternal cell contamination. Whereas the majority of abnormalities in POCs involve numeric changes, the major difficulty is not in the detection of smaller changes undetected by standard cytogenetic studies but rather in cases of no growth of the POC specimen (as is the case in the use of arrays for other prenatal studies or postnatal studies). In cases in which cytogenetic studies have failed because the fetal tissue has not grown in culture, DNA can be directly extracted from the tissue and used for array analysis. Studies have shown that the arrays can be successful even when the tissue has not been viable for cell growth.[23]

One limitation to nongenotyping arrays has been in the detection of cases with triploidy. Although not considered a major problem with postnatal or prenatal analysis, triploidy does have an impact on POC studies, accounting for approximately 15% to 20% of all abnormal spontaneous losses in the first trimester.[24] All arrays, when using their algorithms to determine copy number, take into account the numbers of each chromosome. For example, if there is one chromosome with three copies, the algorithm will compare this with all of the rest of the chromosomes and be able to show that the copy number state of that chromosome is equal to three. However, if all of the chromosomes have three copies, the algorithm will compare all of the chromosomes and indicate that there are only two copies of each chromosome. When a genotyping (SNP) array is used, the algorithm will still indicate that there are two copies of each chromosome, but the allele difference for each chromosome will show the presence of four tracts (not three, as when there are only two chromosomes), indicating that there are in fact three copies of each chromosome, consistent with the presence of triploidy (**Fig. 7**).

Another area that highlights the use of a genotyping array is complete moles. Complete moles have been shown to be of androgenic origin; the majority show complete homozygosity (doubling of one sperm) or a mixture of homozygosity and heterozygosity (the presence of two sperm).[25,26] Traditionally when chromosomes were studied in molar pregnancies, a 46,XX genomic constitution was routinely detected. When a genotyping array is used, the array will demonstrate a 46,XX karyotype, but the genotyping aspect of the array will show a high degree of homozygosity (either complete homozygosity or over 50% homozygosity), indicating the likelihood of a molar pregnancy.

The last aspect in which an SNP genotyping array can add information is in cases in which there may be a mixture of fetal and maternal DNA. The array cannot show if

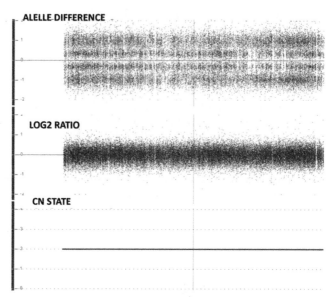

Fig. 7. Use of the GTC software tool with an Affymetrix 6.0 SNP array demonstrating triploidy findings. The CN state is equal to two; the log2 ratio is equal to zero; however, there are four different allele difference tracts (AAA, AAB, ABB, and BBB). The array demonstrates triploidy by showing four genotyping allele tracts for an autosomal chromosome, even though the copy number is only two.

the tissue received is fetal or maternal; however, it can show if there is a mixture of the two types of tissues. If only fetal tissue is present, the array will illustrate any copy number changes, and an examination of the allele difference tract of each individual chromosome will show three tracts in the allele differentiation (if there is a normal amount of genetic material). However, if there is a mixture of maternal and fetal DNA, an examination of the allele difference tracts will show 5 tracts for each chromosome, indicating that a mixture of maternal and fetal tissue is present. If at least 10% of the DNA is fetal, then any copy number alterations can be detected and the analysis will be performed knowing that a mixture does exist (data not shown).

Oncology Studies

The newest field in which arrays have been integrated into routine clinical analysis is oncology. This integration is taking place with both aCGH arrays as well as SNP arrays. In the past 2 years a number of different neoplastic conditions have been studied using a SNP array analysis. These conditions include chronic lymphocytic leukemia (CLL) (see discussion by Schnaiter and colleagues elsewhere in this issue), myelodysplastic syndromes (MDS) (see discussion by Odenike and colleagues elsewhere in this issue), multiple myeloma (see discussion by Slovak elsewhere in this issue), lymphomas (see discussion by Dave and colleagues elsewhere in this issue), and solid tumors (see discussion by Nanjangud and colleagues elsewhere in this issue). Hagenkord and colleagues[27] studied a series of CLL patients with multiple platforms and demonstrated that SNP karyotyping allowed for genome-wide high-resolution detection of copy number changes. In addition, the investigators demonstrated that SNP karyotyping can detect acquired uniparental disomy (aUPD), and both this and copy number changes are associated with established prognostic significance in CLL. Schwartz and colleagues (S. Schwartz, J. Tepperberg, R.D. Burnside, et al, personal communication, 2011) studied 113 patients referred for FISH analysis specific to CLL with an Affymetrix 6.0 array. They noted that approximately one-third of the 13q deletions had a larger deletion that included the retinoblastoma tumor suppressor gene, and that in about 28% of the abnormal FISH cases there were additional abnormalities detected by the array, which allowed the tumor to be classified as having a complex karyotype (>3 abnormalities). In about 5% of these patients, aUPD was detected. All of these findings can be correlated with a poorer prognosis in the patient.

There have been several articles recently published looking at the efficacy of SNP arrays in leading to a better understanding of MDS. Heinrichs and colleagues[28] used an SNP array to study 51 MDS patients. Overall they identified 21 patients (41%) with somatically acquired clonal abnormalities. Of the patients with normal bone marrows (by cytogenetics), 15% had clonal acquired aberrations detected by the array, including 4 with segmental UPD. UPD involving chromosome 7q was identified in 2 patients with a rapidly deteriorating clinical course. Makishima and colleagues[29] also evaluated the effectiveness of SNP array analysis and used standard metaphase analysis, FISH, and a SNP array to study 52 patients with MDS, 7 with MDS/myeloproliferative overlap syndromes, and 15 with acute myeloid leukemia (AML). Based on their study, they indicated that the three techniques are complementary and when applied and interpreted together can improve the diagnostic yield for identifying genetic lesions in MDS and better characterize abnormal karyotypes. In a larger study of 430 patients (250 with MDS, 95 with MDS/myeloproliferative overlap disorder, and 85 with AML from transformed MDS). Tiu and colleagues[30] demonstrated that SNP array studies combined with chromosomal studies provide a much greater diagnostic yield of chromosomal defects compared with cytogenetic analysis alone. The investigators believe that the presence and number of new abnormalities detected by the array studies are independent predictors of overall and event-free survival. In a comparison between patients with aplastic anemia and hypocellular myelodysplastic syndrome, Afable and colleagues[31] found that 36% of patients with MDS and with normal karyotypes had an abnormality by array analysis. In addition, persistent genomic lesions were found in 10 of 33 aplastic anemia patients, suggesting a diagnosis of MDS. As was stated earlier, however, the strength of SNP studies is in the detection of segmental UPD. In a recent study, O'Keefe and colleagues[32] reviewed the biological and clinical features of loss of heterozygosity (LOH) (and segmental UPD) in myeloid disorders. In these malignancies, segmental UPD has been associated with the duplication of oncogenic mutations with concomitant loss of the normal allele. Several examples of this association include the genes JAK2, MPL, c-KIT, and FLT3, and recent investigations have led to the discovery of tumor suppressor genes including CBL and TET2. In their review, the investigators report the involvement of several regions predominantly including 1q, 2p, 2q, 4q, 6p, 7q, 8q, 9p, 10q, 13q, 14q, 17p, 17q, 19q, 21q, and 22q. Based on this initial work they believe that further SNP studies will lead to the discovery of more pathogenic molecular lesions, diagnostic and prognostic markers, and a better understanding of the initiation and progression of hematologic malignancies.

Agnelli and colleagues[33] have taken a similar approach with 45 patients with multiple myeloma and 4 with plasma cell leukemia. The investigators identified a significant number of patients with near tetraploidy, gain of 1q, hyperdiploidy, and deletions of 1p, 13q, 14q, and 22q. SNP array analysis demonstrated the loss of several loci due to the loss of heterozygosity.

Kim and colleagues[34] demonstrated that in 16 of 17 renal cancer tumors that were studied with either an Affymetrix 10K or 250K SNP array they were able to find a recognizable pattern of chromosomal imbalances. From their study they concluded that the specific chromosomal imbalances generated by SNP array analysis were a valuable tool for increasing the unclassifiable renal neoplasms. The investigators considered SNP array analysis a practical technology to use in clinical practice. In a study of 16 microsatellite stable (MSS) and 16 microsatellite instable (MSI) colorectal tumors, 50K SNP array analysis revealed multiple LOH regions in the MSS tumors, whereas multiple deleted and amplified regions were seen in the MSS tumors along with the identification of *MTUS1* as a candidate gene.[35] Hartmann and colleagues[36] studied 47 patients with peripheral T-cell lymphoma, a disorder in which little is known about genomic aberrations, with a 250K SNP analysis. Genomic imbalances involving a variety of changes were detected in 22 patients. Several of these imbalances involved regions containing members of the nuclear factor-kappa B, signaling family as well as genes involved in cell cycle control. The investigators believed that a subgroup of these patients may have involvement of the *REL* gene, and expression of the REL protein may be of pathogenic relevance.

SUMMARY

In this review the use of SNP array technology in clinical diagnostic medicine has been examined. Initially, the methodology of SNP analysis was discussed and examined in detail. SNP array analysis, using both SNP probes (which are polymorphic) and copy number (nonpolymorphic) probes, will allow the detection of both copy number and copy neutral changes. Both SNP and CNP probes can be used to detect copy number changes through quantitative delineation of gain or loss of genetic material. The genotypes for each SNP probe are determined, and this information is additionally used to determine if there is a copy number change.

SNP array analysis has been used successfully for the study of constitutional abnormalities in postnatal populations, prenatal patients, and tissue obtained from products of conception. More recently it has also been used to study somatic changes in a variety of cancer patients. In all of these groups the methodology successfully detected a number of gains and losses of genomic material that were below the level of resolution of cytogenetic analysis. Additionally, in all of these groups copy neutral changes were also detected, where there was also no gain or loss of genetic material.

Whereas all array technology can detect copy number gain and loss, the SNP array can also detect copy neutral changes. In constitutional abnormalities this ability includes both the detection of UPD and consanguinity. In addition to UPD of imprinted chromosomes, a number of recessive diseases have been found by homozygous mapping for both UPD and consanguinity in constitutional abnormalities. A number of instances of segmental UPD have been detected in a variety of neoplastic conditions. When trios (in cases of constitutional samples) are run, the genotype will also allow for the detection of nonpaternity and parent of origin.

This technology is still in its infancy; however, the information presented in this review shows the potential in its use with all specimens. It is an invaluable technique when looking for the causes of constitutional abnormalities or somatic changes.

REFERENCES

1. Tjio HJ, Levan A. The chromosome number of man. Hereditas 1956;42:1–6.
2. Yunis JJ. High resolution of human chromosomes. Science 1976;191:1268–70.

3. Pinkel D, Landegent J, Collins C, et al. Fluorescence in situ hybridization with human chromosome-specific libraries: detection of trisomy 21 and translocations of chromosome 4. Proc Natl Acad Sci U S A 1988;85(23):9138–42.

4. Neill NJ, Torchia BS, Bejjani BA, et al. Comparative analysis of copy number detection by whole-genome BAC and oligonucleotide array CGH. Mol Cytogenet 2010;3:11.

5. Aligent Technologies. Agilent oligonucleotide array-based CGH for genomic DNA analysis. Enzymatic labeling for blood, cells, or tissues (with a high-throughput option) [manual]. Version 6.3. (G4410-90010). Aligent Technologies 5301 Stevens Creek Boulevard, Santa Clara, CA 95051, USA; 2010.

6. DNA Baser Sequence Assembly Software. Single nucleotide polymorphism. Available at: http://www.dnabaser.com/articles/SNP/SNP-single-nucleotide-polymorphism.html. Accessed September 2011.

7. Papenhausen P, Schwartz S, Risheg H, et al. UPD detection using homozygosity profiling with a SNP genotyping microarray. Am J Med Genet A 2011;155A(4): 757–68.

8. Pasion R, Burnside R, Gadi I, et al. An overlooked aspect of SNP array analysis: the importance of detection and counseling for recessive disorders. Available at: http://submissions.miracd.com/acmg/ContentInfo.aspx?conID=2274. Accessed September 2011.

9. McMullan DJ, Bonin M, Hehir-Kwa JY, et al. Molecular karyotyping of patients with unexplained mental retardation by SNP arrays: a multicenter study. Hum Mutat 2009;30(7):1082–92.

10. Gijsbers AC, Lew JY, Bosch CA, et al. A new diagnostic workflow for patients with mental retardation and/or multiple congenital abnormalities: test arrays first. Eur J Hum Genet 2009;17(11):1394–402.

11. Bruno DL, Ganesamoorthy D, Schoumans J, et al. Detection of cryptic pathogenic copy number variations and constitutional loss of heterozygosity using high resolution SNP microarray analysis in 117 patients referred for cytogenetic analysis and impact on clinical practice. J Med Genet 2009;46(2):123–31.

12. Friedman J, Adam S, Arbour L, et al. Detection of pathogenic copy number variants in children with idiopathic intellectual disability using 500 K SNP array genomic hybridization. BMC Genomics 2009;10:526.

13. Bernardini L, Alesi V, Loddo S, et al. High-resolution SNP arrays in mental retardation diagnostics: how much do we gain? Eur J Hum Genet 2010;18(2):178–85.

14. Cottrell C, Mendell J, Hart-Kothari M, et al. Maternal uniparental disomy of chromosome 4 in a patient with limb-girdle muscular dystrophy 2E confirmed by SNP array technology. Clin Genet 2011;Apr 11:doi: 10.1111/j.1399-0004.2011.01681.x. [Epub ahead of print.]

15. Conlin LK, Thiel BD, Bonnemann CG, et al. Mechanisms of mosaicism, chimerism and uniparental disomy identified by single nucleotide polymorphism array analysis. Hum Mol Genet 2010;19(7):1263–75.

16. Papenhausen P, Tepperberg J, Gadi, I. SNP based copy number microarrays provide cues to UPD and recessive allele risk to inbreeding. Available at: http://www.ashg.org/2008meeting/abstracts/fulltext. Accessed September 2011.

17. Schaaf CP, Scott DA, Wiszniewska J, et al. Identification of incestuous parental relationships by SNP-based DNA microarrays. Lancet. 2011;377(9765):555–6. Erratum in: Lancet 2011;377(9768):812.

18. Papić L, Fischer D, Trajanoski S, et al. SNP-array based whole genome homozygosity mapping: a quick and powerful tool to achieve an accurate diagnosis in LGMD2 patients. Eur J Med Genet 2011;54(3):214–9.

19. Faas BH, van der Burgt I, Kooper AJ, et al. Identification of clinically significant, submicroscopic chromosome alterations and UPD in fetuses with ultrasound anomalies using genome-wide 250k SNP array analysis. J Med Genet 2010;47(9):586–94.

20. Srebniak M, Boter M, Oudesluijs G, et al. Application of SNP array for rapid prenatal diagnosis: implementation, genetic counselling and diagnostic flow. Eur J Hum Genet 2011;Jun 22:doi: 10.1038/ejhg.2011.119. [Epub ahead of print.]

21. Harper JC, Harton G. The use of arrays in preimplantation genetic diagnosis and screening. Fertil Steril 2010;94(4):1173–7.

22. Vanneste E, Voet T, Le Caignec CL, et al. Chromosome instability is common in human cleavage-stage embryos. Nat Med 2009;15(5):577–83.

23. Smith JL, Schwartz S, Tepperberg J, et al. Analysis of products of conception by microarray analysis. Cytogenet Genome Res 2010;128:253.

24. Abruzzo MA, Hassold TJ. Etiology of nondisjunction in humans. Environ Mol Mutagen 1995;25(Suppl 26):38–47.

25. Kovacs BW, Shahbahrami B, Tast DE, et al. Molecular genetic analysis of complete hydatidiform moles. Cancer Genet Cytogenet 1991;54(2):143–52.

26. Fujita N, Tamura S, Shimizu N, et al. Genetic origin analysis of hydatidiform mole and non-molar abortion using the polymerase chain reaction method. Acta Obstet Gynecol Scand 1994;73(9):719–25.

27. Hagenkord JM, Monzon FA, Kash SF, et al. Array-based karyotyping for prognostic assessment in chronic lymphocytic leukemia: performance comparison of Affymetrix 10K2.0, 250K Nsp, and SNP6.0 arrays. J Mol Diagn 2010;12(2):184–96.

28. Heinrichs S, Kulkarni RV, Bueso-Ramos CE, et al. Accurate detection of uniparental disomy and microdeletions by SNP array analysis in myelodysplastic syndromes with normal cytogenetics. Leukemia. 2009;23(9):1605–13.

29. Makishima H, Rataul M, Gondek LP, et al. FISH and SNP-A karyotyping in myelodysplastic syndromes: improving cytogenetic detection of del(5q), monosomy 7, del(7q), trisomy 8 and del(20q). Leuk Res 2010;34(4):447–53.

30. Tiu RV, Gondek LP, O'Keefe CL, et al. Prognostic impact of SNP array karyotyping in myelodysplastic syndromes and related myeloid malignancies. Blood 2011;117(17): 4552–60.

31. Afable MG 2nd, Wlodarski M, Makishima H, et al. SNP array-based karyotyping: differences and similarities between aplastic anemia and hypocellular myelodysplastic syndromes. Blood 2011;117(25):6876–84.

32. O'Keefe C, McDevitt MA, Maciejewski JP. Copy neutral loss of heterozygosity: a novel chromosomal lesion in myeloid malignancies. Blood 2010;115(14):2731–9.

33. Agnelli L, Mosca L, Fabris S, et al. A SNP microarray and FISH-based procedure to detect allelic imbalances in multiple myeloma: an integrated genomics approach reveals a wide gene dosage effect. Genes Chromosomes Cancer 2009; 48(7):603–14.

34. Kim HJ, Shen SS, Ayala AG, et al. Virtual-karyotyping with SNP microarrays in morphologically challenging renal cell neoplasms: a practical and useful diagnostic modality. Am J Surg Pathol 2009;33(9):1276–86.

35. Melcher R, Hartmann E, Zopf W, et al. LOH and copy neutral LOH (cnLOH) act as alternative mechanism in sporadic colorectal cancers with chromosomal and microsatellite instability. Carcinogenesis 2011;32(4):636–42.

36. Hartmann S, Gesk S, Scholtysik R, et al. High resolution SNP array genomic profiling of peripheral T cell lymphomas, not otherwise specified, identifies a subgroup with chromosomal aberrations affecting the REL locus. Br J Haematol 2010;148(3):402–12.

Diagnostic Implications of Excessive Homozygosity Detected by SNP-Based Microarrays: Consanguinity, Uniparental Disomy, and Recessive Single-Gene Mutations

Hutton M. Kearney, PhD[a],*, Joseph B. Kearney, PhD[a],
Laura K. Conlin, PhD[b]

KEYWORDS

- Microarray • Single nucleotide polymorphism
- Homozygosity • Autozygosity • Consanguinity
- Uniparental disomy

Single nucleotide polymorphism (SNP)-based microarray analysis provides detection of copy number variations (CNVs) as well as genotype information at multiple polymorphic loci throughout the genome. Although the clinical utility of CNV detection is well accepted,[1,2] information derived from SNP-based microarray analysis has only more recently been utilized in the constitutional cytogenetics laboratory setting.[3,4] In addition to specific genotype data, analysis of SNP allele patterns can provide (1) confirmation of CNV calls, (2) sensitivity for detection of mosaicism, and (3) detection of excessive homozygosity, which is the focus of this review.

Several different SNP-based microarray platforms are currently in clinical use, and this review illustrates similar data obtained from Affymetrix- and Illumina-based microarrays (Affymetrix Inc, Santa Clara, CA, USA; Illumina Inc, San Diego, CA, USA). It is generally not necessary to derive specific genotypes from the microarray data to view the SNP probes as present in a homozygous or heterozygous state. For both platforms, biallelic SNPs are denoted as "A" or "B." Relative allele distribution is typically provided by either allele difference plots or B-allele frequency plots (**Fig. 1**).

Fullerton Genetics Center: data derived from the CytoScan HD was supported in part by Affymetrix, Inc. (arrays and reagents provided in kind for platform R&D).

[a] Fullerton Genetics Center, Mission Health System, 267 McDowell Street, Asheville, NC 28803, USA

[b] Department of Pathology and Laboratory Medicine, The Children's Hospital of Philadelphia, 3615 Civic Center Boulevard, Abramson Research Building, Room 1007B, Philadelphia, PA 19146, USA

* Corresponding author.

E-mail address: hutton.kearney@msj.org

Clin Lab Med 31 (2011) 595–613
doi:10.1016/j.cll.2011.08.003
0272-2712/11/$ – see front matter © 2011 Elsevier Inc. All rights reserved.

labmed.theclinics.com

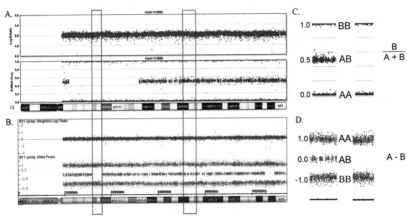

Fig. 1. Allele plots. *(A)* Screenshot of a chromosome 13 from a patient DNA sample run on the Illumina Quad610 array, and visualized in BeadStudio software. *Top:* Log R ratio plot shows a normal copy number state for the chromosome. *Bottom:* B-allele frequency plot shows a large region of homozygosity from bands 13q12.11 to 13q14.3. *(B)* Screenshot of a chromosome 13 from a patient DNA sample run on the Affymetrix CytoScan™ HD array and visualized in Affymetrix Chromosome Analysis Suite (ChAS) software. *Top:* Weighted log$_2$ ratio plot shows a normal copy number state for the chromosome. *Bottom:* Allele difference plot shows 2 regions of homozygosity from bands 13q13.1 to q13.3 and 13q33.2 to q33.3. Panels *C* and *D* represent magnified views of the allele plots for each software, from the boxed regions in panels *A* and *B*. *(C)* B-allele frequency, as plotted in Illumina BeadStudio software. The Y-axis value is determined by the formula given on the right. Alleles are plotted as a frequency, determined by the number of B alleles compared with the total number of alleles (A+B). B-allele frequency of 1 indicates homozygosity for the B allele (2/2), a frequency of 0 indicates homozygosity for the A allele (0/2), and a frequency of 0.5 indicates a heterozygous genotype (1/2). *(D)* Allele difference, as plotted in Affymetrix Chromosome Analysis Suite (ChAS) software. The Y-axis value is determined by the formula given on the right. Alleles are plotted as the difference between the estimated number of A alleles and the estimated number of B alleles (A-B). Each allele corresponds to a value of 0.5. Values near 1 indicate homozygosity for the A allele (AA: [0.5+0.5] – [0] = 1), values near –1 indicate homozygosity for the B allele (BB: [0] – [0.5 + 0.5] = –1), and values near 0 indicate a heterozygous genotype (AB: [0.5] – [0.5] = 0).

Multiple terms are used to describe regions of homozygosity, and each conveys a slightly different meaning (eg, loss of heterozygosity, absence of heterozygosity, runs of homozygosity). Here we use the term *long-contiguous stretch of homozygosity* (LCSH) to describe an uninterrupted region of homozygous alleles with genomic copy number state of 2. The term *LCSH* excludes loss of heterozygosity caused by single copy deletions because these regions exist in a hemizygous state. Minimal thresholds for LCSH calls are generally set around 0.5 to 1 Mb in population genetic analyses[5–7] and more conservatively at 3 to 10 Mb in clinical analyses,[4](Kearney H, Kearney J, and Conlin L, personal communication).

Detection of excessive homozygosity, in and of itself, is not diagnostic of any underlying condition and may be clinically benign. The first step in assessing the clinical relevance of observed LCSH is to distinguish between excessive homozygosity found in multiple regions throughout the genome versus LCSH restricted to a single chromosome. When multiple LCSH regions are found throughout the genome, the findings are generally assumed to represent regions identical by descent (IBD),

Table 1
Correlation between percentage of LCSH and degree of parental relationship

Parental Relationship	Degree	Coefficient of Inbreeding (F)	LCSH (IBD) Predicted in Child (~%)[a]
Parent/child	First	0.25	25
Full siblings	First	0.25	25
Half siblings	Second	0.125	12.5
Uncle/niece or aunt/nephew	Second	0.125	12.5
Double first cousins	Second	0.125	12.5
Grandparent/grandchild	Second	0.125	12.5
First cousins	Third	0.0625	6
First cousins once removed	Fourth	0.03125	3
Second cousins	Fifth	0.015625	1.5
Third cousins	Seventh	0.0039062	<0.5

[a] Assuming outbred population.

with the associated concerns for recessive disorders mapping to the homozygous intervals. When the genomic homozygosity is sufficiently excessive, the finding may trigger a suspicion for parental consanguinity or incest (**Table 1**; **Fig. 2**).[8] One or more regions of LCSH found only on a single chromosome can be a hallmark of uniparental disomy (UPD), either whole-chromosome UPD or segmental UPD,[3,4,9] and may warrant further clinical investigation, particularly when involving chromosomes associated with imprinted gene disorders (**Table 2**). Regardless of mechanism or size, all LCSH segments have the potential to harbor homozygous recessive mutations.

CONSANGUINITY

When LCSH is found distributed throughout the genome, this observation is presumed to represent homozygosity caused by inheritance of genomic regions of IBD. When the parents of a proband share a recent common ancestor, their union is defined as *consanguineous*. The closer the parental relationship, the greater the proportion of shared alleles and, therefore, the greater the risk of the child (proband) inheriting 2 copies of a deleterious gene mutation from his parents.[10–12] Clinical laboratories that perform SNP-based microarray analysis will encounter many cases of presumed parental consanguinity, occasionally with suspicion of abuse/incest because of the degree of consanguinity estimated (**Fig. 2**).[8]

Although this has no immediate clinical utility and represents a pursuit largely of academic or social/ethical/legal interest, an estimate of the total proportion of the LCSH in the genome can be used as a rough assessment of degree of parental relationship (see **Table 1**). A simple method to grossly estimate parental relationship is to add all homozygous regions greater than a defined threshold (eg, 3 Mb), excluding the sex chromosomes (because males are always hemizygous, and X chromosomes in females are often observed with increased LCSH because of more limited recombination). The total autosomal LCSH can then be divided by total autosomal length (2,867,733 kb for hg18) to estimate the percentage of IBD. This estimation can then be correlated with the predicted percentage of IBD for various degrees of relationship (see **Table 1**). It should be noted that this crude calculation is likely to represent an underestimate of the actual homozygous proportion given that

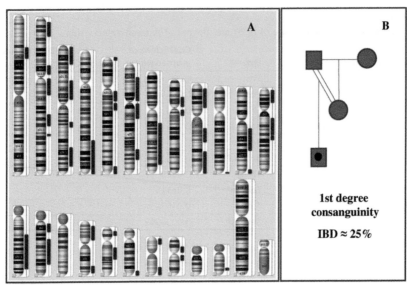

Fig. 2. LCSH patterns seen in consanguinity. *(A)* Male patient with LCSH on multiple chromosomes (Affymetrix Genome-Wide Human SNP 6.0 array data visualized in Affymetrix Chromosome Analysis Suite [ChAS] software). Note that the sex chromosomes are excluded in LCSH modeling. Calculations of total percentage IBD with different minimal LCSH thresholds in this case result in the following estimations: LCSH threshold ≥ 0.5 Mb: 868,341 kb (30% IBD); ≥ 1 Mb: 868,341 kb (30%); ≥ 3 Mb: 866,089 kb (30%); ≥ 5 Mb: 858,676 kb (30%); ≥ 10 Mb: 797,445 kb (28%); ≥ 15 Mb: 700,140 kb (24%), and ≥ 20 Mb: 577,279 kb (20%). These data and those of additional cases suggest that minimal LCSH thresholds between 0.5 and 10 Mb have negligible impact on estimation of percentage of IBD. These data are consistent with first degree consanguinity, as illustrated in panel B (and **Table 1**). *(B)* Pedigree illustrating first-degree consanguinity and predicted percentage IBD. The mother and father of the proband share 50% of their genome (because they are first-degree relatives). There is a one-half probability that the proband will inherit an identical genomic region from both of his parents, making the total estimate of the proband's percentage of IBD in this scenario roughly 25%. Note that other first-degree parental relationships (eg, full siblings) would also yield an estimated 25% IBD in the proband.

(1) only LCSH long enough to be detected by with the array platform/applied threshold will be included and (2) the denominator includes regions of the genome that may not be covered on the microarray (eg, acrocentric short arm and centromeric regions). Although in theory, the background level of population-specific homozygosity in any genome may artificially inflate this observation, in practice, this does not complicate the calculated percentage to any measurable degree, particularly if the threshold used to calculate total LCSH is greater than 1 Mb.[6,7]

Estimating percentage of IBD can be illustrative and suggestive of degree of parental relationship, but if this inference is made at all, it should be accompanied by an appropriate measure of uncertainty. Most importantly, this estimate cannot be taken as evidence of a specific parental relationship. Additionally, this inference assumes a standard 50% distribution of parental alleles in each meiotic division, and unpredictable recombination and chromosome segregation patterns may result in significant deviation from this distribution.[7] Furthermore, consanguinity is very common practice in some populations[13,14]; therefore, it is likely that individuals from

Table 2
UPD chromosomes associated with imprinting disorders

UPD Chromosome	Imprinted Locus	Maternal vs Paternal UPD	Associated Disorder	Major Clinical Features	Known/Proposed Dysregulated Gene(s)
6	q24	Paternal	Diabetes Mellitus, 6q24-related Transient Neonatal[52]	Intrauterine growth retardation, neonatal hyperglycemia	PLAG1, HYMAI
7	p11.2–p12 and q32.2	Maternal	Russell-Silver syndrome[53]	Intrauterine and postnatal growth retardation, triangular facies	GRB10, MEST
11	p15.5	Paternal (segmental)	Beckwith-Wiedemann syndrome[54]	Macrosomia, macroglossia, visceromegaly, omphalocele	IGF2, H19, CDKN1C, KCNQ1, KCNQ1OT1
		Maternal	Russell-Silver syndrome[55]	Intrauterine and postnatal growth retardation, triangular facies	IGF2, H19, CDKN1C, KCNQ1, KCNQ1OT1
14	q32.2	Maternal	Maternal UPD14 syndrome[56–58]	Precocious puberty, hypotonia, joint laxity	RTL1, DLK1
		Paternal	Paternal UPD14 syndrome[56–59]	Skeletal abnormalities, joint contractures, intellectual disability	RTL1, DLK1
15	q11–q13	Paternal	Angelman syndrome[60]	Severe intellectual disability, speech impairment	UBE3A
		Maternal	Prader-Willi syndrome[61]	Hypotonia, hypogonadism, obesity	SNRPN, MKRN, MAGEL2, NDN, U5snoRNAs
20	q13.3	Paternal	Pseudohypoparathyroidism type 1b[62,63]	Neonatal hyperbilirubinemia, parathyroid hormone resistance	GNAS

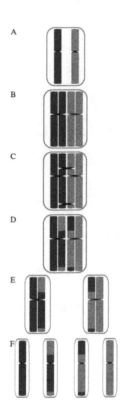

these populations share not just a single recent ancestor but also multiple common ancestors (eg, total genomic homozygosity near or exceeding that seen with first-degree consanguinity, yet the parents have a fairly distant relationship). The laboratory generally has limited or no information regarding the family/social/ethnic situation of the proband; therefore, inferences regarding suspected abuse involving a parent are generally poorly supported; any communications regarding suspicion of abuse should follow appropriate professional guidelines and take place under advisement of one's institutional legal/ethics consult. Currently, there are no professional guidelines for whether concerns for abuse/incest should be revealed after SNP-array analysis and, if so, under what circumstances, although guidance from the American College of Medical Genetics is forthcoming. Regardless of whether consanguinity is suspected, estimated, or even revealed, simply informing the referring physician of increased suspicion for recessive disorders has clinical utility (see Autozygosity Mapping section).

UNIPARENTAL DISOMY

Generally, when isolated LCSH (involving only a single chromosome) is detected, particularly when longer than 10 Mb,[4] uniparental disomy is considered a likely mechanism. UPD is defined as the inheritance of both homologues from a single parent.[15,16] Many excellent reviews have been devoted to UPD,[17–24] and there are informative Web-based resources available as well (Lier lab site, Jena University Hospital[25]; Morrison lab site, University of Otago[26]; Robinson lab site, University of

British Columbia[27]; Jirtle lab site, Duke University[28]). This review will, therefore, not cover the history, exhaustive mechanisms, or specific clinical features of UPD syndromes (see **Table 2** for summary), but will instead focus on the laboratory detection of UPD through SNP-based microarray analysis and appreciation of associated data complexities. Historically, UPD was only suspected when accompanied by a hallmark cytogenetic finding (mosaic trisomy, marker chromosome, or other structural rearrangement, such as a Robertsonian translocation), by clinical manifestation of a disorder of imprinting,[29] or finding homozygosity for a recessive allele with only a single carrier parent.[16] Through the use of SNP-based microarrays, clinical laboratories may now have serendipitous detection of unanticipated UPD events by recognition of hallmark patterns of homozygosity.[4] To appreciate the expected patterns of homozygosity encountered with UPD-involved chromosomes, it is useful to review the various mechanisms known to generate UPD. It is of fundamental importance to first appreciate the basic concepts of meiosis and meiotic recombination, which are summarized in **Fig. 3**.

There are 2 primary mechanisms by which UPD involving a whole chromosome may be generated: (1) trisomy rescue, the most frequently observed mechanism and (2) monosomy rescue.[23] Gamete complementation has also been proposed as a UPD mechanism,[15] but this is thought to be a very rare event. Additionally, segmental UPD (involving only part of a chromosome) may also be generated through somatic events.[17] Given that the majority of these mechanisms generate UPD with full or partial homozygosity of parental markers (**Figs. 4–6**), SNP-based microarrays are very useful for detecting LCSH patterns that may be predictive (but not diagnostic) of UPD.[3,4,9,24] Uniparental *isodisomy* refers to inheritance of 2 identical chromosomes from a single parent, whereas uniparental *heterodisomy* refers to inheritance of 2 homologous chromosomes from the same parent. Because of meiotic recombination, even UPD events involving an entire chromosome are usually not purely isodisomic or heterodisomic, but instead often have a mixture of both types of segments.

Trisomy Rescue

Zygotes with nonmosaic trisomy for most chromosomes are usually not compatible with life (exceptions are trisomies involving chromosomes 13, 18, 21, and sex chromosomes). Those zygotes that do survive have typically either lost the trisomy entirely, have experienced a structural reduction of the trisomic chromosome (usually conversion to a marker or ring chromosome), or are mosaic. These events are collectively known as *trisomy rescue*.[21] Restoration to euploid state can occur through mitotic nondisjunction, which produces a normal (euploid) daughter cell and an aneuploid daughter cell (with monosomy, which presumably does not survive) or by anaphase lag, in which one of the aneuploid chromosomes is not incorporated into the new-forming nucleus and is subsequently lost. By chance alone, two-thirds of the

←

Fig. 3 Normal meiosis. (*A*) A pair of homologous chromosomes illustrated before chromosome replication; shading differences represent general heterozygosity. (*B*) Chromosome replication resulting in identical sister chromatids. (*C*) Recombination between nonsister chromatids (note that involvement of only 2 chromatids is depicted for clarity, yet crossover events may collectively involve 2, 3, or 4 chromatids). (*D*) Resulting genetic exchange from meiotic recombination. (*E*) First division (meiosis I), with separation of chromosome homologues into 2 daughter cells. (*F*) Second division (meiosis II), with each daughter cell (gamete or polar body) containing 1 chromatid.

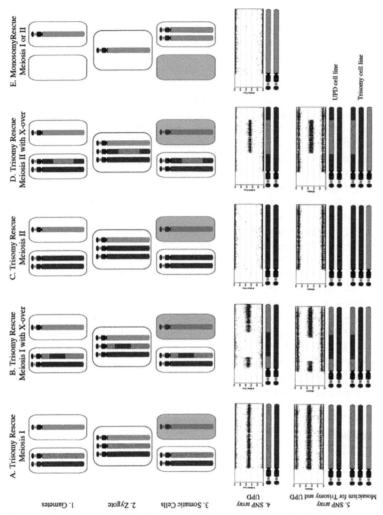

Fig. 4. Uniparental disomy resulting from meiotic errors. Columns *A–E* each represent 1 type of meiotic error, including (*A*) trisomy resulting from a meiosis I error without recombination and (*B*) with recombination, (*C*) a meiosis II error without recombination and (*D*) with recombination, and (*E*) a monosomy rescue resulting from either meiosis I or II error. Rows 1–3 model the chromosome involved in the uniparental disomy cells through various stages of development. Row 4 shows a theoretical allele plot for each of these scenarios as plotted in Illumina BeadStudio software. Row 5 shows a theoretical allele plot involving mosaicism for a uniparental disomy cell line and a trisomic cell line for each of the mechanisms. Predicted chromosomal compositions in the sampled tissue are illustrated below the allele plots. Plot A4 shows array data resulting from complete uniparental heterodisomy. This chromosome does not contain any LCSH and cannot be distinguished from a chromosome with normal biparental inheritance. Plots C4 and E4 show array data resulting from complete uniparental isodisomy; there are no heterozygous SNP alleles. These 2 plots are indistinguishable from one another; therefore, unless mosaicism is present (C5), the mechanism cannot be inferred. Plots B4 and D4 show chromosomes with mixed isodisomy and heterodisomy. The placement of the detected LCSH can be used to infer meiosis I errors (B4) from meiosis II errors (D4). Note that not all of the data modeled in this illustration represent confirmed cases of UPD; some of the data are modeled to illustrate concepts.

time a "rescue" event results in a disomic line with biparental inheritance, whereas one-third of the time UPD occurs. For topical relevance, the remainder of the discussion of trisomy rescue will presume that the rescue results in UPD. Depending on the origin of the trisomy (eg, meiosis I or II) and the stochastic arrangement of recombination events, the UPD chromosomes may be completely heterodisomic, completely isodisomic, or mixed hetero- and isodisomic (see **Fig. 4**). Importantly, the location of isodisomy (homozygosity) relative to any imprinted loci has no clinical relevance when considering UPD involving an entire chromosome. For example, as illustrated in **Fig. 5**, an individual with Prader-Willi syndrome caused by maternal UPD15 may have uniparental heterodisomy (heterozygous allele calls) across the critical region at 15q11.2–q13. This concept will be further supported in the following discussions of UPD mechanism.

First, consider trisomy rescue in the absence of recombination (see **Fig. 4**A). If the original segregation error occurred in meiosis I, the resulting gametes would either be nullisomic or contain both chromosome homologues (heterodisomic). Fertilization of the heterodisomic gamete followed by trisomy rescue to generate UPD would result in uniparental heterodisomy for the entire chromosome. This is a very important scenario to understand, given that this UPD event would not generate any regions of homozygosity detectable by SNP-based microarray yet would be pathogenic if involving an imprinted chromosome. If the initiating segregation error originated in meiosis II (see **Fig. 4**C), the resulting gametes would be normal, nullisomic, or contain 2 copies of identical chromosomes (isodisomic). Fertilization of the isodisomic gamete followed by trisomy rescue to generate UPD would result in uniparental isodisomy (homozygosity) for the entire chromosome and would be readily detectable by SNP-based microarray. When whole chromosome homozygosity is encountered, UPD can be reasonably presumed.

Now, let us consider trisomy rescue involving chromosomes with meiotic recombination events (crossing over) (see **Fig. 4**B, D). As before, a trisomic zygote can be corrected by a subsequent mitotic event (either nondisjunction or anaphase lag). Those rescued trisomies resulting from meiosis I errors will result in heterodisomy around the centromere, whereas those from meiosis II errors will result in isodisomy around the centromere. The remaining distribution of hetero- and isodisomy is dependent on the number and position of meiotic crossover events.

Monosomy Rescue

Zygotes with monosomy for a chromosome (other than the X chromosome) are not compatible with life and can be rescued only by duplication of the monosomic chromosome. This can occur through a mitotic nondisjunction, resulting in a daughter cell with nullisomy and a daughter cell with restored euploidy. This mechanism can only result in whole-chromosome uniparental isodisomy (see **Fig. 4**E).

Mitotic Errors of Chromosome Segregation to Generate UPD

In addition to uniparental disomy as a result of meiotic error, UPD can be a consequence of somatic events. When nondisjunction or anaphase lag occurs in a euploid somatic cell, the resulting daughter cells would be aneuploid. A second nondisjunction or anaphase lag could correct this event, resulting in a euploid cell again; however, this may result in daughter cells with incorrect distribution of the parental chromosomes, with UPD as a result (see **Fig. 6**B). This UPD would always be isodisomic for the entire chromosome (LKC, unpublished data).[30]

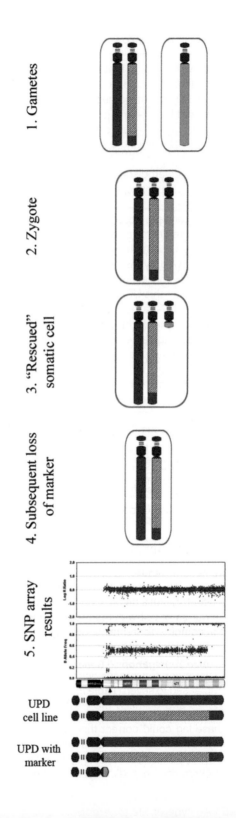

Segmental UPD

Segmental isodisomy, in which only a portion of a chromosome shows uniparental inheritance with the remainder of the chromosome showing biparental inheritance, can also occur somatically. One mechanism to generate segmental UPD is nonsister (homologous) chromatid exchange during mitosis (**Fig. 6A**). This would result in 2 daughter cells containing complementary segmental uniparental isodisomies. Because most cases of segmental UPD have only one abnormal cell line detected (reviewed in Kotzot[17]), one of the resulting daughter cells may not be compatible with survival. Alternatively, these events may represent chromosomal breakage and repair (break-induced replication) using the homologous chromosome as a template.[31] The resulting UPD from either mechanism (assuming a single break or exchange) would affect only one arm of the chromosome and should extend from the break/exchange to the telomere. Segmental UPD is unlikely if the homozygosity is interstitial or present at the termini of both arms, as these findings are not consistent with a single mitotic break/exchange event.[18] In rare cases, if 2 mitotic exchanges occurred, the segmental UPD would be interstitially located.[32] Because segmental UPD mechanisms generate only uniparental isodisomy, the location of the LCSH (isodisomy) relative to any imprinted loci should be considered.[28] In contrast to whole-chromosome UPD, only the loci involved in the isodisomic segment are at risk for imprinted disorders if segmental UPD is confirmed as the mechanism underlying the LCSH (see Follow-up testing to confirm UPD).

Whole-genome UPD

Chimeric individuals with whole-genome UPD have been reported in a handful of cases, with both maternal and paternal whole-genome UPD.[3,33–37] These individuals are chimeric for 2 cell lines: one cell line with normal biparental inheritance and one cell line with uniparental isodisomy of the entire genome. The presence of paternal whole-genome UPD (androgenetic chimerism) can result in the clinical presentation of known paternally imprinted disorders, such as Beckwith-Wiedemann syndrome, whereas the presence of maternal whole-genome UPD (parthenogenetic chimerism) can present with Prader-Willi or other maternally imprinted disorders (**Table 2**). Although several mechanisms have been hypothesized for these chimeric whole-genome UPD observations, the most plausible is endoreduplication of 1 parental genome before pronuclei fusion in the fertilized egg.[18,38]

Fig. 5. Trisomy rescue resulting in a mosaic marker chromosome and UPD. SNP-array data (Illumina Quad610 array, visualized in BeadStudio software) seen in a patient with Prader-Willi syndrome, with proposed mechanisms illustrated. (1) Gametes, with an ovum containing 2 chromosomes 15 as a result of a meiosis I error. (2) Zygote, with trisomy for chromosome 15. (3) A trisomy rescue event resulting in a small marker derived from the paternal chromosome 15. (4) Subsequent mosaic loss of the marker, resulting in whole-chromosome maternal UPD. (5) SNP array results show heterodisomy for the majority of the chromosome, with isodisomy only at the q terminus. A mosaic duplication is detected near the centromere, showing a pattern consistent with a mosaic marker. The imprinted region at 15q11.2 to q13 associated with Prader-Willi syndrome is indicated on the chromosome ideogram. Note that the marker chromosome does not contain this genomic region; therefore, both cell lines exhibit UPD of the relevant chromosomal region. Note also that the imprinted region is within a region of heterodisomy, but is fully uniparental (see also **Fig. 4**-A5).

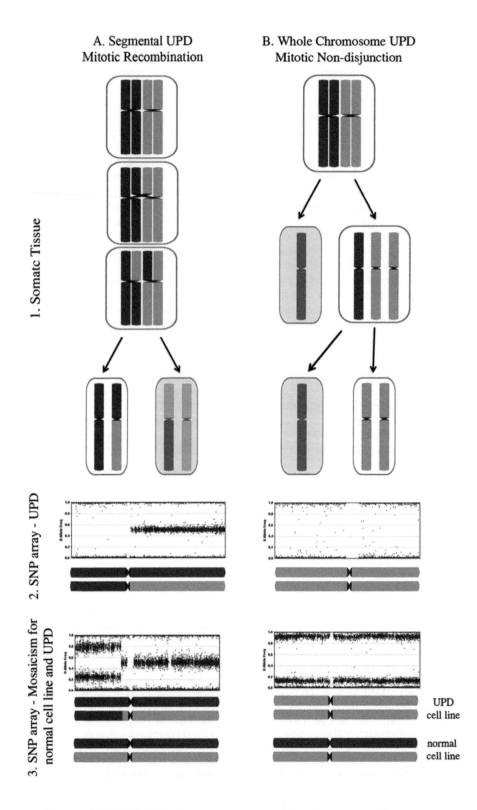

Inferences Regarding Origin of UPD Derived from Detection of Mosaicism

Mosaicism for a trisomic cell line, a cell line with a marker/derivative chromosome, or a cell line with normal biparental inheritance is an additional line of evidence by which one may infer the origin of the UPD (see **Figs. 4–6**). If a trisomic cell line is present either in the same tissue as the UPD or in other tissues (such as placenta), the origin of the UPD is most likely a trisomy rescue (see **Fig. 4A–D**). Mosaicism involving a normal biparental cell line with a segmental UPD cell line or a whole chromosome uniparental isodisomy cell line most likely indicates a mitotic origin (see **Fig. 6**), although other more rare and esoteric chromosomal arrangements are possible.[17,18] SNP arrays have been used successfully to detect mosaicism for segmental UPD in cases of Beckwith-Wiedemann syndrome[3,38] and in revertant skin in patients with ichthyosis.[39]

The presence of homozygosity for an entire chromosome is most likely associated with a monosomy rescue (see **Fig. 4E-4**); however, chromosome segregation errors in meiosis II without the presence of crossovers (see **Fig. 4C-4**) and mitotic segregation errors (see **Fig. 6B-2**) may also result in uniparental isodisomy for the whole chromosome. The finding of mosaicism for a monosomic cell line (consistent with monosomy rescue), a trisomic cell line (consistent with trisomy rescue), or a normal biparental cell line (consistent with mitotic nondisjunction) may clarify the mechanism of the UPD event (see **Figs. 4E, 4C-5,** and **6B-3**). Note that the presence of a monosomic cell line in a monosomy rescue event would have to be ascertained by decreased log2 values across the chromosome (suggesting low-level monosomy), or traditional cytogenetic methods. SNP allele patterns would be unaffected in this scenario.

Follow-up Testing to Confirm UPD

As outlined previously, failure to detect LCSH by SNP microarray analysis does not exclude the possibility of UPD (see **Fig. 4A**). For this reason, SNP microarrays cannot be considered a diagnostic assay for UPD when analyzing the proband alone. Similarly, the finding of LCSH involving a single chromosome should not be considered diagnostic of UPD. Large isolated regions of LCSH (even those larger than 10 Mb) may still represent IBD with distant consanguinity. Regions of LSCH greater than 1 Mb have been found in outbred populations, typically attributed to recombination "cold spots" leading to SNP markers in linkage disequilibrium.[4,6,7] Additionally,

---

←

Fig. 6. Uniparental disomy resulting from mitotic errors. Row 1 illustrates a potential model of somatic events consistent with the SNP data shown. Row 2 shows patient allele plots (Illumina Quad610 array, visualized in BeadStudio software). Row 3 shows patient allele plots involving mosaicism for a UPD cell line and a normal cell line. Models for chromosome composition responsible for the data shown are illustrated below the allele plots. (*A*) Segmental uniparental disomy resulting from mitotic recombination. Homologous chromatid exchange during somatic development is illustrated with crossing over on the short arm of chromosome 7. The 2 potential daughter cells resulting from this exchange are shown; however, only one of these cell lines is detected in this individual (the shaded cell is not detected). Alternatively, the SNP data shown are consistent with break-induced replication at the site of exchange (not illustrated). (*B*) Mitotic nondisjunction resulting in whole chromosome isodisomy. Sequential mitotic nondisjunction and selection events can result in cells with isodisomy for an entire chromosome. Note that here only trisomy rescue is illustrated, but one could also model rescue of the monosomic cell line created by the first mitotic error.

structural elements such as translocation or inversion breakpoints are known to inhibit recombination[40]; therefore, it is possible that some families may be cosegregating very large (even >10 Mb) contiguous haplotypes surrounding these rare elements.

When an LCSH detected by SNP-based microarray suggests UPD, further molecular analysis is necessary for UPD confirmation and determination of parent of origin. LCSH involving a chromosome associated with an imprinting disorder (summarized in **Table 2**) should be strongly considered for UPD confirmatory testing, particularly when the clinical features of the patient are consistent with the syndrome of interest.

In principle, definitive UPD testing requires the demonstration of uniparental inheritance of multiple informative markers for the chromosome in question. Testing typically involves genotyping microsatellite polymorphisms distributed along the length of the putative UPD chromosome in the mother, father, and proband (trio analysis).[41,42] In cases of suspected UPD for imprinted chromosomes, specific diagnostic testing of methylation patterns for the corresponding imprinting disorder may also be available.[43]

Established clinical guidelines for *whole-chromosome* UPD molecular testing[44] require at least 2 fully informative markers to establish either uniparental or biparental inheritance of a chromosome. Informative markers distinguish maternal and paternal alleles such that the parent (or parents) of origin for a chromosome segment in the proband can be unambiguously determined. Because nonpaternity can confound UPD test results, it is recommended that parentage be established by demonstrating paternal inheritance of at least 1 marker on a non-UPD chromosome. Guidelines for the analysis of *segmental* UPD have not been established. Although numerous well-defined microsatellite markers exist, this technique may not be suited for detection of segmental UPD, given that the established (clinically validated) assay may not have sufficient markers within the specific region of isodisomy to confirm a small segmental UPD. Microarray-based SNP genotyping of trios has been used to detect both whole-chromosome and segmental UPD.[45,46] This option seems especially suited for follow-up of incidental LCSH findings detected by SNP-based microarray analysis, given that this analysis already genotypes thousands of SNPs distributed along the proband's putative UPD chromosome. Were it not cost prohibitive, this technique might be used to replace the relatively inexpensive microsatellite UPD analysis.

AUTOZYGOSITY MAPPING

Regardless of whether LCSH is present as a result of consanguinity, UPD, or undetermined origin, the potential for recessive disease may be significant. The term *autozygosity* refers to homozygosity of alleles that are identical by descent (inherited from a common ancestor), as contrasted with homozygosity identical by state (random inheritance). Autozygosity mapping has been used successfully to discover the genetic basis of numerous recessive disorders in consanguineous families.[47–49] Although it is generally outside the scope of a routine diagnostic laboratory investigation to pursue gene discovery efforts, autozygosity mapping restricted to known disease genes remains a feasible and useful diagnostic tool.[50,51] When the clinical indication for study is very specific and the differential diagnosis is limited to genetically well-characterized recessive disorders, mapping candidate genes to determine location relative to LCSH segments is relatively straightforward.[48,50] Finding a gene of interest in an LCSH, although certainly not diagnostic of a homozygous mutation in that gene, may help to prioritize follow-up testing for multigenic disorders. The utility of this exercise is illustrated in the following case (Kearney H , unpublished data). SNP microarray testing for a patient with a clinical diagnosis of Usher syndrome (unknown type) revealed 4 regions of LCSH (each 3–10 Mb in length, totaling approximately 0.8% of the autosomal length). Given that Usher syndrome can result from mutations in multiple genes, all known disease-causing genes were investigated, and only one, *USH2A*, was found in an LCSH. This finding was followed by referral for *USH2A* gene sequencing, which resulted in successful identification of a homozygous pathogenic mutation in the patient (**Fig. 7**).

For cases of excessive homozygosity in which the genetic basis for the patient features is unclear, or in which limited phenotypic information is communicated to the laboratory, the referring physician can be provided with a list of candidate genes in the homozygous intervals. Further consideration of those genes associated with recessive disorders may prompt the physician to consider disorders that may not have

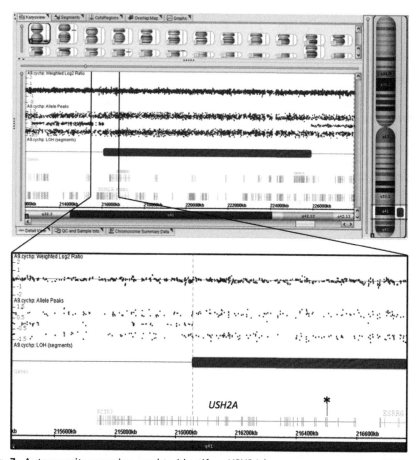

Fig. 7. Autozygosity mapping used to identify a *USH2A* homozygous mutation. *(A)* Screen shot of a 10-Mb LCSH (purple bar) on chromosome 1q seen in a patient with clinical features of Usher syndrome. This segment spans 85 genes, including *USH2A*, one of several known genes involved in the etiology of Usher syndrome. Vertical lines denote area of zoom highlighted in lower panel. *(B)* Zoomed view shows that the 1q LCSH spans only a portion of the *USH2A* gene (underscoring the utility of high-density SNP arrays for autozygosity mapping). Subsequent referral for *USH2A* gene sequencing identified a pathogenic homozygous recessive mutation (position of mutation shown as an *asterisk*).

been obvious during the initial clinical evaluation. Personal laboratory experience suggests that causative recessive gene mutations are detected through autozygosity mapping and sequence confirmation in approximately 10% of the cases reported of LCSH (Kearney and colleagues unpublished data).

SUMMARY

Given its widespread clinical use and high sensitivity for CNV detection, chromosomal microarray analysis has become an indispensible component of constitutional cytogenetic laboratory testing. SNP-based microarrays, with their added ability to detect genome-wide allele states, can also detect LCSH. Although a stand-alone finding of LCSH rarely results in a definitive diagnosis, it can trigger additional testing, potentially leading to a diagnosis of an imprinting syndrome or rare genetic recessive disorder not recognized in the original clinical differential. In addition, SNP data allow for inferences regarding complex cytogenetic mechanisms, furthering our understanding of uniparental disomy. As SNP-based arrays gain more widespread diagnostic use and more patient series are published, the clinical impact of LCSH detection will be more fully realized.

REFERENCES

1. Miller DT, Adam MP, Aradhya S, et al. Consensus statement: chromosomal microarray is a first-tier clinical diagnostic test for individuals with developmental disabilities or congenital anomalies. Am J Hum Genet 2010;86(5):749–64.
2. Manning M, Hudgins L. Array-based technology and recommendations for utilization in medical genetics practice for detection of chromosomal abnormalities. Genet Med 2010;12(11):742–5.
3. Conlin LK, Thiel BD, Bonnemann CG, et al. Mechanisms of mosaicism, chimerism and uniparental disomy identified by single nucleotide polymorphism array analysis. Hum Mol Genet 2010;19(7):1263–75.
4. Papenhausen P, Schwartz S, Risheg H, et al. UPD detection using homozygosity profiling with a SNP genotyping microarray. Am J Med Genet A 2011;155(4):757–68.
5. Nothnagel M, Lu TT, Kayser M, et al. Genomic and geographic distribution of SNP-defined runs of homozygosity in Europeans. Hum Mol Genet 2010;19(15):2927–35.
6. Gibson J, Morton NE, Collins A. Extended tracts of homozygosity in outbred human populations. Hum Mol Genet 2006;15(5):789–95.
7. McQuillan R, Leutenegger AL, Abdel-Rahman R, et al. Runs of homozygosity in European populations. Am J Hum Genet 2008;83(3):359–72.
8. Schaaf CP, Scott DA, Wiszniewska J, et al. Identification of incestuous parental relationships by SNP-based DNA microarrays. Lancet 2011;377(9765):555–56.
9. Jinawath N, Zambrano R, Wohler E, et al. Mosaic trisomy 13: understanding origin using SNP array. J Med Genet 2011;48(5):323–6.
10. Modell B, Darr A. Science and society: genetic counselling and customary consanguineous marriage. Nat Rev Genet 2002;3(3):225–9.
11. Stoll C, Alembik Y, Dott B, et al. Parental consanguinity as a cause of increased incidence of birth defects in a study of 131,760 consecutive births. Am J Med Genet 1994;49(1):114–17.
12. Stoltenberg C, Magnus P, Skrondal A, et al. Consanguinity and recurrence risk of birth defects: a population-based study. Am J Med Genet 1999;82(5):423–8.
13. Bittles AH, Black ML. Evolution in health and medicine Sackler colloquium: Consanguinity, human evolution, and complex diseases. Proc Natl Acad Sci U S A 2010;107 (Suppl 1):1779–86.

14. Leutenegger AL, Sahbatou M, Gazal S, et al. Consanguinity around the world: what do the genomic data of the HGDP-CEPH diversity panel tell us? Eur J Hum Genet 2011;19(5):583–7.
15. Engel E. A new genetic concept: uniparental disomy and its potential effect, isodisomy. Am J Med Genet 1980;6(2):137–43.
16. Spence JE, Perciaccante RG, Greig GM, et al. Uniparental disomy as a mechanism for human genetic disease. Am J Hum Genet 1988;42(2):217–26.
17. Kotzot D. Complex and segmental uniparental disomy (UPD): review and lessons from rare chromosomal complements. J Med Genet 2001;38(8):497–507.
18. Kotzot D. Complex and segmental uniparental disomy updated. J Med Genet 2008;45(9):545–56.
19. Yamazawa K, Ogata T, Ferguson-Smith AC. Uniparental disomy and human disease: an overview. Am J Med Genet C Semin Med Genet 2010;154C(3):329–34.
20. Liehr T. Cytogenetic contribution to uniparental disomy (UPD). Mol Cytogenet 2010; 3:8.
21. Robinson WP. Mechanisms leading to uniparental disomy and their clinical consequences. Bioessays 2000;22(5):452–9.
22. Engel E. Uniparental disomy revisited: the first twelve years. Am J Med Genet 1993;46(6):670–4.
23. Engel E. A fascination with chromosome rescue in uniparental disomy: Mendelian recessive outlaws and imprinting copyrights infringements. Eur J Hum Genet 2006; 14(11):1158–69.
24. Lapunzina P, Monk D. The consequences of uniparental disomy and copy number neutral loss-of-heterozygosity during human development and cancer. Biol Cell 2011;103(7):303–17.
25. Liehr T. Cases with uniparental disomy (UPD). Available at: www.med.uni-jena.de/fish/sSMC/00START-UPD.htm. Accessed July 8, 2011.
26. Morison I. Catalogue of parent of origin effects. Available at: http://igc.otago.ac.nz/home.html. Accessed July 8, 2011.
27. Robinson W. Chromosomal mosaicism; uniparental disomy. Available at: www.medgen.ubc.ca/wrobinson/mosaic/clinical/prenatal/upd.htm. Accessed July 8, 2011.
28. Jirtle RL. Geneimprint. Available at: www.geneimprint.com/site/genes-by-species. Homo+sapiens. Accessed July 8, 2011.
29. Nicholls RD, Knoll JH, Butler MG, et al. Genetic imprinting suggested by maternal heterodisomy in nondeletion Prader-Willi syndrome. Nature 1989;342(6247):281–5.
30. Kotzot D, Utermann G. Uniparental disomy (UPD) other than 15: phenotypes and bibliography updated. Am J Med Genet A 2005;136(3):287–305.
31. O'Keefe C, McDevitt MA, Maciejewski JP. Copy neutral loss of heterozygosity: a novel chromosomal lesion in myeloid malignancies. Blood 2010;115(14):2731–9.
32. Moynahan ME, Jasin M. Mitotic homologous recombination maintains genomic stability and suppresses tumorigenesis. Nat Rev Mol Cell Biol 2010;11(3):196–207.
33. Yamazawa K, Nakabayashi K, Kagami M, et al. Parthenogenetic chimaerism/mosaicism with a Silver-Russell syndrome-like phenotype. J Med Genet 2010;47(11): 782–5.
34. Strain L, Warner JP, Johnston T, et al. A human parthenogenetic chimaera. Nat Genet Oct 1995;11(2):164–9.
35. Romanelli V, Nevado J, Fraga M, et al. Constitutional mosaic genome-wide uniparental disomy due to diploidisation: an unusual cancer-predisposing mechanism. J Med Genet 2011;48(3):212–16.

36. Winberg J, Gustavsson P, Lagerstedt-Robinson K, et al. Chimerism resulting from parthenogenetic activation and dispermic fertilization. Am J Med Genet A 2010; 152A(9):2277–86.

37. Yamazawa K, Nakabayashi K, Matsuoka K, et al. Androgenetic/biparental mosaicism in a girl with Beckwith-Wiedemann syndrome-like and upd(14)pat-like phenotypes. J Hum Genet 2011;56(1):91–3.

38. Romanelli V, Meneses HN, Fernandez L, et al. Beckwith-Wiedemann syndrome and uniparental disomy 11p: fine mapping of the recombination breakpoints and evaluation of several techniques. Eur J Hum Genet 2011;19(4):416–21.

39. Choate KA, Lu Y, Zhou J, et al. Mitotic recombination in patients with ichthyosis causes reversion of dominant mutations in KRT10. Science 2010;330(6000):94–7.

40. Morel F, Laudier B, Guerif F, et al. Meiotic segregation analysis in spermatozoa of pericentric inversion carriers using fluorescence in-situ hybridization. Hum Reprod 2007;22(1):136–41.

41. Carpenter NJ, May K, Roa B, et al. Developmental disabilities. In: Leonard DGB, editor. Molecular pathology in clinical practice. 1st edition. New York: Springer; 2006. p. 73–86.

42. Giardina E, Peconi C, Cascella R, et al. A multiplex molecular assay for the detection of uniparental disomy for human chromosome 15. Electrophoresis 2008;29(23): 4775–9.

43. Pagon RA. GeneTests: an online genetic information resource for health care providers. J Med Libr Assoc 2006;94(3):343–8.

44. Shaffer LG, Agan N, Goldberg JD, et al. American College of Medical Genetics statement of diagnostic testing for uniparental disomy. Genet Med 2001;3(3):206–11.

45. Altug-Teber O, Dufke A, Poths S, et al. A rapid microarray based whole genome analysis for detection of uniparental disomy. Hum Mutat 2005;26(2):153–9.

46. Bruce S, Leinonen R, Lindgren CM, et al. Global analysis of uniparental disomy using high density genotyping arrays. J Med Genet 2005;42(11):847–51.

47. Lander ES, Botstein D. Homozygosity mapping: a way to map human recessive traits with the DNA of inbred children. Science 1987;236(4808):1567–70.

48. Alkuraya FS. Homozygosity mapping: one more tool in the clinical geneticist's toolbox. Genet Med 2010;12(4):236–39.

49. Sheffield VC, Nishimura DY, Stone EM. Novel approaches to linkage mapping. Curr Opin Genet Dev 1995;5(3):335–41.

50. Alkuraya FS. Autozygome decoded. Genet Med 2010;12(12):765–71.

51. Jiang Z. Wierenga K. Genomic oligoarray and SNP array evaluation tool v1.0. Available at: www.ccs.miami.edu/cgi-bin/ROH/ROH_analysis_tool.cgi. Accessed July 8, 2011.

52. Temple IK, Mackay DJG. Diabetes mellitus, 6q24-related transient neonatal. 1993. Available at: http://www.ncbi.nlm.nih.gov/pubmed/20301706. Accessed July 9, 2011.

53. Saal HM. Russell-Silver syndrome. 1993. Available at: http://www.ncbi.nlm.nih.gov/pubmed/20301499. Accessed July 9, 2011.

54. Shuman C, Beckwith JB, Smith AC, et al. Beckwith-Wiedemann syndrome. 1993. Available at: http://www.ncbi.nlm.nih.gov/pubmed/20301568. Accessed July 9, 2011.

55. Bullman H, Lever M, Robinson DO, et al. Mosaic maternal uniparental disomy of chromosome 11 in a patient with Silver-Russell syndrome. J Med Genet 2008;45(6): 396–99.

56. Sutton VR, Shaffer LG. Search for imprinted regions on chromosome 14: comparison of maternal and paternal UPD cases with cases of chromosome 14 deletion. Am J Med Genet 2000;93(5):381–7.
57. Murphy SK, Wylie AA, Coveler KJ, et al. Epigenetic detection of human chromosome 14 uniparental disomy. Hum Mutat 2003;22(1):92–7.
58. Kagami M, Sekita Y, Nishimura G, et al. Deletions and epimutations affecting the human 14q32.2 imprinted region in individuals with paternal and maternal upd(14)-like phenotypes. Nat Genet 2008;40(2):237–42.
59. Cotter PD, Kaffe S, McCurdy LD, et al. Paternal uniparental disomy for chromosome 14: a case report and review. Am J Med Genet 1997;70(1):74–9.
60. Dagli AI, Williams CA. Angelman syndrome. 1993. Available at: http://www.ncbi.nlm.nih.gov/pubmed/20301323. Accessed July 9, 2011.
61. Cassidy SB, Schwartz S. Prader-Willi syndrome. 1993. Available at: http://www.ncbi.nlm.nih.gov/pubmed/20301505. July 9, 2011.
62. Bastepe M, Lane AH, Juppner H. Paternal uniparental isodisomy of chromosome 20q—and the resulting changes in GNAS1 methylation—as a plausible cause of pseudohypoparathyroidism. Am J Hum Genet 2001;68(5):1283–9.
63. Lecumberri B, Fernandez-Rebollo E, Sentchordi L, et al. Coexistence of two different pseudohypoparathyroidism subtypes (Ia and Ib) in the same kindred with independent Gs{alpha} coding mutations and GNAS imprinting defects. J Med Genet 2010;47(4):276–80.

Laboratory Aspects of Prenatal Microarray Analysis

Allen N. Lamb, PhD[a,b,*]

KEYWORDS

- Array comparative genomic hybridization
- Prenatal microarrays • Maternal cell contamination
- Amniocytes • Chorionic villi • Abnormal ultrasound

The recent development and clinical implementation of array comparative genomic hybridization (aCGH) or microarrays has resulted in the most rapid and significant changes in the field of cytogenetics since the development of reliable chromosome banding techniques in the 1970s. aCGH detects gains and losses, which are referred to as copy number variations (CNVs), the size of which is determined by the array design[1] (see "Prenatal Array Design" section).

The widespread use of arrays for postnatal cases has revealed many additional abnormalities that were not detectable by G-banded analysis and has altered the view of the extent of the causes of developmental delay, intellectual disability, multiple congenital anomalies, and autism. This has led to the recognition of new microdeletion and microduplication syndromes (see the article by Deak and colleagues elsewhere in this issue), and that the segmental duplication structure of the genome results in nonallelic homologous recombination (NAHR) that causes these genomic disorders.[2–5] Analysis of multiple published studies shows that arrays increase the detection rate of clinically significant abnormalities above standard karyotyping by 10% to 15%[6] and has led to the recommendation that microarray analysis should be a first-tier test.[6,7] Microarrays also have an added benefit of providing a quantitative assessment of the genome, as opposed to the more subjective, qualitative approach with the historical standard of G-banded karyotypes, thus reducing errors or false-negative results. These false-negative

The author was an employee of Signature Genomics, a PerkinElmer, Inc. company that performs prenatal and postnatal microarray analysis, when the majority of this review was written.

[a] Cytogenetics and Genomic Microarray Laboratory, ARUP Institute for Clinical and Experimental Pathology, Salt Lake City, UT, USA

[b] Department of Pathology, University of Utah Health Sciences Center, Salt Lake City, UT 84108, USA

* Corresponding author. ARUP Laboratories, MS 115-H01, 500 Chipeta Way, Salt Lake City, UT 84108-1221.

E-mail address: allen.n.lamb@aruplab.com

results occur more frequently than most clinicians are aware of and are seen in both postnatal and prenatal studies.

The current use of prenatal aCGH has been mostly limited to follow-up of a normal traditional karyotype in cases with an abnormal ultrasound, usually associated with multiple congenital anomalies, and for the further definition of cytogenetic abnormalities, such as unbalanced translocations, marker chromosomes, and checking for losses/gains at the breakpoints of reciprocal translocations. However, the yield for specific ultrasound abnormalities and other indications, such as maternal serum screen positive cases and advanced maternal age (AMA), has not been defined. Therefore, more studies are needed before aCGH becomes a first-tier test for prenatal genetic diagnosis. There is no consensus on what are we trying to achieve in prenatal genetic diagnosis owing to these recent changes in technology. Until recently, the range of genetic abnormalities had been defined by maternal serum screening programs, which includes trisomy 21 and other major aneuploidies. This large-genome-rearrangement view has led some to argue for the use of more rapid aneuploidy screens (fluorescence in situ hybridization [FISH], quantitative fluorescent polymerase chain reaction [QF-PCR], multiplex ligation-dependent probe amplification [MLPA]), and even forgoing traditional karyotype analysis if ultrasound findings are normal, as a cost-effective and adequate testing strategy in the current climate of increasing health care costs.[8,9] But this approach does not allow detection of the newer microdeletion/microduplication syndromes that have been discovered recently, and thus will not impact many of the cases of developmental delay, intellectual disability, multiple congenital anomalies, and autism that are seen in the postnatal population.[2] There is currently no way to find and concentrate these newer abnormalities in the prenatal population, as maternal serum screening has done for trisomy 21 and other aneuploidies.

One of the major concerns for the use of aCGH in the prenatal genetic diagnosis is the findings of variants of unknown/uncertain/unclear significance[10,11] (the term variant of unknown significance [VUS] is used in this article). Many clinicians and genetic counselors would like to keep the VUS to a minimum in prenatal cases. Unlike prenatal cases, postnatal cases with a VUS can wait for the accumulation of evidence that can demonstrate correlation or greatly reduce the likelihood of clinical significance over several months or years as additional studies are completed and published. One of the key steps for determining the clinical significance of a postnatal VUS is not the determination of inheritance, but rather the comparison of the frequencies of a CNV in a patient and normal control populations.[3,4] However, with current databases this approach is at present not possible for many CNVs, and it may not be efficient with the limited time available in the context of prenatal diagnosis.

There have been several recent reviews on the role of aCGH in prenatal studies and the reader may wish to consult these for other details not covered in this review.[10,12–14]

PRENATAL SAMPLE TYPES AND LABORATORY PROCESSING

Amniotic fluid cells, or amniocytes, obtained by amniocentesis, and chorionic villus cells, obtained by transcervical or transabdominal sampling, are the main source of cells for prenatal chromosome and microarray analysis.[15,16] The cells obtained may be used for direct analysis or set up in culture to get dividing cells and to increase the total number of cells available for testing.

There are expectations that prenatal aCGH will result in more rapid turnaround time (TAT) by eliminating the need for tissue culture and decreasing the labor involved when compared to traditional cytogenetic analysis. Although TAT will be more rapid for the majority of cases by direct analysis, culturing will be needed on a percentage of cases. Cultures will be needed when direct extractions yield insufficient or poor quality DNA. In addition, some cases may require FISH follow-up to visualize the rearrangement; for example, determining a tandem versus insertional event for a gain, or an unbalanced translocation or derivative chromosome versus a separate gain and loss.

Therefore, laboratories may want to develop protocols to have backup cultures and then discard them if not needed (which incurs added expense in time and materials), or alternatively, to hold material and set up in culture only if needed (which results in longer TAT).

For cases with direct analysis, if results of adequate quality are obtained and FISH is needed, a preliminary report may be issued as it would take additional time before cells can be grown and harvested for FISH analysis to be performed. In the early months and years of a laboratory's experience with prenatal aCGH, a number of cases and a comfort level may need to be reached before culturing becomes a minor part of the prenatal aCGH process.

Amniocytes

The experience gained over the years for use in traditional chromosome and FISH analyses for uncultured and cultured cells is very useful for aCGH studies.[17] Amniocyte quantity is assessed after centrifugation and by gross examination of the cell pellet. This also allows for the assessment of the amount of blood present in the sample, usually of maternal origin. Based on examination of samples used for classic cytogenetics and for rapid aneuploidy assays, the cell pellet size varies from sample to sample and by gestational age (generally increasing with increasing gestational age).

For traditional cytogenetic analysis, cell culture of amniocytes is needed. Only a subset of the total cell population will attach and grow in culture. Amniocyte cultures usually yield a better quality and quantity of DNA for aCGH as compared to extraction of direct amniocytes.

Experience with prenatal aCGH demonstrates that 7 to 10 mL of amniotic fluid should provide enough amniocytes to yield a sufficient quantity and quality of DNA to perform aCGH on the direct extraction for most cases. However, samples and DNA yields from extractions are variable and at times an insufficient quantity or quality of DNA is obtained. This may be particularly challenging for samples less than 16 weeks gestational age. Therefore, for a certain percentage of cases (not yet defined due to the limited number of published cases on directs), amniocytes must be grown in culture to provide adequate material to perform aCGH and provide material for metaphase FISH analysis.

Chorionic Villi

For chorionic villus sampling (CVS), careful dissection of villi from maternal decidua is important. Villi are composed of (1) an outer layer with trophoblasts that are spontaneously dividing and used for direct chromosome analysis and (2) inner core of mesenchymal cells that are enzymatically separated (digested) and grown in culture.

There is an important distinction between a direct study for a traditional chromosome analysis and a direct for a microarray analysis with CVS. For a cytogenetic analysis, the direct uses the spontaneously dividing trophoblasts, and the culture uses the mesenchymal core cells. For aCGH, the direct is a proteinase K digestion of both the trophoblastic and mesenchymal core cells. This difference in a direct for traditional cytogenetic analysis and for an array analysis is important to remember when abnormal results are obtained and explanations and additional testing are being considered.

The trophoblasts are not as closely representative of the fetus as are the mesenchymal core cells. In addition, both layers may also have chromosomal changes that are not seen in the fetus, referred to as confined placental mosaicism (CPM).[18] For cytogenetic analysis, if there are discrepancies between the direct and culture results, an amniocentesis is often performed, as amniocytes are usually more representative of the fetus. The algorithm to use for possible mosaicism or CPM with aCGH has not been established because of limited published studies with CVS, but the lessons learned from classic cytogenetics are likely to be the most important guide (eg, see Refs.[19,20]).

MATERNAL CELL CONTAMINATION

Maternal cell contamination (MCC) has only rarely been a problem in traditional cytogenetic analysis with cultured amniocytes, but there has been an increased concern in cultured CVS. MCC has been of more concern in assays that use uncultured amniocytes and direct CVS. Direct amniotic fluid has a greater chance of MCC because of the presence of blood (usually of maternal origin), and direct CVS may also have some contaminating maternal decidua present.

For amniocytes, the amount of maternal blood is best visualized when cells are centrifuged. Occasionally, maternal fibroblasts may also be present, but cannot be visually detected (usually picked up during the amniocentesis, and if the first part of draw is not omitted, these maternal cells may end up with the fetal cells). Once amniocytes are cultured, the maternal blood does not present problems from an MCC perspective; however, maternal fibroblasts, although not usually presenting problems for in situ culture techniques owing to the low level, may become a problem when expanded with subculturing.

For CVS, samples vary in the ease to clean maternal decidua from the villi, and laboratories vary in the skill of performing this identification and cleaning. In general, with good technique, MCC is rarely an issue during cytogenetic analysis for most laboratories. However, if subculturing is needed, a very low level of maternal cells may be expanded and interfere with obtaining the correct diagnosis.

In contrast to classic cytogenetic analysis, DNA-based testing for MCC (usually STR-based markers) is routinely performed in many laboratories for molecular mutation detection of single genes in prenatal diagnosis. The risk for MCC is especially of concern when PCR-based tests are involved, owing to the risk of preferential amplification and over-representation of maternal DNA.[21,22]

As many view aCGH as a cytogenetic test, there has been a tendency to rarely request MCC on most prenatal aCGH tests, especially those involving amniocytes. ACGH is currently performed after traditional cytogenetic analysis and requires the additional expansion of cultures to obtain sufficient DNA, and the length of time in culture and the amount of subculturing can significantly expand an initial low level of maternal cells. **Table 1** presents some data from our laboratory (Signature Genomics) over a period of several months and shows that the rate of MCC was approximately 1% for amniocyte cultures and approximately 4% for CVS cultures. As expected, there is a higher level of MCC in CVS cultures than in amniocyte cultures.

Does the presence of any level of MCC potentially invalidate the aCGH result or can copy number gains or losses still be detected accurately in the presence of various levels of MCC? There are no published studies that systematically examine the effects of different levels of MCC on different sized CNVs in aCGH. A potential source of information is studies of mosaicism, and these suggest that levels of a second cell line

Table 1		
Detection of MCC in 466 prenatal samples		
	Total Cases	MCC Detected (%)
Cultured amniocytes	327	3 (0.9)
Cultured CVS	139	6 (4.3)

as low as 10% may be occasionally be detected; however, more consistent detection is in the 20% to 30% range.[23–25] This information implies that if an abnormality is present, it may still be detected even in the presence of significant MCC. But a more important question may be at what level of MCC is an abnormality covered up and not detected? Does this differ for deletions versus duplications and for CNVs of different sizes? For example, is a smaller deletion covered up by a lower percentage of MCC than a larger deletion?

Preliminary unpublished studies performed in our laboratory (Signature Genomics) suggest that a large deletion of 2.5 Mb (eg, the DiGeorge syndrome [DGS]/velocardiofacial syndrome [VCFS] region) can be detected at a higher level of MCC than the same size duplication. This is expected owing to the differences in the log 2 ratio shifts for a deletion (2:1) compared to a duplication (2:3); therefore, a duplication is covered up by a lower level of MCC.

Small deletions in the range of 75 to 100 kb are covered up by lower levels of MCC than are larger deletions. Although the lower limits of size and level of MCC have not been systematically determined for duplications, preliminary data suggest this is likely to be in the 15% to 20% range. The lower limits may also be somewhat variable depending on the quality of the DNA and the experimental noise, so once the MCC level is above 10% there is always the possibility that a small, clinically significant duplication within a gene could be missed. Levels of MCC less than 10% appear not to interfere with detection of small abnormalities, but as platforms become more gene- and exon-centric, this low level may be of concern with prenatal use.

An MCC assay that is quantitative, as some laboratories have validated for opposite sex bone marrow transplants, is more useful as opposed to a simple presence/absence approach. If there is less than 10% MCC present, there is probably little concern, as seen in our preliminary unpublished studies. There is more concern when the amount approaches the 15% to 20% range, and the aCGH results should probably be considered invalidated.

Although most clinicians acknowledge the need for MCC studies for female fetuses, they often do not order the testing for a male fetus, as it is assumed that aCGH testing will readily detect the presence of any maternal DNA. However, preliminary data suggest that we may not be able to detect 10% to 15% MCC in a male fetus in some experiments, seen as a shift in the X and Y chromosome plots (potentially a low-level mosaic gain of X and loss of Y probes). This is the range of MCC that could possibly cover up the presence of a small duplication, which is especially concerning if completely within a gene. Therefore, although this risk may be low, it appears that something clinically significant could potentially be missed in a male fetus and we would not be aware of the contaminating MCC.

The preceding discussion is based on the assumption that a DNA amplification step is not involved. However, SNP-based arrays that use an amplification step will be more sensitive to small amounts of contaminating maternal DNA. This may limit the testing on direct samples with a SNP-based platform, as the presence of any contaminating maternal DNA would invalidate the array results. It could also present problems for testing for some CVS cultures that have been repeatedly expanded.

MCC should be performed on the same DNA extraction as used for the array; if the array needs to be repeated on a new DNA extraction, then the MCC analysis should also be performed on the new extraction as maternal cells may be expanded with additional subculturing.

Samples from pregnancies with oligohydramnios appear to have a higher risk for MCC, where approximately 10% of cases obtained by amniocentesis may have overwhelming MCC.[26] Such samples usually do not show evidence of blood contamination and the origin and type of maternal cell is not clear.

PRENATAL ARRAY DESIGN

An optimal design for a prenatal array has not been agreed upon. Most laboratories now use an oligonucleotide-based array. The size, number, and spacing of probes both within genes and for intergenic regions determine the size of CNVs that can be detected. Most platforms tend to have coverage that is denser in regions of known microdeletion and microduplication syndromes, and for genes known to be associated with clinical disease. Some platforms also provide more coverage in telomeric and around centromeric regions. Platforms often differ by the density of oligonucleotide probe coverage in the intergenic regions and the regions between known syndromes, but this most likely does not result in major differences in the ability to detect clinically significant CNVs. Some off-the-shelf platforms have equally dense spacing throughout the genome and do not vary the spacing by biological importance.

There is a desire to balance the ability to detect small clinically significant copy number changes and minimize the finding of VUS.[10,11] This balance is difficult to achieve because of the general observation that as the resolution of the array increases so do the number of VUS. It may be useful to have more than one basic platform design depending on the clinical indication. If there is a higher likelihood of detecting a small clinically significant CNV, then a design with denser probe coverage may be a better choice, for example, for ultrasound abnormalities or a known cytogenetic rearrangement. However, the higher density array will have a potentially higher VUS detection rate. For an indication with a lower likelihood of a significant CNV, such as advanced maternal age or for a couple with a low tolerance for results of unknown significance, then a less dense design may be more appropriate to minimize the detection of a VUS.

As a demonstration of different density platforms, **Table 2** shows the detection rate for clinically significant findings and for VUS for prenatal cases run over several months in our laboratory (Signature Genomics) on a dense platform (135K features) and for a less dense platform (55K). This shows that by reducing the coverage in the backbone, fewer VUS are encountered. The goal is to reduce

Table 2			
Detection rate (%) for clinically significant findings and VUS on two different density platforms			
	No. of Cases	Abnormal, Clinically Significant (%)	VUS (%)
55K	203	7 (3.4)	11 (5.4)
135K	362	20 (5.5)	34 (9.4)

further the number of VUS encountered without reducing the detection of small, clinically significant CNVs. This will require a platform with the flexibility to move the oligonucleotide probes around, or with the ability to mask data from certain probes if the basic platform is not flexible. The occurrence of a VUS cannot be eliminated completely because the clinical significance is not known for the reciprocal duplication of some microdeletion syndromes. For example, while the phenotype of the 15q13.3 microdeletion syndrome is established, the clinical significance of the reciprocal duplication is not.[27]

LIMITATIONS OF ACGH

SNP-based platforms can provide genotypic information and will provide detection of triploids and tetraploids, which will be important when aCGH replaces the traditional karyotype as a first-tier test. Copy number only platforms cannot detect female triploids, whereas male triploids can be detected as a partial gain of the X chromosome and a partial loss of the Y chromosome; these appear to be low level mosaicism of the sex chromosomes, and would lead to additional studies to define the observation further. Mosaicism should potentially be easier to detect with an SNP platform. However, whether an SNP platform is also capable of detecting low levels of MCC has not yet been systematically evaluated.

Neither copy number nor SNP platforms can detect balanced rearrangements, such as reciprocal translocations and inversions, but they should detect any gain or losses near the breakpoints.

DETERMINING THE SIGNIFICANCE OF CNVs

The interpretation of the clinical significance of CNVs is based on the experience gained from postnatal cases. These studies have discovered and characterized new microdeletion/microduplication syndromes and identified single dosage sensitive genes.[2,3] Various algorithms for determining the clinical significance of unknown CNVs have been published (eg, Ref.[6]), but these are generally of limited help as not much is known about the role of most of the genes in the genome in causing human disease. A lack of information about genes does not mean that the gene has no role in causing human disease, but that its role is currently unknown. Most algorithms include parental studies as a key to determining clinical significance. However, experience now shows that inheritance does not determine the significance of a CNV for the individual case, but requires the comparison of the frequency of the CNV in a patient population to that in a control population.[3] The difficulty in determining the clinical significance of CNVs is the reason many clinicians favor a design for microarrays that will minimize the detection of a VUS in prenatal studies.[10,11] Databases are good for collating both pathogenic and common CNVs, but until the numbers of patient and control samples are very large, these will be less helpful for helping us decide the clinical significance of rare CNVs.

VALIDATION AND GUIDELINES FOR PRENATAL aCGH

Validation guidelines are currently available only for postnatal arrays,[28] and these will have to serve as a guide until prenatal guidelines are developed. Separate validations should be performed for different sample types and this would include validation studies for cultured amniocytes and cultured CVS, as well as direct (uncultured) amniocytes and direct CVS. Other less common prenatal sample types include cystic hygroma fluid, fetal urine from a bladder tap, and fluid from a plural effusion. As these specimens are only rarely seen in the cytogenetics laboratory, it would be difficult to obtain a sufficient number of cases to perform the same level of validation as for the more common sample types. As amniocytes are a mixed population of cells from many sources,[17] these rarer sample types may be best viewed as an amniotic fluid sample, and depending on whether done as a direct or as a culture. Fetal blood would be considered the same sample type as postnatal blood samples and should not require a separate validation study, but other College of American Pathologists/American College of Medical Genetics guidelines require evidence of fetal origin.

American College of Obstetricians and Gynecologists (ACOG) has issued guidelines for the use of aCGH in prenatal studies.[29] Based on the limited published experience, these recommend arrays only after traditional cytogenetic analysis on pregnancies with abnormal anatomic findings by ultrasound or in cases of fetal demise and congenital anomalies where a traditional karyotype has failed. However, if cells fail to grow in culture, will the DNA quality be adequate for aCGH?

PUBLISHED LITERATURE ON PRENATAL MICROARRAYS

The total number of prenatal cases in the published literature is still fewer than 1000 cases, with the single largest study of 300. Most of these studies are covered in a recent review with a meta-analysis and can be consulted for more detailed information.[30] This is currently the best summary to attempt to glean information about which clinical indications will yield abnormal results for aCGH until a large National Institute of Child Health and Human Development (NICHD) funded prospective study with more than 4000 patients undergoing concurrent karyotyping and microarray analysis is completed in late-2011.[31] Other recent prenatal microarray summaries may be found in Refs.[32,33]

Some of these individual prenatal array studies and the abnormality detection rates are listed in **Table 3**. These studies differ in the percentage of cases with various indications, as well as with the classification of CNVs that are clinically significant and of unknown clinical significance, making all but general conclusions difficult. Even the large meta-analysis tends to favor the assumption that inherited CNVs are benign whereas the de novo ones are more likely clinically significant.[30] However, experience now shows that the issues surrounding CNV inheritance are much more complex and that penetrance, variable expression, and second hits or point mutations in other genes also may play a role, so determination of inheritance does not tend to be informative for most CNVs in individual cases.[3,4]

Based on the meta-analysis,[30] these studies suggest that the additional abnormality detection rate beyond traditional karyotyping for all clinical indications is 3.6% (95% confidence interval [CI], 1.5–8.5), and may be as high as 5.2% (95% CI, 1.9–13.9) if just structural abnormalities detected by ultrasound are considered.

Table 3
Published prenatal microarray studies and clinically significant detection rates

References	No. of Cases	Pathogenic CNVs (%)
Sahoo et al[34]	98	5 (5.1)
Shaffer et al[35]	151	2 (1.3)
van der Veyver et al[36]	289	4 (1.4)
Coppinger et al[37]	244	7 (2.9)
Kleeman et al[38]	50	1 (2)
Tyreman et al[39]	106	10 (9.4)

Results of unknown significance are listed as approximately 1% overall and 2% in cases of ultrasound abnormalities, which are most likely biased underestimates.

It is hoped that the NICHD study[31] will provide sufficient information for the detection rates for many of the indications, such as AMA, abnormal maternal serum screen, and some specific ultrasound abnormalities. However, more studies are needed to provide rates for some of the less frequent ultrasound findings.

It is currently thought that many of the microdeletion/microduplication cases will not have associated ultrasound abnormalities. However, knowing a clinically significant CNV is present in a fetus may lead to more careful and focused ultrasound examinations based on what is known about the postnatal phenotype associated with the CNV. The prenatal presentation may also have unexpected findings owing to the broad range of variable features that may be associated with different syndromes.

PRODUCTS OF CONCEPTION

There are insufficient studies on products of conception (POCs) to determine how significant smaller CNVs will be, in addition to the major aneuploidies, in playing a role in pregnancy loss.[12,13] It is also hoped that aCGH will be successful on a higher percentage of cases than traditional cytogenetic analysis, as many POC cases fail to grow in culture due to cell death and contamination. However, it has not yet been shown that DNA quality will be adequate for aCGH to be successful on a significant proportion of these growth failure cases.

GENETIC COUNSELING ISSUES

The issues arising from prenatal aCGH are more complicated than traditional karyotyping because of the reporting of a variant of unknown significance. These cause concerns for the clinician, genetic counselor, and patient. Even with known microdeletion/microduplication syndromes, the counseling issues are complicated because of the large number of these syndromes that have highly variable features.[2,3] These uncertainties were encountered much less frequently with traditional cytogenetics and FISH, with examples provided by the 22q11.2 duplication and with mosaicism, especially for sex chromosomes and supernumerary marker chromosomes. These issues will become more comfortable in prenatal genetic counseling, as it is for those doing postnatal counseling, as experience and familiarity is gained with these syndromes and issues. Some of the counseling issues have been more fully explored,[40] but additional studies are needed in this area.

SUMMARY

Medical science is at an interesting stage for the introduction of aCGH in prenatal genetic diagnosis. The value of aCGH after traditional chromosome analysis has been demonstrated for the indications of abnormal ultrasound and as follow-up to an abnormal karyotype that needs further characterization (for examples, see **Figs. 1–4**). Sufficient data is not available to make aCGH a first-tier test for prenatal genetic diagnosis as it is for postnatal cases, but it is expected that sufficient data will be collected over the upcoming months that will allow recommendations to be made. Most of the lessons learned from traditional cytogenetics and FISH will be important to build upon and provide guidance over the next couple of years as more experience is gained with prenatal microarrays.

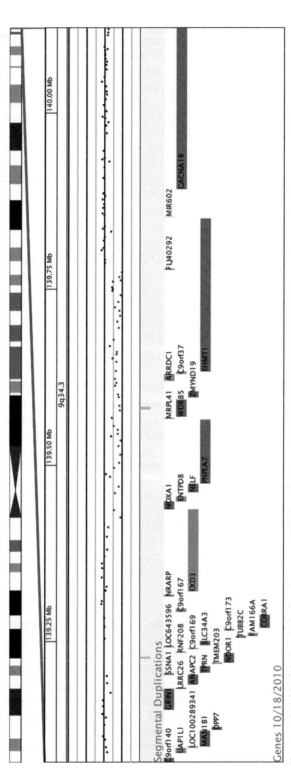

Fig. 1. A 348-kb deletion includes the gene *EHMT1* at 9q34 : arr 9q34.3(139,426,567-139,774,589)x1. Abnormal ultrasound with findings of bilateral clubbing, two vessel cord, and choroid plexus cysts in a male fetus with a normal karyotype. DNA was isolated from cultured amniocytes. For clinical information associated with a deletion of *EHMT1*, see Ref.[41] and OMIM 607001. (*Courtesy of* Signature Genomics, Inc., Spokane, WA)

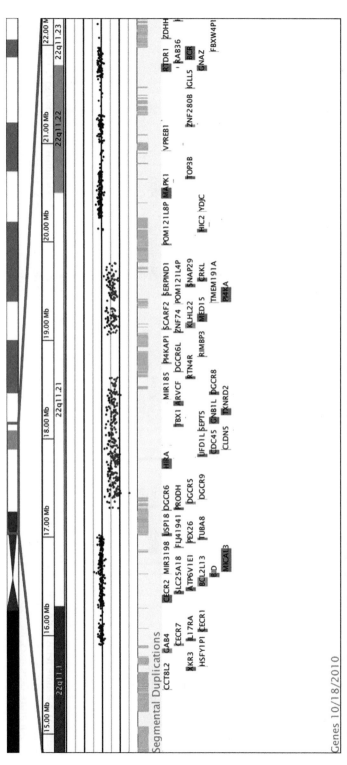

Fig. 2. The commonly observed deletion of the DGS/VCFS region at 22q11.21: arr22q11.21(17,299,469-19,790,658)x1. Abnormal ultrasound findings of lemon sign, small cerebellum, and prominent lateral ventricle in a male fetus with a normal karyotype. DNA was isolated from cultured amniocytes. This clinical finding would not lead to the ordering of a FISH probe to the DGS/VCFS region. (*Courtesy of Signature Genomics, Inc., Spokane, WA*)

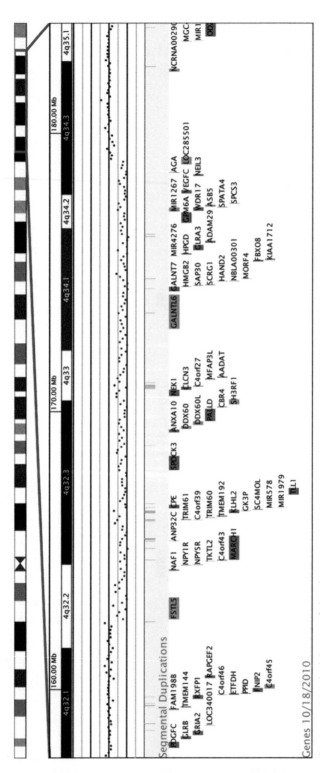

Fig. 3. A 16.5-Mb deletion of the chromosome 4 long arm: arr 4q32.2q34.3(162,531,081-178,999,152)x1. Abnormal ultrasound findings of anasarca (edema) in a male fetus. DNA was isolated from cultured amniocytes. Karyotype was reported as normal, but the deletion is large enough to be seen on a 400–450 G-banded analysis. There is an extensive literature available for this region to provide clinical information for counseling: see Ref.[42] (Courtesy of Signature Genomics, Inc., Spokane, WA)

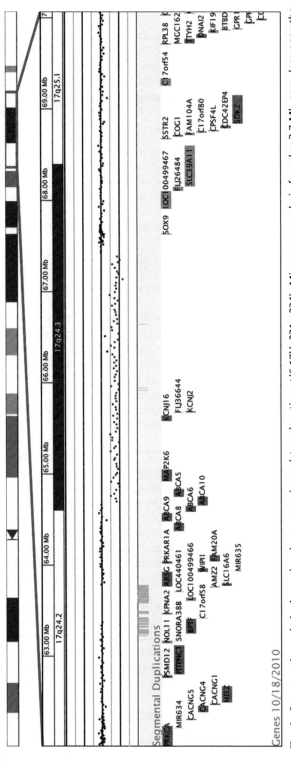

Fig. 4. Cytogenetic analysis showed a de novo reciprocal translocation: t(6;17)(q221;q?24). Microarray analysis found a 2.7-Mb copy loss near the chromosome 17 breakpoint: arr 17q24.3(64,700,993-67,389,251)x1. Abnormal ultrasound findings of micrognathia in a female fetus. DNA from cultured CVS. The deleted region is just proximal to SOX9 and is a control region that affects expression of this gene; some interruptions of this region have been associated with campomelic dysplasia (CD). For clinical information associated with CD, see Ref.[43] and OMIM 608160 and 114290. (*Courtesy of Signature Genomics, Inc., Spokane, WA*)

ACKNOWLEDGMENTS

The author's experience and some of the data presented in this review were developed while employed as a Laboratory Director at Signature Genomics, a PerkinElmer company in Spokane, Washington. The author is grateful for many discussions with the laboratory staff, genetic counselors, and laboratory directors at Signature Genomics, especially Justine Coppinger for many discussions and the preliminary data in **Tables 1** and **2** and Dr Beth Torchia for technical discussions.

REFERENCES

1. Lee C, Scherer SW. The clinical context of copy number variation in the human genome. Expert Rev Mol Med 2010;12:e8.
2. Mefford HC, Eichler EE. Duplication hotspots, rare genomic disorders, and common disease. Curr Opin Genet Dev 2009;19:196–204.
3. Girirajan S, Eichler E. Phenotypic variability and genetic susceptibility to genomic disorders. Hum Mol Genet 2010;19:R176–87.
4. Sharp AJ. Emerging themes and new challenges in defining the role of structural variation in human disease. Hum Mutat 2009;30:135–44.
5. Stankiewicz P, Lupski JR. Structural variation in the human genome and its role in disease. Annu Rev Med 2010;61:437–55.
6. Miller DT, Adam MP, Aradhya S, et al. Consensus statement: chromosomal microarray is a first-tier clinical diagnostic test for individuals with developmental disabilities or congenital anomalies. Am J Hum Genet 2010;86:749–64.
7. Manning M, Hudgins L. Array based technology and recommendations for utilization in medical genetics practice for detection of chromosomal abnormalities (ACMG Practice Guidelines). Genet Med 2010;12:742–5.
8. Ogilvie CM, Yaron Y, Beaudet AL. Currrent controversies in prenatal diagnosis: 3: For prenatal diagnosis, should we offer less or more than metaphase karyotyping? Prenat Diag 2009;29:11–4.
9. Gerkas J, van den Berg DG, Durand A, et al. Rapid testing versus karyotyping in Down's syndrome screening: cost-effectiveness and detection of clinically significant chromosome abnormalities. Eur J Hum Genet 2011;19:3–9.
10. Friedman JM. High-resolution array genomic hybridization in prenatal diagnosis. Prenat Diagn 2009;29:20–8.
11. Pergament E. Controversies and challenges of array comparative genomic hybridization in prenatal genetic diagnosis. Genet Med 2007;9:596–9.
12. Veermeech JR. Prenatal diagnosis by microaray analysis. In: Milunsky A, Milunsky J, editors. Genetic disorders and the fetus. 6th edition. West Sussex (UK): Wiley-Blackwell; 2010. p. 365–79.
13. Savage MS, Mourad MJ, Wapner RJ. Evolving applications of microarray analysis in prenatal diagnosis. Curr Opin Obstet Gynecol 2011;23:103–8.
14. Fruhman G, van der Veyver IB. Applications of Array comparative genomic hybridization in obstetrics. Obstet Gynecol Clin North Am 2010;37:71–85.
15. Elias S. Amniocentesis and fetal blood sampling. In: Milunsky A, Milunsky J, editors. Genetic disorders and the fetus. 6th edition. West Sussex (UK): Wiley-Blackwell; 2010. p. 63–93.
16. Monni G, Ibba RM, ZoppiMA. Prenatal genetic diagnosis through chorionic villous sampling. In: Milunsky A, Milunsky J, editors. Genetic disorders and the fetus. 6th edition. West Sussex (UK): Wiley-Blackwell; 2010. p. 160–93.

17. van Dyke DL. Amniotic fluid cell culture. In: Milunsky A, Milunsky J, editors. Genetic disorders and the fetus. 6th edition. West Sussex (UK): Wiley-Blackwell; 2010. p. 138–59.

18. Kalousek DK, Vekemans M. Confined placental mosaicism. J Med Genet 1996;33: 529–33.

19. Hahnemann JM, Vejerslev LO. Accuracy of cytogenetic findings on chorionic villus sampling (CVS)—Diagnostic consequences of CVS mosaicism and non-mosaic discrepancy in centres contributing to EUCROMIC 1986–1992. 1997;17:801–20.

20. Smith K, Lowther G, Maher E, et al. The predictive value of findings of the common aneuploidies, trisomies 13, 18, and 21, and numerical sex chromosome abnormalities at CVS: experience from the ACC U.K. collaborative study. Prenat Diag 1999;19:817–26.

21. Nagan N, Faulkner NE, Curtis C, et al. Laboratory guidelines for detection, interpretation, and reporting of maternal cell contamination in prenatal analyses a report of the association for molecular pathology. J Mol Diagn 2011;13:7–11.

22. Schrijver I, Cherny SC, Zehnder JL. Testing for maternal cell contamination in prenatal samples: a comprehensive survey of current diagnostic practices in 35 molecular diagnostic laboratories. J Mol Diagn 2007;9:394–400.

23. Ballif BC, Rorem EA, Sundin K, et al. Detection of low-level mosaicism by array CGH in routine diagnostic specimens. Am J Med Genet A 2006;140:2757–67.

24. Cheung SW, Shaw CA, Scott DA, et al. Microarray-based CGH detects chromosomal mosaicism not revealed by conventional cytogenetics. Am J Med Genet A 2007;143: 1679–86.

25. Scott SA, Cohen N, Brandt T, et al. Detection of low-level mosaicism and placental mosaicism by oligonucleotide array comparative genomic hybridization. Genet Med 2010;12:85–92.

26. Estabrooks LL, Sanford Hanna J, Lamb AN. Overwhelming maternal cell contamination in amniotic fluid samples from patients with oligohydramnios can lead to false prenatal interphase FISH results. Prenat Diagn 1999;19:179–81.

27. van Bon BW, Mefford HC, Menten B, et al. Further delineation of the 15q13 microdeletion and duplication syndromes: a clinical spectrum varying from non-pathogenic to a severe outcome. J Med Genet 2009;46:511–23.

28. Shaffer LG, Beaudet AL, Brothman AR, et al. Microarray analysis for constitutional cytogenetic abnormalities. Genet Med 2007;9:654–62.

29. ACOG Committee Opinion No. 446: Array comparative genomic hybridization in prenatal diagnosis. Obstet Gynecol 2009;114:1161–3.

30. Hillman SC, Pretlove S, Coormarasamy A, et al. Additional information from array comparative hybridization technology over conventional karyotyping in prenatal diagnosis: a systematic review and meta-analysis. Ultrasound Obstet Gynecol 2011; 37:6–14.

31. Savage MS, Mourad MJ, Wapner RJ. Evolving applications of microarray analysis in prenatal diagnosis. Curr Opin Obstet Gynecol 2011;23:103–8.

32. Veermeesch JR. Prenatal diagnosis by microarray analysis. In: Milunsky A, Milunsky J, editors. Genetic disorders and the fetus. 6th edition. West Sussex (UK): Wiley-Blackwell; 2010. p. 365–79.

33. Fruhman G, van den Veyver IB. Applications of array comparative genomic hybridization in obstetrics. Obstet Gynecol Clin North Am 2010; 37:71–85.

34. Sahoo T, Cheung SW, Ward P, et al. Prenatal diagnosis of chromosomal abnormalities using array-based comparative genomic hybridization. Genet Med 2006; 8:719–27.

35. Shaffer LG, Coppinger J, Alliman S, et al. Comparison of microarray-based detection rates for cytogenetic abnormalities in prenatal and neonatal specimens. Prenat Diagn 2008; 28:789–95.

36. Van den Veyver IB, Patel A, Shaw CA, et al. Clinical use of array comparative genomic hybridization (aCGH) for prenatal diagnosis in 300 cases. Prenat Diagn 2009;29:29–39.

37. Coppinger J, Alliman S, Lamb AN, et al. Whole-genome microarray analysis in prenatal specimens identifies clinically significant chromosome alterations without increase in results of unclear significance compared to targeted microarray. Prenat Diagn 2009; 29:1156–66.

38. Kleeman L, Bianchi D, Shaffer LG, et al. Use of array comparative genomic hybridization for prenatal diagnosis of fetuses with sonographic anomalies and normal metaphase karyotype. Prenat Diagn 2009;29:1213–7.

39. Tyreman M, Abbott KM, Willatt LR, et al. High resolution array analysis: diagnosing pregnancies with abnormal ultrasound findings. J Med Genet 2009;46:531–41.

40. Darilek S, Ward P, Pursley A, et al. Pre- and postnatal genetic testing by array-comparative genomic hybridization: genetic counseling issues. Genet Med 2008;10: 13–8.

41. Kleefstra T, van Zelst-Stams WA, Nillesen WM, et al. Further clinical and molecular delineation of the 9q subtelomeric deletion syndrome supports a major contribution of EHMT1 haploinsufficiency to the core phenotype. J Med Genet 2009;46:598–606.

42. Tzaschach A, Menzel C, Erdogan F, et al. Characterization of an interstitial 4q32 deletion in a patient with mental retardation and a complex chromosome rearrangement. Am J Med Genet 2010;152A:1008–12.

43. Leipoldt M, Erdel M, Bien-Willner GA, et al. Two novel translocation breakpoints upstream of SOX9 define borders of the proximal and distal breakpoint cluster region in campomelic dysplasia. Clin Genet 2007;71:67–75.

Acute Lymphoblastic Leukemia

Christine J. Harrison, PhD, FRCPath

KEYWORDS
- Acute lymphoblastic leukemia • Childhood • Adult
- Diagnosis • Prognosis • Genetics

Acute lymphoblastic leukemia (ALL) is characterized by the accumulation of malignant immature lymphoid cells in the bone marrow. It is predominantly a childhood disease, occurring rarely in adults. In fact, it is the most common malignancy in children, representing one third of pediatric cancers. The annual incidence is approximately 1 case per 100,000 in the general population, ranging from 4 cases to 1 case per 100,000 in children and adults, respectively. The peak incidence occurs between the ages of 2 and 5 years, with a smaller peak over 50 years of age.

ALL is classified broadly as B-lineage and T-lineage.[1] B cell precursor ALL (BCP-ALL) is a malignancy of the lymphoblasts committed to the B cell lineage. It is generally associated with a good outcome in children with a cure rate of approximately 85%, whereas in adults the overall survival is less than 50%. Those features associated with an adverse outcome in BCP-ALL are cytogenetics, infancy, age under 10 years, high white blood cell count, slow response to initial therapy, and the presence of minimal residual disease after first therapy.

T-lineage ALL (T-ALL) is a malignancy of the thymocytes that accounts for approximately 15% of childhood and 25% of adult ALL. It is most common in adolescents and more frequent in males than females. T-ALL is generally considered to be an aggressive high-risk disease. In these patients the presence of minimal residual disease is a strong prognostic factor. Recently, intensified treatment has improved outcome of T-ALL patients.[2]

Many important chromosomal abnormalities have been reported in both BCP-ALL and T-ALL. It is of interest that a number have been shown to arise prenatally, long before the onset of leukemia is diagnosed.[3] In childhood ALL, the incidences of individual chromosomal abnormalities are well-established (**Fig. 1**). It is also known that their distribution varies according to age (**Fig. 2**).[4] Especially in BCP-ALL, these chromosomal abnormalities are strong independent indicators of risk of relapse,[5] whereas in T-ALL they contribute significantly to the understanding of the biology of

Disclosure: This work was supported by Leukaemia and Lymphoma Research, UK.
Leukaemia Research Cytogenetics Group, Northern Institute for Cancer Research, Newcastle University, Level 5 Sir James Spence Institute, Royal Victoria Infirmary, Newcastle-upon-Tyne NE1 4LP, UK
E-mail address: christine.harrison@newcastle.ac.uk

Clin Lab Med 31 (2011) 631–647
doi:10.1016/j.cll.2011.08.016
0272-2712/11/$ – see front matter © 2011 Elsevier Inc. All rights reserved.

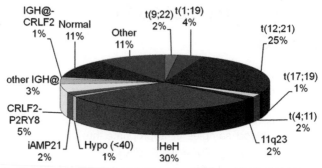

Fig. 1. The distribution of cytogenetic changes in childhood BCP-ALL. Hypo, near-haploid and low-hypodiploid karyotypes with < 40 chromosomes grouped together; HeH, high hyperdiploidy with 51–65 chromosomes; 11q23, patients with translocations of the *MLL* gene other than t(4;11); iAMP21, intrachromosomal amplification of chromosome 21.

the disease. These genetic features provide the focus for this article in which those changes with the greatest significance in relation to their biological and clinical relevance are presented. The main abnormalities and their associated genes are summarized for BCP-ALL in **Table 1** and T-ALL in **Table 2**. For a detailed catalog of chromosomal abnormalities in ALL, the reader is referred to Harrison and Johansson.[6] In the author's opinion, within the current era, the definition of cytogenetics, at least for ALL, must be inclusive of genomic abnormalities detected at the DNA level.

B CELL PRECURSOR ALL
Poor Risk Abnormalities

Philadelphia chromosome
Particularly in childhood BCP-ALL, chromosomal abnormalities are important for risk stratification for treatment. The most well-known is the translocation between

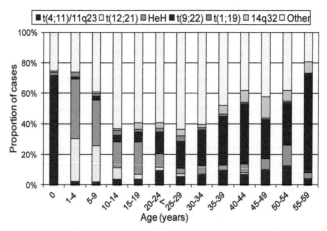

Fig. 2. The distribution of the common established chromosomal abnormalities according to age. Note the highest incidence of other abnormalities in the older children/adolescent age group. HeH, high hyperdiploidy (51–65 chromosomes); 14q32, *IGH@* translocations.

Table 1
Genetic abnormalities of known prognostic significance in BCP-ALL

Abnormality Risk	Abnormality Type	Specific Aberration	Molecular Genetic Features	Age Group
Poor risk abnormalities	Philadelphia chromosome	t(9;22)(q34;q11)	BCR, ABL1	Mainly adults, some children
	MLL rearrangement	t(4;11)(q21;q23)	MLL, AFF1	Mainly infants, some children and adults
		t(6;11)(q27;q23)	MLLT4, MLL	All
		t(9;11)(p21;q23)	MLLT3, MLL	All
		t(11;19)(q23;p13.3)	MLLT1, MLL	Mainly infants, some children and adults
	TCF3 rearrangement	t(1;19)(q23;p13.3)	TCF3, PBX1	All
		t(17;19)(q22;p13)	TCF3, HLF	All
	Near-haploidy	24–29 chromosomes	Whole chromosome gains onto the haploid set, often with doubling of chromosome number	Children
	Low hypodiploidy	31–39 chromosomes	Whole chromosome gains onto the haploid set, often with doubling of chromosome number	Adults
	IGH translocation	t(14;19)(q32;q13)	CEBPA, IGH@	Older children and adults
		t(14;20)(q32;q13)	CEBPB, IGH@	Older children and adults
		t(8;14)(q11;q32)	CEBPD, IGH@	Older children and adults
		inv(14)(q11q32)	CEBPE, IGH@	Older children and adults
		t(14;14)(q11;q32)	CEBPE, IGH@	Older children and adults
		t(6;14)(p22;q32)	ID4, IGH@	Older children and adults
		t(14;19)(q32;p13)	EPOR, IGH@	
		t(X;14)(p22;q32)	CRLF2, IGH@	
		t(Y;14)(p11;q32)	CRLF2, IGH@	
	iAMP21	Grossly abnormal chromosome 21	?RUNX1 and other genes on chromosome 21	Older children
	Gene deletion	IKZF1	IKZF1	All
	Gene mutation	CREBBP	CREBBP	Children
Good risk abnormalities	Cryptic translocation	t(12;21)(p13;q22)	ETV6, RUNX1	Young children
	High hyperdiploidy	51–65 chromosomes	Whole chromosome gains, FLT3, NRAS, KRAS, PTPN11, PAX5 mutations	Mostly children, some adults

Table 2
Significant genetic abnormalities in T-ALL

Type of Aberration	Aberration	Molecular Genetic Features
Aberrant expression of transcription factors and related genes	t(1;7)(p34;q34)	LCK, TRB@
	TAL1 deletion	TAL1, STIL
	t(6;7)(q23;q34)	MYB, TRB@
	t(7;9)(q34;q32)	TAL2, TRB@
	t(7;9)(q34;q34.3)	NOTCH1, TRB@
	t(7;11)(q34;p13)	LMO1, TRB@
	t(7;11)(q34;p15)	LMO2, TRB@
	t(7;12)(q34;p13.3)	CCND2, TRB@
	t(7;19)(q34;p13)	LYL1, TRB@
	t(8;14)(q24;q11)	MYC, TCRA/D@
	t(11;14)(p13;q11)	LMO1, TRA@/TRD@
	t(11;14)(p15;q11)	LMO2, TRA@/TRD@
	t(12;14)(p13;q11)	CCND2, TRA@.
	inv(14)(q11q32)	BCL11B, TRD@
	t(14;14)(q11;q32)	BCL11B, TRD@
	NKX2-1 rearrangements	NKX2-1
	NKX2-2 rearrangements	NKX2-2
	MEF2C rearrangements	MEF2C
	t(14;21)(q11;q22)	OLIG2, TRA@
Abnormalities of homeodomain genes	t(7;10)(q34;q24)	TLX1, TRB@
	t(10;14)(q24;q11)	TLX1, TRA@/TRD@
	t(5;14)(q35;q32)	TLX3, BCL11B
Abnormalities of the HOXA cluster	inv(7)(p15q34)	HOXA@, TRB@
	t(7;7)(p15;q34)	HOXA@, TRB@
	t(7;14)(p15;q11)	HOXA@, TRD@
	t(7;14)(p15;q32)	HOXA@, BCL11B
Fusion transcripts	t(6;11)(q27;q23)	MLLT4, MLL
	t(9;9)(q34;q34)	NUP214, ABL1
	t(9;14)(q34;q32)	EML1, ABL1
	t(10;11)(p12;q14)	PICALM, MLLT10
Copy number changes	MYB duplication	MYB
	del(9p)	CDKN2A
	del(18)(p11)	PTPN2
Mutations	NOTCH1 mutations	NOTCH1
	FBXW7 mutations	FBXW7
	PFH6 mutations	PFH6

chromosomes 9 and 22, t(9;22)(q34;q11), otherwise known as the Philadelphia chromosome (Ph), which is the hallmark chromosomal change of chronic myeloid leukemia (**Fig. 3**A). The translocation gives rise to the *BCR-ABL1* fusion with constitutive activation of the tyrosine kinase, BCR-ABL1. The translocation accounts for approximately 2% of BCP-ALL in children and has been associated with a dismal

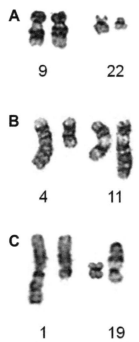

9   22

4   11

1   19

Fig. 3. Partial karyotypes from patients with (A) t(9;22)(q34;q11) or the Philadelphia chromosome, (B) t(4;11)(q21;q23), and (C) t(1;19)(q23;p13.3). The chromosomes are numbered underneath each pair, and within each pair the abnormal chromosome is on the right hand side.

outcome. More recently, treatment with the tyrosine kinase inhibitor imatinib has significantly increased disease-free survival, although it is as yet too early to know if this result will translate into improvements in overall survival.[7] Trials are in progress to determine whether the new-generation tyrosine kinases, for example dasatinib and nilotinib, can further improve outcome.

MLL rearrangements
Chromosomal abnormalities involving the chromosomal band 11q23, resulting in rearrangements of the *MLL* gene, account for approximately 2% of childhood BCP-ALL. The translocation, t(4;11)(q21;q23) giving rise to the *MLL-AFF1* fusion (previously known as *MLL-AF4*), is the most common (**Fig. 3**B). However, more than 80 *MLL* partners have been reported, with more than 50 of them characterized at the molecular level.[8] Childhood BCP-ALL patients with t(4;11) have also been classified as high-risk, although this statistic is currently under review because the outcome seems to be age-dependent.[5]

TCF3 rearrangements
Among patients with *TCF3* rearrangements, those with t(1;19)(q23;p13.3)/*TCF3-PBX1* fusion (**Fig. 3**C) were originally regarded as high-risk on some treatment protocols. However, on modern therapy they are classified as standard risk.[9] In contrast, the rare variant, t(17;19)(q22;p13)/*HLF-TCF3* fusion, has a dismal outcome on all therapies.[10] Thus, accurate identification is important for appropriate risk stratification.

Near-haploidy and low hypodiploidy

Near-haploidy (24–29 chromosomes) and low hypodiploidy (31–39 chromosomes) are rare abnormalities comprising less than 1% each of childhood BCP-ALL. These abnormalities are associated with a poor treatment response, and patients who have them are stratified as high-risk. The abnormalities represent numerical chromosomal changes in ploidy level characterized by the gain of specific chromosomes onto the haploid chromosome set. In the majority of patients, a population of cells with an exact doubling of this chromosome number is present, producing tetrasomies of the gained chromosomes.[11,12] The doubling of a near-haploid population results in a karyotype with over 50 chromosomes, which is easily mistaken for high hyperdiploidy (see high hyperdiploidy section below). The presence of tetrasomies rather than trisomies of the gained chromosomes distinguishes near-haploid doubling from the classical form of high hyperdiploidy. It is important that these differences are identified because of the poor outcome of the near-haploid doubling compared with the good prognosis associated with high hyperdiploidy.

IGH@ Translocations

Translocations involving the immunoglobulin heavy chain locus, *IGH@*, at 14q32 with a range of partner genes are emerging as a significant subgroup in childhood BCP-ALL.[13–16] The partners include five of the *CEBP* gene family members[13] and the cytokine receptors: *EPOR* and *CRLF2*.[15,16] The latter is a cryptic translocation involving *IGH@* and the *CRLF2* gene, which is located within the pseudoautosomal region (PAR1) of both sex chromosomes, t(X;14)(p22;q32) or t(Y;14)(p11;q32).[16] All *IGH@* translocations occur more frequently in older children and adolescents and, although numbers are small, these translocations seem to have an inferior outcome.

iAMP21

The cytogenetic subgroup, intrachromosomal amplification of chromosome 21 (iAMP21), was identified during routine screening for the presence of the *ETV6-RUNX1* fusion by fluorescence in situ hybridization (FISH).[17,18] Patients are negative for the *ETV6-RUNX1* fusion but show multiple copies of *RUNX1* (3 or more additional signals). In metaphase, multiple signals are seen in tandem duplication along an abnormal chromosome 21.[19] In interphase, the signals are clustered together. Cytogenetics, FISH, and genomic approaches have shown that the morphology of the abnormal chromosome 21 is highly variable between patients (**Fig. 4**). The commonly amplified region always includes the *RUNX1* gene.[19–21] More recent studies have confirmed that iAMP21 is a primary genetic change and that the mechanisms leading to instability of the abnormal chromosome 21 are inherent within the chromosome structure.[22]

iAMP21 was originally described as poor risk,[23] although the outcome has since been shown to be protocol-dependent.[24] Thus its accurate detection is important in order to guide therapy.

Good Risk Abnormalities

ETV6-RUNX1 fusion

A significant structural abnormality is the cryptic translocation, t(12;21)(p13;q22)/ *ETV6-RUNX1* fusion (**Fig. 5**). This abnormality occurs in approximately 25% of younger children with BCP-ALL.[25] These patients have an extremely good prognosis.

High hyperdiploidy

High hyperdiploidy (51–65 chromosomes) is an important numerical abnormality.[26] It accounts for approximately 30% of childhood BCP-ALL and is characterized by the

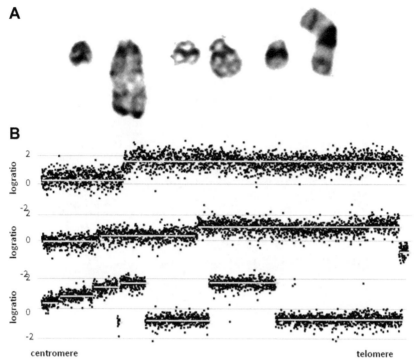

Fig. 4. Cytogenetics and array-based comparative genomic hybridization (aCGH) from different iAMP21 patients indicating the variability of the abnormal chromosome 21. (*A*) Partial karyotypes of 3 pairs of chromosomes 21 from 3 different patients with iAMP21. Within each pair the normal chromosome 21 is on the left and the abnormal iAMP21 chromosome on the right. (*B*) Three aCGH profiles of iAMP21 from 3 different patients showing the variable copy number gain and loss along chromosome 21.

gain of specific chromosomes. High hyperdiploidy is also associated with an excellent outcome in children. It is largely unknown why both abnormalities are linked to a good prognosis. The reasons may be in part age-related because, overall, younger children have the best treatment response, and these abnormalities occur predominantly in younger children.

Submicroscopic Abnormalities

A significant discovery was that the disruption of genes involved in B cell development, through deletions, amplifications, point mutations, and structural rearrangements, played an important role in leukemogenesis in childhood BCP-ALL.[27] Approximately 40% of these patients had abnormalities of genes involved in the B cell development and differentiation pathway, including: *PAX5, TCF3, EBF1, LEF1, IKZF1* and *IKZF3*. Other genes frequently affected were those controlling cell cycle progression including: *CDKN2A, CDKN1B,* and *RB1* (**Fig. 6**A).[28,29] Whether there is a link between these abnormalities and outcome has become a critical question. Alterations of *IKZF1* (which encodes the lymphoid transcription factor, IKAROS) are common in *BCR-ABL1*-positive ALL, known to have a poor outcome.[30] However, *IKZF1* deletions have also been found to be a marker of poor prognosis in Ph-negative BCP-ALL

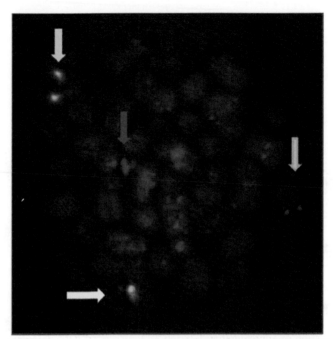

Fig. 5. A metaphase showing the t(12;21)(p13;q22)/*ETV6-RUNX1* fusion. The chromosomes are counterstained with DAPI (*blue*) There is one red signal indicating the normal copy of *RUNX1* on the normal chromosome 21 (*red arrow*), a green signal indicating the normal copy of *ETV6* on the normal chromosome 12 (*green arrow*), and a yellow signal indicating the presence of the *ETV6-RUNX1* fusion on the derived chromosome 21 (*yellow arrow*). The second red signal (*pale blue arrow*) indicates part of the *RUNX1* signal on the derived chromosome 12.

patients.[31-33] Currently this observation is being further validated in prospective independent and unselected trial-based patient cohorts.

In addition to the cryptic translocation, t(X;14)(p22;q32) or t(Y;14)(p11;q32), creating *IGH@-CRLF2*, as mentioned earlier, a deletion within PAR1, giving rise to the *P2RY8-CRLF2* fusion, has also been reported.[16,34–36] Both rearrangements lead to overexpression of CRLF2, which has been defined as a novel significant abnormality in BCP-ALL. *CRLF2* alterations, including activating mutations of the *CRLF2* receptor itself,[37] are associated with activating *JAK2* mutations, which together result in constitutive activation of the JAK-STAT signalling pathway.[16,35,36] Activation of this pathway has been associated with an intermediate[38] or worse prognosis[39] in children, particularly those of Hispanic origin[40] and has been highlighted as an important consideration for targeted therapy.

Mutations

Somatic mutations affecting key genes involved in pathways relating to the development of BCP-ALL have been known for a few years.[41] The first comprehensive mutational screen of the key exons of genes deregulating the RAS-RAF-MEK-ERK pathway: *NRAS, KRAS2, PTPN11, FLT3,* and *BRAF,* showed that these somatic mutations constituted one of the most common genetic aberrations in childhood ALL.

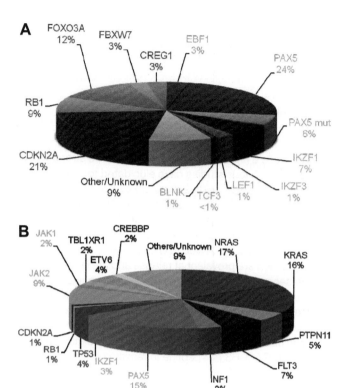

Fig. 6. The relative incidences of (A) deletions and (B) mutations in the key signaling pathways in childhood BCP-ALL. The genes are color-coded according to the pathway to which they belong: B cell differentiation and development, blue; TP53/RB1, red; Ras signaling, purple; JAK/STAT, green, noncanonical pathways and other/unknown genes, black. (A) Deletions are shown for the B cell differentiation and development and TP53/RB1 pathways only. The PAX5 mutation rate stated by Mullighan and colleagues[27] is given (PAX5 mut). The relative incidences of the mutations in the lower chart are estimated from Zhang and colleagues.[42]

Moreover, these mutations were implicated in progression to relapse in some patients. However, for many of the mutations, the clinical and biological significance, as well as their relationship to one another and other genetic changes, remained unknown. Recently, Zhang and colleagues[42] have reported the first large-scale sequence analysis in ALL, from which they identified that the most frequently mutated genes were *NRAS, KRAS, PAX5,* and *JAK2,* each mutated in more than 10% of childhood high-risk BCP-ALL patients (**Fig. 6**B). When these mutations were combined with copy number alterations,[32] the following four known cancer signaling pathways, B cell development and differentiation, Ras signaling, JAK/STAT signaling, and the TP53/RB1 tumor suppressor pathway were found to be involved in 68%, 54%, 11%, and 54% of cases, respectively.

In addition to these mutations in key pathways, inactivating mutations were observed in other noncanonical pathways, including *ETV6* and *CREBBP*. These findings endorse the value of comprehensive evaluation of sequence alterations toward yielding additional biological insights into childhood high-risk BCP-ALL. How these mutations relate to cytogenetics and submicroscopic abnormalities in terms of their clinical relevance remains to be elucidated.

Relapse

Although the cure rate in childhood BCP-ALL is high, 20% of patients relapse. Relapsed ALL is a significant clinical challenge because survival post relapse remains poor.[43] Thus, it is important that those patients at high risk of relapse are identified at the time of diagnosis. Diagnosis is difficult because patients with relapsed ALL are clinically diverse and have a highly heterogeneous outcome strongly linked to the site and timing of relapse.[43] Previous studies have elucidated four principal origins for the relapse clone: (a) evolved from ancestral clone, (b) evolved from diagnostic clone, (c) recurrence of diagnosis clone, and (d) unrelated clone. Backtracking studies indicated that the relapse clones were often present at diagnosis as minor clones, suggesting that they had been selected for during treatment.[44] Evidence from the literature indicates that deletions of genes involved in B cell development and differentiation as well as cell cycle regulation are prevalent at relapse and are likely to play a causal role. However, these are secondary abnormalities that may be gained or lost at relapse.[44] From targeted sequencing studies it has recently been reported that there is a strong association between mutations in the histone acetyltransferase gene, *CREBBP*, and relapsed BCP-ALL.[45] Although these studies have been very informative at the biological level, none have yet resulted in any change to the management of relapsed patients.

Adults

In adult ALL, the role of cytogenetics in patient management has largely been centered on the Ph chromosome. Although the overall incidence of Ph-positive ALL in adults is approximately 25%, it is correlated with age and rises to more than 50% among patients over age 55. As indicated earlier for childhood Ph-positive ALL, the presence of the Ph chromosome is associated with a poor outcome and has also been used to direct therapy in adult patients. Because Ph-negative adult ALL is rare and the frequency of recurrent chromosomal abnormalities is low, little is known about their prognostic relevance. In a large study of adult Ph-negative ALL,[46] high hyperdiploidy was found in a low percentage (10%), whereas deletions of the short arm of chromosome 9 (9p) and the translocation, t(4;11)(q21;q23), were found in a higher percentage of adult patients (9% each) when compared with childhood ALL. High hyperdiploidy and deletions of 9p were associated with an improved outcome. As in children, the improved outcome for patients with high hyperdiploidy may be age-related, because this abnormality arises more frequently in the younger adults. Near-haploidy is rarely observed in adults, whereas low hypodiploidy (31–39 chromosomes) occurs at a higher incidence (4%) than found in children (<1%). As indicated earlier, low hypodiploidy often presents with doubling of the hypodiploid chromosome number comprising 68 to 78 chromosomes, known as near-triploidy.[47] Low hypodiploidy/near-triploidy and complex karyotype, consisting of 5 or more unrelated chromosomal abnormalities (5% incidence), are independent prognostic indicators associated with an inferior event-free and overall survival. Thus these observations have provided compelling evidence of the importance of cytogenetics in the prediction of prognosis in adult ALL, and cytogenics are now being used for risk stratification for treatment.

Adolescents

Adolescents with ALL have an inferior outcome compared with younger children. This outcome is reflected in part by the increased frequency of T-ALL and, in BCP-ALL, by differences in their cytogenetic profile. Adolescents have a higher incidence of Ph-positive ALL and a lower incidence of the good risk abnormalities: high hyperdiploidy and *ETV6-RUNX1* fusion. A higher incidence of *IGH@* translocations has also been noted in this age group. The inferior prognosis of adolescents prompted a review of survival of patients in this age group treated on pediatric versus adult clinical treatment trials. Consistently, those treated on childhood protocols had improved outcome,[48] which has led to major revisions in the treatment of adolescent ALL.

Infants

ALL in infants under 1 year of age is rare. The biological features are different from ALL in older children, with infants having an immature B cell phenotype (proB ALL), lacking CD10 expression and a high tumor load at presentation.[49] It has been known for some time that at the genetic level, infant ALL is characterized by a high frequency of approximately 80% of patients with rearrangements of the *MLL* gene involving all partners, of which over 50% have t(4;11)(q21;q23).[50,51] Overall, event-free survival rate is considerably lower for infants compared with older children with ALL,[52] whereas among infants outcome is heterogeneous.[53] Event-free survival varies according to *MLL* status, CD10 expression, age at diagnosis, presenting white blood cell count, central nervous system involvement, coexpression of myeloid markers, and early response to prednisone.[49] A subset of approximately 20% of infants with ALL do not have rearrangements of *MLL (MLL* germline), a small number of whom have the common cytogenetic abnormalities found in older children with ALL. These *MLL* germline patients have been shown to have an improved prognosis, with approximately 3-fold decreased risk of an event compared with *MLL* rearranged cases.[51]

Down Syndrome

Children with Down syndrome have a markedly increased risk of acute leukemia, both ALL and acute myeloid leukemia. The cytogenetic profile differs from non-Down syndrome ALL. Although a significant proportion of Down syndrome ALL has the typical BCP-ALL abnormalities, incidence varies markedly. For example, the frequency of high hyperdiploidy was 11% compared with approximately 30% in non-Down syndrome childhood BCP-ALL. Similarly, the incidence of *ETV6-RUNX1* was lower; 10% versus 25%. Specific genetic subtypes of Down syndrome ALL were implicated by the significant overrepresentation of cases with gain of an X chromosome, the translocation t(8;14)(q11;q32) involving *IGH@* with *CEBPD*,[13] and deletion of 9p.[54] As already noted, Down syndrome patients have a high incidence of CRLF2 deregulation and *JAK2* mutations.[16,36,55,56] As seen in non-Down syndrome patients, Down syndrome ALL patients have additional submicroscopic deletions in key genes, including *ETV6*, *CDKN2A*, and *PAX5*. Collectively, these results infer a different yet complex molecular pathogenesis for Down syndrome ALL leukemogenesis, with trisomy 21 as a first event followed by chromosome gains, gene deletions, and activating *JAK2* mutations as complementary genetic events.

T CELL PRECURSOR ALL

T-ALL is a malignancy of thymocytes. The leukemic transformation is caused by a multistep pathogenesis involving a large number of genetic changes that allow uncontrolled cell growth. Although no changes to treatment have been implemented in relation to genetic changes in T-ALL, the study of genetics has improved our knowledge of the biology. The genetic abnormalities observed in T-ALL are largely distinct from those observed in BCP-ALL, and many are cryptic at the cytogenetic level.[57] The abnormalities have been variously classified according to cytogenetics, genomic copy number changes, and gene expression profiling, as reviewed by Van Vlierberghe and colleagues.[58] The significant ones are outlined here.

Translocations involving the T cell receptor loci are found in approximately 35% of T-ALL.[59] These translocations usually result in oncogenes becoming juxtaposed to the promoter and enhancer elements of the *TCR* genes, leading to their aberrant expression and the development of T-ALL. Alternatively, aberrant expression of oncogenic transcription factors in T-ALL may result from loss of the upstream transcriptional mechanisms that normally down-regulate the expression of these oncogenes during T cell development.[60,61] Aberrant expression of one or more transcription factors is a critical component of the molecular pathogenesis of T-ALL. These transcription factors include the class B basic helix-loop-helix (*bHLH*) genes *TAL1, TAL2, LYL1, OLIG2,* and *MYC*, as well as genes involved in transcription regulation, for example, the cysteine-rich LIM-only domain, *LMO1* and *LMO2* genes. Abnormalities also affect the homeodomain genes, *TLX1* and *TLX3*, and members of the *HOXA* cluster, usually through translocations or deletions. The formation of oncogenic fusion transcripts is rare in T-ALL. Translocations of this type include *MLL* fusions and *PICALM-MLLT10*, as well some rare rearrangements involving the tyrosine kinase gene, *ABL1*. The *NUP214-ABL1* fusion is of interest because in the majority of cases it is formed as the result of episomal amplification.[62] This fusion is a secondary abnormality found in only a proportion of cells.[63] T-ALL cells with *NUP214-ABL1* amplification have shown response to tyrosine kinase inhibitors in culture, providing hope for the improved treatment of patients with this abnormality.[64]

Mutations, particularly those involving *NOTCH1* and *FBXW7*, are significant in T-ALL, together being found in approximately 70% of cases. Mutations and deletions of the X-linked tumor suppressor gene *PHF6*[65] and *PTPN2*[66] have recently been reported; the latter has been identified as a modulator of response to treatment. Chromosomal rearrangements and amplification of *MYB* at 6q23 have been found in approximately 8% of T-ALL, which represents an interesting molecular target for therapy.[67,68]

De Keersmaecker and colleagues[69] classified the different T-ALL–specific abnormalities into subgroups that defined four pathways based on different classes of mutations that (1) provide a proliferative advantage, (2) impair differentiation and survival, (3) affect the cell cycle, and (4) provide self-renewal capacity. The majority of T-ALL patients harbor a minimum of one abnormality from each group. More recently, genetic abnormalities in T-ALL have been classified as Types A and B.[58] Type A delineates specific subgroups in T-ALL and functions mainly by facilitating differentiation arrest at specific stages of T cell development. Type B abnormalities are shared between T-ALL subgroups and target cellular processes, including cell cycle, *NOTCH1* pathway, and TCR signalling. Interlaced with these four major classes of mutations is the molecular classification, which has emerged from gene expression profiling.[70] Profiling has identified several gene expression signatures indicative of arrest at specific stages of thymocyte development; an *LYL1*-positive signature represents immature thymocytes (pro-T), *TLX1*-positive represents early cortical thymocytes, and *TAL1* correlates with late cortical thymocytes. Recently, by integrated transcript and genomic analysis, two new T-ALL subtypes were identified, each in approximately 20% of T-ALL which lacked rearrangements of previously known oncogenes.[71] One subtype was associated with cortical arrest, expression of cell cycle genes, and ectopic expression of NKX2-1 and NKX2-2, for which rearrangements were identified. The second was associated with immature T cell development and high expression of the MEF2C transcription factor activated by rearrangements of *MEF2C*, transcription factors that target *MEF2C*- or MEFC-associated cofactors, highlighting *NKX2-1, NKX2-2,* and *MEF2C* as defining oncogenic pathways in T-ALL oncogenes. Molecular analysis has shown its capacity to elucidate significant pathways relevant to the future treatment of T-ALL. These findings have indicated that continued genetic analysis in T-ALL is important to further classify this heterogeneous disease.[58,71]

This article has been dedicated to cytogenetics and genomic studies of ALL; however, the impact of transcriptome studies in the classification of ALL cannot be ignored. Global gene expression profiling has identified distinct subgroups of ALL associated with the established cytogenetic subgroups, other genomic changes, and outcome.[72,73] In future, these approaches may be used to stratify patients for treatment. Consideration must also be given to the role of microRNA expression[74] as well as epigenetic factors such as DNA methylation,[75] and their influence on prognosis and biology of the disease when correlated with the already complex interactions observed at the genomic level. Within the next few years, with these and advancing technologies of next-generation and whole genome sequencing, we are likely to see an explosion of novel genetic anomalies. Potentially individualized targeted therapy is on the horizon.

SUMMARY

Precursor B-ALL (BCP-ALL) is associated with a good outcome in children. Cytogenetics is one of the gold standards for risk stratification for treatment that has contributed to improved survival. Although in T-ALL genetic analysis has not been used to guide therapy, it has contributed significantly to the understanding of the biology. State-of-the-art technologies in genomic and high throughput targeted sequencing are revealing novel genetic changes linked to biological and clinical features including outcome. A number of new biomarkers provide the potential for molecular targets for therapy with promise for further improvements in survival and quality of life for ALL sufferers.

REFERENCES

1. Swerdlow SH, Campo E, Harris NL, et al. WHO classification of Tumours of Haematopoietic and Lymphoid Tissue. 4th edition. Lyon (France): International Agency for Research on Cancer; 2008.
2. Silverman LB, Stevenson KE, O'Brien JE, et al. Long-term results of Dana-Farber Cancer Institute ALL Consortium protocols for children with newly diagnosed acute lymphoblastic leukemia (1985–2000). Leukemia 2010;24:320–34.
3. Greaves M. In utero origins of childhood leukaemia. Early Hum Dev 2005;81:123–9.
4. Harrison CJ. Cytogenetics of paediatric and adolescent acute lymphoblastic leukaemia. Br J Haematol 2009;144:147–56.
5. Moorman AV, Ensor HM, Richards SM, et al. Prognostic effect of chromosomal abnormalities in childhood B-cell precursor acute lymphoblastic leukaemia: results from the UK Medical Research Council ALL97/99 randomised trial. Lancet Oncol 2010;11:429–38.
6. Harrison CJ, Johansson B. Acute lymphoblastic leukaemia. In: Heim S, Mitelman F, editors. Cancer cytogenetics. 3rd edition. Hoboken (NJ): Wiley-Blackwell; 2009 p. 233–96.

7. Schultz KR, Bowman WP, Aledo A, et al. Improved early event-free survival with imatinib in Philadelphia chromosome-positive acute lymphoblastic leukemia: a children's oncology group study. J Clin Oncol 2009;27:5175–81.

8. Meyer C, Schneider B, Jakob S, et al. The MLL recombinome of acute leukemias. Leukemia 2006;20:777–84.

9. Kager L, Lion T, Attarbaschi A, et al. Incidence and outcome of TCF3-PBX1-positive acute lymphoblastic leukemia in Austrian children. Haematologica 2007; 92:1561–4.

10. Hunger SP. Chromosomal translocations involving the E2A gene in acute lymphoblastic leukemia: clinical features and molecular pathogenesis. Blood 1996;87: 1211–24.

11. Nachman JB, Heerema NA, Sather H, et al. Outcome of treatment in children with hypodiploid acute lymphoblastic leukemia. Blood 2007;110:1112–5.

12. Harrison CJ, Moorman AV, Broadfield ZJ, et al. Three distinct subgroups of hypodiploidy in acute lymphoblastic leukaemia. Br J Haematol 2004;125:552–9.

13. Akasaka T, Balasas T, Russell LJ, et al. Five members of the CEBP transcription factor family are targeted by recurrent IGH translocations in B-cell precursor acute lymphoblastic leukemia (BCP-ALL). Blood 2007;109:3451–61.

14. Russell LJ, Akasaka T, Majid A, et al. t(6;14)(p22;q32): a new recurrent IGH translocation involving ID4 in B-cell precursor acute lymphoblastic leukemia (BCP-ALL). Blood 2008;111:387–91.

15. Russell LJ, De Castro DG, Griffiths M, et al. A novel translocation, t(14;19)(q32; p13), involving IGH and the cytokine receptor for erythropoietin. Leukemia 2009; 23:614–7.

16. Russell LJ, Capasso M, Vater I, et al. Deregulated expression of cytokine receptor gene, CRLF2, is involved in lymphoid transformation in B-cell precursor acute lymphoblastic leukemia. Blood 2009;114:2688–98.

17. Harrison CJ, Moorman AV, Barber KE, et al. Interphase molecular cytogenetic screening for chromosomal abnormalities of prognostic significance in childhood acute lymphoblastic leukaemia: a UK Cancer Cytogenetics Group Study. Br J Haematol 2005;129:520–30.

18. Soulier J, Trakhtenbrot L, Najfeld V, et al. Amplification of band q22 of chromosome 21, including AML1, in older children with acute lymphoblastic leukemia: an emerging molecular cytogenetic subgroup. Leukemia 2003;17:1679–82.

19. Harewood L, Robinson H, Harris R, et al. Amplification of AML1 on a duplicated chromosome 21 in acute lymphoblastic leukemia: a study of 20 cases. Leukemia 2003;17:547–53.

20. Robinson HM, Harrison CJ, Moorman AV, et al. Intrachromosomal amplification of chromosome 21 (iAMP21) may arise from a breakage-fusion-bridge cycle. Genes Chromosomes Cancer 2007;46:318–26.

21. Strefford JC, Van Delft FW, Robinson HM, et al. Complex genomic alterations and gene expression in acute lymphoblastic leukemia with intrachromosomal amplification of chromosome 21. Proc Natl Acad Sci USA 2006;103:8167–72.

22. Rand V, Parker H, Russell LJ, et al. Genomic characterization implicates iAMP21 as a likely primary genetic event in childhood B-cell precursor acute lymphoblastic leukemia. Blood 2011;117:6848–55.

23. Moorman AV, Richards SM, Robinson HM, et al. Prognosis of children with acute lymphoblastic leukemia (ALL) and intrachromosomal amplification of chromosome 21 (iAMP21). Blood 2007;109:2327–30.

24. Attarbaschi A, Mann G, Panzer-Grumayer R, et al. Minimal residual disease values discriminate between low and high relapse risk in children with B-cell precursor acute lymphoblastic leukemia and an intrachromosomal amplification of chromosome 21: the Austrian and German acute lymphoblastic leukemia Berlin-Frankfurt-Munster (ALL-BFM) trials. J Clin Oncol 2008;26:3046–50.

25. Romana SP, Poirel H, Leconiat M, et al. High frequency of t(12;21) in childhood B-lineage acute lymphoblastic leukemia. Blood 1995;86:4263–9.

26. Moorman AV, Richards SM, Martineau M, et al. Outcome heterogeneity in childhood high-hyperdiploid acute lymphoblastic leukemia. Blood 2003;102:2756–62.

27. Mullighan CG, Goorha S, Radtke I, et al. Genome-wide analysis of genetic alterations in acute lymphoblastic leukaemia. Nature 2007;446:758–64.

28. Kuiper RP, Schoenmakers EF, van Reijmersdal SV, et al. High-resolution genomic profiling of childhood ALL reveals novel recurrent genetic lesions affecting pathways involved in lymphocyte differentiation and cell cycle progression. Leukemia 2007;21: 1258–66.

29. Strefford JC, Worley H, Barber K, et al. Genome complexity in acute lymphoblastic leukemia is revealed by array-based comparative genomic hybridization. Oncogene 2007;26:4306–18.

30. Mullighan CG, Miller CB, Radtke I, et al. BCR-ABL1 lymphoblastic leukaemia is characterized by the deletion of Ikaros. Nature 2008;453:110–4.

31. Den Boer ML, van Slegtenhorst M, De Menezes RX, et al. A subtype of childhood acute lymphoblastic leukaemia with poor treatment outcome: a genome-wide classification study. Lancet Oncol 2009;10:125–34.

32. Mullighan CG, Su X, Zhang J, et al. Deletion of IKZF1 and prognosis in acute lymphoblastic leukemia. N Engl J Med 2009;360:470–80.

33. Kuiper RP, Waanders E, van der Velden VH, et al. IKZF1 deletions predict relapse in uniformly treated pediatric precursor B-ALL. Leukemia 2011;24:1258–64.

34. Mullighan CG, Collins-Underwood JR, Phillips LA, et al. Rearrangement of CRLF2 in B-progenitor- and Down syndrome-associated acute lymphoblastic leukemia. Nat Genet 2009;41:1243–6.

35. Yoda A, Yoda Y, Chiaretti S, et al. Functional screening identifies CRLF2 in precursor B-cell acute lymphoblastic leukemia. Proc Natl Acad Sci USA 2009;107:252–7.

36. Hertzberg L, Vendramini E, Ganmore I, et al. Down syndrome acute lymphoblastic leukemia: a highly heterogeneous disease in which aberrant expression of CRLF2 is associated with mutated JAK2: a report from the iBFM Study Group. Blood 2010; 115:1006–17.

37. Chapiro E, Russell L, Lainey E, et al. Activating mutation in the TSLPR gene in B-cell precursor lymphoblastic leukemia. Leukemia 2010;24:642–5.

38. Ensor HM, Schwab C, Russell LJ, et al. Demographic, clinical, and outcome features of children with acute lymphoblastic leukemia and CRLF2 deregulation: results from the MRC ALL97 clinical trial. Blood 2010;117:2129–36.

39. Cario G, Zimmermann M, Romey R, et al. Presence of the P2RY8-CRLF2 rearrangement is associated with a poor prognosis in non-high-risk precursor B-cell acute lymphoblastic leukemia in children treated according to the ALL-BFM 2000 protocol. Blood 2010;115:5393–7.

40. Harvey RC, Mullighan CG, Chen IM, et al. Rearrangement of CRLF2 is associated with mutation of JAK kinases, alteration of IKZF1, Hispanic/Latino ethnicity, and a poor outcome in pediatric B-progenitor acute lymphoblastic leukemia. Blood 2010;115: 5312–21.

41. Case M, Matheson E, Minto L, et al. Mutation of genes affecting the RAS pathway is common in childhood acute lymphoblastic leukemia. Cancer Res 2008;68:6803–9.

42. Zhang J, Mullighan CG, Harvey RC, et al. Key pathways are frequently mutated in high risk childhood acute lymphoblastic leukemia: a report from the Children's Oncology Group. Blood 2011. [Epub ahead of print].

43. Bailey LC, Lange BJ, Rheingold SR, et al. Bone-marrow relapse in paediatric acute lymphoblastic leukaemia. Lancet Oncol 2008;9:873–83.

44. Mullighan CG, Phillips LA, Su X, et al. Genomic analysis of the clonal origins of relapsed acute lymphoblastic leukemia. Science 2008;322:1377–80.

45. Mullighan CG, Zhang J, Kasper LH, et al. CREBBP mutations in relapsed acute lymphoblastic leukemia. Nature 2011;471:235–9.

46. Moorman AV, Harrison CJ, Buck GA, et al. Karyotype is an independent prognostic factor in adult acute lymphoblastic leukemia (ALL): analysis of cytogenetic data from patients treated on the Medical Research Council (MRC) UKALLXII/Eastern Cooperative Oncology Group (ECOG) 2993 trial. Blood 2007;109:3189–97.

47. Charrin C, Thomas X, Ffrench M, et al. A report from the LALA-94 and LALA-SA groups on hypodiploidy with 30 to 39 chromosomes and near-triploidy: 2 possible expressions of a sole entity conferring poor prognosis in adult acute lymphoblastic leukemia (ALL). Blood 2004;104:2444–51.

48. Ramanujachar R, Richards S, Hann I, et al. Adolescents with acute lymphoblastic leukaemia: outcome on UK national paediatric (ALL97) and adult (UKALLXII/E2993) trials. Pediatr Blood Cancer 2007;48:254–61.

49. Biondi A, Cimino G, Pieters R, et al. Biological and therapeutic aspects of infant leukemia. Blood 2000;96:24–33.

50. Heerema NA, Arthur DC, Sather H, et al. Cytogenetic features of infants less than 12 months of age at diagnosis of acute lymphoblastic leukemia: impact of the 11q23 breakpoint on outcome: a report of the Childrens Cancer Group. Blood 1994;83:2274–84.

51. Pieters R, Schrappe M, De LP, et al. A treatment protocol for infants younger than 1 year with acute lymphoblastic leukaemia (Interfant-99): an observational study and a multicentre randomised trial. Lancet 2007;370:240–50.

52. Chessells JM, Harrison CJ, Watson SL, et al. Treatment of infants with lymphoblastic leukaemia: results of the UK Infant Protocols 1987–1999. Br J Haematol 2002;117:306–14.

53. Chessells JM, Harrison CJ, Kempski H, et al. Clinical features, cytogenetics and outcome in acute lymphoblastic and myeloid leukaemia of infancy: report from the MRC Childhood Leukaemia working party. Leukemia 2002;16:776–84.

54. Forestier E, Izraeli S, Beverloo B, et al. Cytogenetic features of acute lymphoblastic and myeloid leukemias in pediatric patients with Down syndrome: an iBFM-SG study. Blood 2008;111:1575–83.

55. Kearney L, Gonzalez De Castro D, Yeung J, et al. Specific JAK2 mutation (JAK2R683) and multiple gene deletions in Down syndrome acute lymphoblastic leukemia. Blood 2009;113:646–48.

56. Bercovich D, Ganmore I, Scott LM, et al. Mutations of JAK2 in acute lymphoblastic leukaemias associated with Down's syndrome. Lancet 2008;372:1484–92.

57. Harrison CJ. Genetics of T-cell acute lymphoblastic leukemia. Hematology Education. p. 154–60. Available at: http://onlinehaematologica.org/supplements/Hematology_Education_2007.pdf. 2007

58. Van Vlierberghe P, Pieters R, Beverloo HB, et al. Molecular-genetic insights in paediatric T-cell acute lymphoblastic leukaemia. Br J Haematol 2008;143:153–68.

59. Bergeron J, Clappier E, Cauwelier B, et al. HOXA cluster deregulation in T-ALL associated with both a TCRD-HOXA and a CALM-AF10 chromosomal translocation. Leukemia 2006;20:1184–7.

60. Ferrando AA, Herblot S, Palomero T, et al. Biallelic transcriptional activation of oncogenic transcription factors in T-cell acute lymphoblastic leukemia. Blood 2004; 103:1909–11.
61. van Vlierberghe P, van GM, Beverloo HB, et al. The cryptic chromosomal deletion del(11)(p12p13) as a new activation mechanism of LMO2 in pediatric T-cell acute lymphoblastic leukemia. Blood 2006;108:3520–9.
62. Graux C, Cools J, Melotte C, et al. Fusion of NUP214 to ABL1 on amplified episomes in T-cell acute lymphoblastic leukemia. Nat Genet 2004;36:1084–9.
63. Graux C, Stevens-Kroef M, Lafage M, et al. Heterogeneous patterns of amplification of the NUP214-ABL1 fusion gene in T-cell acute lymphoblastic leukemia. Leukemia 2009;23:125–33.
64. Quintas-Cardama A, Tong W, Manshouri T, et al. Activity of tyrosine kinase inhibitors against human NUP214-ABL1-positive T cell malignancies. Leukemia 2008;22: 1117–24.
65. Van Vlierberghe P, Palomero T, Khiabanian H, et al. PHF6 mutations in T-cell acute lymphoblastic leukemia. Nat Genet 2010;42:338–42.
66. Kleppe M, Lahortiga I, El Chaar T, et al. Deletion of the protein tyrosine phosphatase gene PTPN2 in T-cell acute lymphoblastic leukemia. Nat Genet 2010;42:530–5.
67. Clappier E, Cuccuini W, Kalota A, et al. The C-MYB locus is involved in chromosomal translocation and genomic duplications in human T-cell acute leukemia (T-ALL), the translocation defining a new T-ALL subtype in very young children. Blood 2007;110: 1251–61.
68. Lahortiga I, De Keersmaecker K, Van Vlierberghe P, et al. Duplication of the MYB oncogene in T cell acute lymphoblastic leukemia. Nat Genet 2007;39:593–5.
69. De Keersmaecker K, Marynen P, Cools J. Genetic insights in the pathogenesis of T-cell acute lymphoblastic leukemia. Haematologica 2005;90:1116–27.
70. Ferrando AA, Look AT. Gene expression profiling in T-cell acute lymphoblastic leukemia. Semin Hematol 2003;40:274–80.
71. Homminga I, Pieters R, Langerak AW, et al. Integrated transcript and genome analyses reveal NKX2-1 and MEF2C as potential oncogenes in T cell acute lympho-blastic leukemia. Cancer Cell 2011;19:484–97.
72. Harvey RC, Mullighan CG, Wang X, et al. Identification of novel cluster groups in pediatric high-risk B-precursor acute lymphoblastic leukemia with gene expression profiling: correlation with genome-wide DNA copy number alterations, clinical char-acteristics, and outcome. Blood 2010;116:4874–84.
73. Yeoh EJ, Ross ME, Shurtleff SA, et al. Classification, subtype discovery, and predic-tion of outcome in pediatric acute lymphoblastic leukemia by gene expression profiling. Cancer Cell 2002;1:133–43.
74. Gefen N, Binder V, Zaliova M, et al. Hsa-mir-125b-2 is highly expressed in childhood ETV6/RUNX1 (TEL/AML1) leukemias and confers survival advantage to growth inhib-itory signals independent of p53. Leukemia 2010;24:89–96.
75. Milani L, Lundmark A, Kiialainen A, et al. DNA methylation for subtype classification and prediction of treatment outcome in patients with childhood acute lymphoblastic leukemia. Blood 2010;115:1214–25.

Genetics of Chronic Lymphocytic Leukemia

Andrea Schnaiter, MD, Daniel Mertens, PhD, Stephan Stilgenbauer, MD*

KEYWORDS

• CLL • Genetics • *TP53* • *ATM* • *IGHV* • FISH

In general, chronic lymphocytic leukemia (CLL) is easy to diagnose; a peripheral blood sample for blood count, blood smear, and flow cytometry are sufficient. Whereas morphology and the immunophenotype of CLL cells are quite homogenous, there is a marked heterogeneity in the clinical course. The majority of patients do not require extended therapy, and the disease impacts them minimally; a distinct subgroup of patients, however, experiences rapid progression and insufficient response to treatment. The Binet and Rai staging systems [1,2] are accepted prognostic factors in CLL but these systems are not able to differentiate between good and bad prognosis,[3] especially in the early stage. Cytogenetics provides a better insight into the pathogenesis of the disease and helps to estimate a patient's prognosis more accurately. The discovery of different genomic aberrations that are associated with the prognosis has been very meaningful.[4] Furthermore, the mutation status of the variable segments of the immunglobulin heavy chain genes (*IGHV*) has become one of the most important prognostic factors in CLL.[5,6]

Classical cytogenetics includes chromosome banding analysis, which had been difficult to achieve in the mostly nondividing CLL cells. Only recently have dedicated stimulation techniques brought forward this method and made it suitable for CLL diagnostics. In contrast, fluorescence in situ hybridization is also applicable in nondividing cells and has, therefore, found its way into CLL routine diagnostics.[7] Analysis of chromosomal aberrations led to the discovery of important genes involved in CLL tumorigenesis such as *TP53* and *ATM*.[8,9] A closer look at recurrent chromosomal changes is provided by more advanced methods, with higher resolution like comparative genomic hybridization (CGH) and single nucleotide polymorphism (SNP) array analysis. Moreover, DNA sequencing techniques have changed over the years, and today there are high-throughput methods of particular sensitivity that are embraced by the term "next generation sequencing."

The authors have nothing to disclose.

Department of Internal Medicine III, University of Ulm, Albert Einstein Allee 23, 89081 Ulm, Germany

* Corresponding author.

E-mail address: stephan.stilgenbauer@uniklinik-ulm.de

Clin Lab Med 31 (2011) 649–658

doi:10.1016/j.cll.2011.07.006

labmed.theclinics.com

0272-2712/11/$ – see front matter © 2011 Elsevier Inc. All rights reserved.

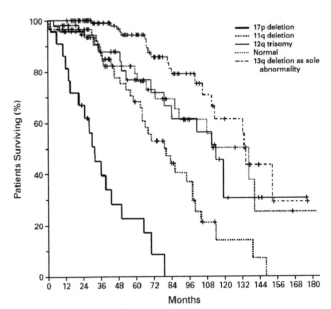

Fig. 1. The hierarchical model of chromosomal abnormalities in CLL: Probability of survival related to the time after diagnosis among the genetic subgroups.[4]

FLUORESCENCE IN SITU HYBRIDIZATION

Fluorescence in situ hybridization (FISH) is used to detect specific DNA sequences on chromosomes of dividing (metaphase) and nondividing (interphase) cells so that numerical as well as structural chromosomal aberrations can be delineated. Interphase FISH has become a standard technique in CLL due to the fact that the majority of CLL cells are arrested in the G0/early G1 phase of the cell cycle and rarely divide in vitro.

In a comprehensive study, at least one chromosomal aberration was detected by FISH in 268 of 325 cases of CLL (82%).[4] The most common aberrations were deletion in 13q (55%), deletion in 11q (18%), trisomy of 12q (16%), deletion in 17p (7%), and deletion in 6q (6%). Correlation of the cytogenetic data with clinical and laboratory findings led to a hierarchical model of 5 major categories with different prognostic outcome: 17p deletion, 11q deletion without 17p deletion, 12q trisomy without 17p deletion or 11q deletion, normal karyotype and 13q deletion as the sole abnormality (**Fig. 1**). Patients with 17p deletion have the worst prognosis. This deletion affects the tumor suppressor gene *TP53* and is associated with refractoriness to conventional chemotherapy with fludarabine. The ataxia teleangiectasia mutated (*ATM*) gene is located on the long arm of chromosome 11. Its deletion has been shown to be associated with poorer outcome and marked lymphadenopathy.[4] In a large randomized, open-label, phase 3 trial (CLL8 trial of the GCLLSG, NCT00281918) on FCR (fludarabine, cyclophosphamied, rituximab) as first-line treatment, the negative prognostic effect of the 17p deletion was not abrogated with chemoimmunotherapy, whereas the rate of complete remissions in 11q deleted cases was increased by more than times. This interesting result suggests that the bad prognostic significance of the 11q deletion might be overcome by this effective regimen and that a specific first-line treatment might change the natural course of the disease.[10]

There is consensus to use interphase FISH in routine practice in CLL at the time of treatment, mainly to detect patients with a 17p deletion who will not respond to conventional chemotherapy and who will experience early progression and short survival after therapy.[7,11] These patients might benefit from agents that act independently of p53 like alemtuzumab, flavopiridol, and allogeneic stem cell transplantation.[12,13] Moreover, as the cytogenetic profile can change over the course of the disease,[14] these diagnostics might be repeated before subsequent therapies.

TP53 *Mutation*

The deletion of 17p13 in CLL affects the tumor suppressor gene *TP53*. In 80–90% of the cases, a deletion of 17p is associated with a mutated *TP53* gene on the remaining copy.[15] This is considered one reason why p53 pathway-based therapies like fludarabine or its combinations such as fludarabine/cyclophosphamid (FC), fludarabine/cyclophosphamide/rituximab (FCR), etc, are not effective in patients with 17p deletion. *TP53* mutations have been found in 4% to 15% of patients in early stage untreated CLL and are associated with a poorer outcome.[15–17] Mutations of *TP53* independently of a 17p deletion have been shown in 4.5% of the cases in a recent analysis of the randomized prospective CLL4 trial of the GCLLSG (randomized fludarabine vs fludarabine/cyclophosphamide [FC] as first-line treatment). Progression-free survival and overall survival of patients with a sole *TP53* mutation is similar to those of patients with 17p deletion (**Fig. 2**).[15]

ATM *Mutation*

The kinase *ATM* is activated by DNA double-strand breaks and targets *P53*, among others. The *ATM* gene is localized in the minimal consensus region in bands 11q22.3 to 11q23.1. Deletion of 11q has been shown in 18% of CLL patients.[4] In about one third of 11q-deleted patients, a simultaneous mutation of *ATM*[18] has been found. Overall survival is shorter in patients with an 11q deletion combined with an *ATM* mutation of the remaining allele compared to a sole 11q deletion (**Fig. 3**). Deletion of 11q as well as *ATM* mutations are associated with poorer outcome.[4] Furthermore, an association between mutation of the *ATM* gene and unmutated *IGHV* genes has been shown.[19]

CHROMOSOME BANDING ANALYSIS

Compared to FISH, chromosome banding analysis (CBA) provides an overview of the whole genome but is limited to dividing cells during metaphase. Chronic lymphocytic leukemia cells have a low mitotic activity and, therefore, this technique has not been applicable until recently.[20]

However, stimulation with CD40 ligand or the combination of CpG-oligonucleotides and IL-2 has achieved an increase in metaphase spreads.[21] Balanced and unbalanced translocations were seen in 34% of the patients. Most of them had not been previously described and were not recurrent in the cohort. In a large study on 506 CLL samples, 98.8% were successfully stimulated by the immunostimulatory CpG-oligonucleotide DSP30 and IL-2. Chromosome banding analysis detected 83% aberrations compared to 78.4% found by FISH. In addition, a subgroup with a complex aberrant karyotype was seen, which was associated with an unmutated *IGHV*-status and expression of CD38.[22] Chromosome banding analysis, therefore, detects additional abnormalities and might complement FISH-generated data. However, further studies are needed to determine the value of CBA for prognosis and treatment.

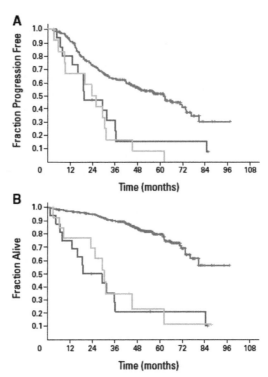

Fig. 2. Outcome of patients with sole *TP53* mutation (*yellow*) and patients with 17p deletion (*gray*) compared to the remaining patients (*blue*)[15]: (*A*) The median progression free survival was significantly shorter for patients with sole *TP53* mutation (23.3 months) or 17p deletion (19.2 months) compared to the remaining patients (61.8 months, *P*<.001). (*B*) The median overall survival was significantly shorter for patients with sole *TP53* mutation (30.2 months) or 17p deletion (19.2 months) compared to the remaining patients (median OS not reached, *P*<.001).

COMPARATIVE GENOMIC HYBRIDIZATION

Comparative genomic hybridization was developed during the 1990s. The method detects copy number changes (gains and losses) but not balanced chromosomal changes. Tumor DNA and normal tissue DNA are labelled with a different fluorescence dye and hybridized to normal metaphase chromosomes or to an array/matrix of specific DNA probes. The distribution of the fluorescence markers shows gains and losses of the tumor DNA compared to the normal tissue DNA.

Analysis of 106 B-CLL cases by array-based comparative genomic hybridization (matrix-CGH) showed high specificity and sensitivity of the method. Previously unrecognized, recurrent genomic imbalances were discovered: trisomy 19 associated with trisomy 12 and *IGHV* hypermutation, and the gain of the *MYC* oncogene on chromosome 2p24 accompanied by an increased expression of MYCN mRNA.[23]

Representational oligonucleotide microarray analysis (ROMA) is a type of high-resolution CGH to detect copy number changes. In a study of 58 CLL patient samples, at least 1 genomic alteration was detected in each CLL sample compared to previous studies using other techniques like FISH that report alterations in only

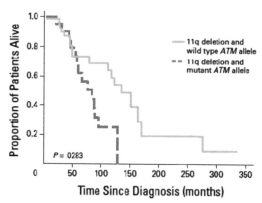

Fig. 3. Overall survival from diagnosis of patients with 11q deletion and wild type *ATM* allele compared to patients with 11q deletion and mutant *ATM* allele: The overall survival was significantly shorter for patients with 11q deletion and *ATM* mutation compared to patients with 11q deletion and wild type *ATM* allele (*P* = .0283).[18]

80% of the cases. Furthermore, previously undescribed alterations were identified (8p21.2-p12 and 2q37.1) and subclones of CLL within the same patient were seen.[24]

SINGLE NUCLEOTIDE POLYMORPHISM ARRAYS

Single nucleotide polymorphisms (SNPs) are the most frequent type of variation in the human genome and are highly conserved within a population. Single nucleotide polymorphism arrays are a type of DNA microarray designed to detect SNPs within a population or between different samples. Single nucleotide polymorphism arrays detect copy number gains and losses and copy number neutral regions with loss of heterozygosity (copy neutral LOH or "uniparental disomy") at high resolution genome-wide. In contrast, FISH is limited to chromosomal changes specific to the probes used, and chromosome banding analysis in stimulated CLL cells is of lower resolution so that submicroscopic findings are overlooked.

A study of 70 CLL cases evaluated the diagnostic potential of 10k and 50k Affymetrix SNP arrays. Matched-pair analysis of intra/individual normal genomes was conducted via buccal swabs as nontumor controls. Chromosomal imbalances were found in 65.6% and 81.5%. Aberrations were detected at the expected frequency. Additionally, 24 regions of LOH were found in 14 cases that are not detectable by alternative methods.[25]

In a more recent study in 178 CLL patient samples of CD19-sorted tumor cells and buccal cells as nontumor controls, a 50kXbaI SNP array platform was used. The samples were derived from 139 untreated and 39 previously treated patients. Genomic complexity scores were delineated and a correlation to "time to first therapy" (TTFT) or "time to subsequent therapy" (TTST) was done. An increasing complexity score was correlated to a short time to first therapy in previously untreated patients and to a short time to subsequent therapy in previously treated patients. Genomic complexity was found to be an independent risk factor for TTFT and TTST.[26]

Another study (in 171 cases) examined loss of heterozygosity and subchromosomal copy losses on chromosome 13. The major finding of that study was the heterogeneity of the 13q14 deletion—meaning that different subtypes of the deletion exist. Two types of deletion were defined: Type I aberrations in 60% of the del(13)(q14) cases that show a

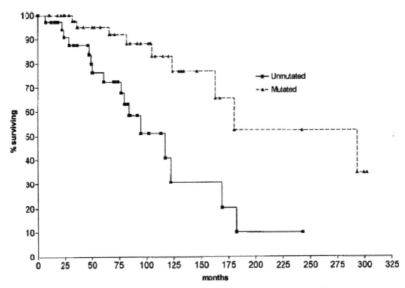

Fig. 4. Overall survival from diagnosis of patients with unmutated VH genes compared to patients with mutated VH genes. The median survival of patients with unmutated VH genes (117 months) was significantly shorter than the median survival of patients with mutated VH genes (293 months, P<.001).[28]

loss of *Rb* and breaks close to the miR16/15a locus; and type II alterations in 40% of the cases that include *Rb*. Expression analysis revealed a lower expression of miR15 and miR16a variably accompanied by biallelic loss of miR15/16a in about 15 % of the CLL cases.[27] It is important to evaluate the power of the SNP array analysis for prognostication in comparison to FISH in prospective trials.

IGHV REARRANGEMENT AND MUTATION STATUS

The presence or absence of somatic hypermutation within the variable segments of the clonally rearranged immunoglobulin heavy chain variable genes (*IGHV*) is an important prognostic factor in CLL. A study of 84 patients showed an unmutated *IGHV* status in 45.2% of the cases, as well as an association between advanced stage/progressive disease and the use of the immunoglobulin VH genes *V1-69*, *D3-3*, and isolated trisomy 12. Survival was significantly lower than in cases with mutated *IGHV* status (**Fig. 4**).[28] A concurrent study found an association with unmutated *IGHV* status and the expression of CD38 (**Fig. 5**). Clinical data showed worse response to chemotherapy and shorter survival.[5]

Immunoglobulin heavy chain variable genes status is determined by DNA sequencing. The search for surrogate markers led to CD38 and 70, whose expression correlates with *IGHV* mutation status. ZAP70 is usually involved in T-cell receptor signalling. A correlation between ZAP70 expression in CLL cells and *IGHV* status, disease progression, and survival was found in a study of 56 CLL patients. All of the patients who showed at least 20% of ZAP70-positive cells had an unmutated *IGHV* status, whereas *IGHV* was mutated in 21 of 24 patients with less than 20% of ZAP70 positive cells.[29] A more recent study showed a high association of mutated *IGHV* status and ZAP70 expression in CLL without high-risk features like 17p deletion, 11q

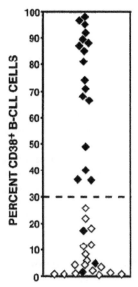

Fig. 5. Percentages of CD38 expressing CLL cells of 37 patient samples. All cases with ≥30% CD38 positive cells are *IGHV* unmutated (<2% difference from the most similar germline gene).[5]

deletion, and usage of the VH gene *V3-21,* but a marked discordance in cases where those high-risk markers were present.[30] Nevertheless, ZAP70 determination is still difficult due to unstandardized flow cytometric methods.

NEXT GENERATION SEQUENCING

DNA sequencing has long been dominated by the automated Sanger method.[31] Meanwhile, a number of new techniques summarized as "next generation sequencing" (NGS) have been developed that are suitable for high-throughput analysis. Next generation sequencing produces large volumes of sequence data of a whole genome or exome.

Rare abnormalities can be identified and quantified without prior functional knowledge of a particular gene. Exome sequencing provides additional information about alternative splicing and sequence variation in identified genes.[32]

A recent study combining next generation whole-exome sequencing with genome-wide high-density SNP array analysis revealed candidate tumor-specific nonsynonymous mutations. Thirty-six mutations corresponding to 36 distinct genes were found by screening an independent panel of 48 CLL DNAs. The coding genome of CLL contains, on average, 14 somatic gene alterations per case. Further studies are needed to delineate the importance of these alterations for pathogenesis and therapy.[33] Another study concentrated on functional mutations in the Wnt pathway. Two novel nonsynonymous mutations in the Wnt pathway, members *DKK2* and *BCL9*, were found by Illumina sequencing of 2 genomes and 4 exomes from patients with advanced CLL. Based on these findings, the dysregulation of the Wnt pathway in CLL was shown by gene expression analysis and further functional assays.[34]

Sequencing-based methods can, in principle, replace most nucleic acids-based technologies like microarrays analyses (gene expression profiling and mCGH, as noted above), and other methods not intuitively associated with sequencing—like chromosome banding to identify translocations (NGS of paired-end tags, PET-seq).[35] However, while experimental protocols are well optimized, post-experiment aspects—especially of data handling and analysis—are challenging and are subject of further development.

SUMMARY

Genetic analyses have contributed greatly in dissecting CLL into different pathogenic and prognostic subgroups. Fluorescence in situ hybridization is increasingly recommended as the standard diagnostic test at diagnosis, and particularly before the initiation of therapy. Particularly, patients with a 17p deletion have to be detected before treatment initiation. They should be offered p53 independent therapeutic regimens. The *IGHV* mutation status is one of the most important prognostic factors detected by mutation analysis. Newer cytogenetic techniques provide more and more high-resolution analysis. Today, it is possible to analyze not only selective gene loci but the whole genome or exome. Further investigations are required to find new prognostic factors, explore signalling pathways, and locate new therapeutic targets. It is likely that comprehensive and sensitive "whole genome" approaches such as NGS will lead to the discovery of novel abnormalities of pathogenic and prognostic relevance and will, ultimately, be used in a clinical diagnostic setting.

REFERENCES

1. Rai KR, Sawitsky A, Cronkite EP, et al. Clinical staging of chronic lymphocytic leukemia. Blood 1975;46:219–34.
2. Binet JL, Auquier A, Dighiero G, et al. A new prognostic classification of chronic lymphocytic leukemia derived from a multivariate survival analysis. Cancer 1981;48: 198–206.
3. Zwiebel JA, Cheson BD. Chronic lymphocytic leukemia: staging and prognostic factors. Semin Oncol 1998;25:42–59.
4. Dohner H, Stilgenbauer S, Benner A, et al. Genomic aberrations and survival in chronic lymphocytic leukemia. N Engl J Med 2000;343:1910–6.
5. Damle RN, Wasil T, Fais F, et al. Ig V gene mutation status and CD38 expression as novel prognostic indicators in chronic lymphocytic leukemia. Blood 1999;94:1840–7.
6. Krober A, Seiler T, Benner A, et al. V(H) mutation status, CD38 expression level, genomic aberrations, and survival in chronic lymphocytic leukemia. Blood 2002;100: 1410–6.
7. Hallek M, Cheson BD, Catovsky D, et al. Guidelines for the diagnosis and treatment of chronic lymphocytic leukemia: a report from the International Workshop on Chronic Lymphocytic Leukemia updating the National Cancer Institute-Working Group 1996 guidelines. Blood 2008;111:5446–56.
8. Dohner H, Stilgenbauer S, Fischer K, et al. Cytogenetic and molecular cytogenetic analysis of B cell chronic lymphocytic leukemia: specific chromosome aberrations identify prognostic subgroups of patients and point to loci of candidate genes. Leukemia 1997;11(Suppl 2):S19–24.
9. Starostik P, Manshouri T, O'Brien S, et al. Deficiency of the ATM protein expression defines an aggressive subgroup of B-cell chronic lymphocytic leukemia. Cancer Res 1998;58:4552–7.
10. Hallek M, Fischer K, Fingerle-Rowson G, et al. Addition of rituximab to fludarabine and cyclophosphamide in patients with chronic lymphocytic leukaemia: a randomised, open-label, phase 3 trial. Lancet 2010;376:1164–74.

11. Gribben JG. How I treat CLL up front. Blood 2010;115:187–97.
12. Byrd JC, Lin TS, Dalton JT, et al. Flavopiridol administered using a pharmacologically derived schedule is associated with marked clinical efficacy in refractory, genetically high-risk chronic lymphocytic leukemia. Blood 2007;109:399–404.
13. Stilgenbauer S, Zenz T, Winkler D, et al. Subcutaneous alemtuzumab in fludarabine-refractory chronic lymphocytic leukemia: clinical results and prognostic marker analyses from the CLL2H study of the German Chronic Lymphocytic Leukemia Study Group. J Clin Oncol 2009;27:3994–4001.
14. Stilgenbauer S, Sander S, Bullinger L, et al. Clonal evolution in chronic lymphocytic leukemia: acquisition of high-risk genomic aberrations associated with unmutated VH, resistance to therapy, and short survival. Haematologica 2007;92:1242–5.
15. Zenz T, Eichhorst B, Busch R, et al. TP53 mutation and survival in chronic lymphocytic leukemia. J Clin Oncol 2010;28:4473–9.
16. Dohner H, Fischer K, Bentz M, et al. p53 gene deletion predicts for poor survival and non-response to therapy with purine analogs in chronic B-cell leukemias. Blood 1995;85:1580–9.
17. el Rouby S, Thomas A, Costin D, et al. p53 gene mutation in B-cell chronic lymphocytic leukemia is associated with drug resistance and is independent of MDR1/MDR3 gene expression. Blood 1993;82:3452–9.
18. Austen B, Skowronska A, Baker C, et al. Mutation status of the residual ATM allele is an important determinant of the cellular response to chemotherapy and survival in patients with chronic lymphocytic leukemia containing an 11q deletion. J Clin Oncol 2007;25:5448–57.
19. Austen B, Powell JE, Alvi A, et al. Mutations in the ATM gene lead to impaired overall and treatment-free survival that is independent of IGHV mutation status in patients with B-CLL. Blood 2005;106:3175–82.
20. Juliusson G, Oscier DG, Fitchett M, et al. Prognostic subgroups in B-cell chronic lymphocytic leukemia defined by specific chromosomal abnormalities. N Engl J Med 1990;323:720–4.
21. Mayr C, Speicher MR, Kofler DM, et al. Chromosomal translocations are associated with poor prognosis in chronic lymphocytic leukemia. Blood 2006;107:742–51.
22. Haferlach C, Dicker F, Schnittger S, et al. Comprehensive genetic characterization of CLL: a study on 506 cases analysed with chromosome banding analysis, interphase FISH, IgV(H) status and immunophenotyping. Leukemia 2007;21:2442–51.
23. Schwaenen C, Nessling M, Wessendorf S, et al. Automated array-based genomic profiling in chronic lymphocytic leukemia: development of a clinical tool and discovery of recurrent genomic alterations. Proc Natl Acad Sci USA 2004;101:1039–44.
24. Grubor V, Krasnitz A, Troge JE, et al. Novel genomic alterations and clonal evolution in chronic lymphocytic leukemia revealed by representational oligonucleotide microarray analysis (ROMA). Blood 2009;113:1294–303.
25. Pfeifer D, Pantic M, Skatulla I, et al. Genome-wide analysis of DNA copy number changes and LOH in CLL using high-density SNP arrays. Blood 2007;109:1202–10.
26. Kujawski L, Ouillette P, Erba H, et al. Genomic complexity identifies patients with aggressive chronic lymphocytic leukemia. Blood 2008;112:1993–2003.
27. Ouillette P, Erba H, Kujawski L, et al. Integrated genomic profiling of chronic lymphocytic leukemia identifies subtypes of deletion 13q14. Cancer Res 2008;68:1012–21.
28. Hamblin TJ, Davis Z, Gardiner A, et al. Unmutated Ig V(H) genes are associated with a more aggressive form of chronic lymphocytic leukemia. Blood 1999;94:1848–54.
29. Crespo M, Bosch F, Villamor N, et al. ZAP-70 expression as a surrogate for immunoglobulin-variable-region mutations in chronic lymphocytic leukemia. N Engl J Med 2003;348:1764–75.

30. Krober A, Bloehdorn J, Hafner S, et al. Additional genetic high-risk features such as 11q deletion, 17p deletion, and V3-21 usage characterize discordance of ZAP-70 and VH mutation status in chronic lymphocytic leukemia. J Clin Oncol 2006;24:969–75.
31. Sanger F, Nicklen S, Coulson AR. DNA sequencing with chain-terminating inhibitors. Proc Natl Acad Sci USA 1977;74:5463–7.
32. Metzker ML. Sequencing technologies - the next generation. Nat Rev Genet 2010; 11:31–46.
33. Fabbri G, Trifonov V, Rossi D, et al. The Genome of Chronic Lymphocytic Leukemia. ASH Annual Meeting Abstracts 2010;116:51.
34. Wang L, Pochet N, Cibulskis K, et al. Whole genome sequencing identifies functional mutations in the wnt pathway in CLL. ASH Annual Meeting Abstracts 2010;116:693.
35. Campbell PJ, Stephens PJ, Pleasance ED, et al. Identification of somatically acquired rearrangements in cancer using genome-wide massively parallel paired-end sequencing. Nat Genet 2008;40:722–9.

Acute Myeloid Leukemia: Conventional Cytogenetics, FISH, and Moleculocentric Methodologies

Jennifer J.D. Morrissette, PhD[a], Adam Bagg, MD[b],*

KEYWORDS

• AML • Cytogenetics • FISH • Molecular genetic
• Classification

Acute myeloid leukemia (AML) is a heterogeneous group of malignancies that account for 1 of 4 broad subtypes of leukemia, neoplasms typically originating in the bone marrow and manifesting in the peripheral blood. AML is most common in the elderly population, with an incidence of approximately 3.4 per 100,000 per year,[1] and a median age of 70 years at diagnosis. The morphologic hallmark of AML is an excessive accumulation (typically >20%) of blasts and other defined immature cells affecting 1 or more "myeloid" lineages, which includes myeloid, monocytic, erythroid, and megakaryocytic precursors. The fundamental defect leading to this accumulation is maturation arrest. AML historically has been categorized by not only the lineages that are affected but also by the stage and degree of differentiation at which the block occurred. The outcome of this block in the normal physiologic progression of maturation is loss of normal hematopoietic differentiation, with an accumulation of blasts, leading to thrombocytopenia, neutropenia, and anemia.

There have been different attempts to classify AML into reproducible, clinically relevant groups. The French American British (FAB) scheme classified the subtypes of AML based on morphologic, immunophenotypic, and cytochemical features, using designations from M0 to M7. This system was remarkably prescient, in that some subtypes were subsequently associated with specific recurrent chromosome abnormalities [eg, FAB M3 with t(15;17)]. More recently (initially in 2001, updated in 2008), the World Health Organization (WHO) has incorporated genetic features into the

Adam Bagg is supported, in part, by the Leukemia and Lymphoma Society of America and the J.P. McCarthy Foundation.

[a] Department of Pathology and Laboratory Medicine, University of Pennsylvania, 201 John Morgan Building, 3620 Hamilton Walk, Philadelphia, PA 19104-4283, USA
[b] Department of Pathology and Laboratory Medicine, University of Pennsylvania, 7.103 Founders Pavilion, 3400 Spruce Street, Philadelphia, PA 19104-4283, USA
* Corresponding author.
E-mail address: adambagg@mail.med.upenn.edu

Clin Lab Med 31 (2011) 659–686
doi:10.1016/j.cll.2011.08.006
0272-2712/11/$ – see front matter © 2011 Elsevier Inc. All rights reserved.

classification of subtypes of AML. Indeed, approximately 60% of AMLs are now genetically classified,[2] although less than one-half of these are cytogenetically defined, highlighting the expansion of those characterized by molecular abnormalities that are not discernible by conventional cytogenetics. The WHO categorizes AML into 4 main groupings: (1) AML with recurrent genetic abnormalities, (2) AML with myelodysplasia-related changes, (3) therapy-related myeloid neoplasms, and (4) AML not otherwise specified.[3] This review focuses on the first group and highlights the central role of cytogenetics in the second and third groups; throughout, the emphasis will be on initial diagnosis and not on the topic of tracking minimal residual disease.

In addition, other recurrent cytogenetic defects and many of the important submicroscopic molecular genetic defects will also be noted. Indeed, the development of AML requires multiple events with the suggestion of at least 2 hits necessary for leukemogenesis. The 2 pathways currently purported to be involved in the development of AML are those that are necessary for proliferation and survival (class I mutations) and others that prevent normal hematopoiesis by blocking differentiation (class II mutations).[4,5] Examples of class I mutations include those affecting *FLT3*, *KIT*, and *NRAS*, whereas examples of class II mutations include t(8;21) and inv(16)/t(16;16).

SAMPLE SUBMISSION

Bone marrow is the preferred specimen to detect abnormalities seen in AML. Ideally, samples for cytogenetic studies should be drawn before treatment to maximize the potential for cell growth in the laboratory. Most laboratories request 1 to 3 mL of spiculated bone marrow specimen, ideally from the first draw from a heparinized needle into a sodium heparin tube. If the first draw of bone marrow is unavailable, resetting the needle or turning the bevel 180° is recommended, so as not to have blood contamination of the marrow specimen. The specimen should be kept at room temperature if setup can occur within 24 to 48 hours, otherwise storage at 4°C is recommended. A sample stored for up to 3 to 4 days at 4°C may yield good results, because neoplastic myeloid cells are typically more tolerant than neoplastic lymphoid cells, but prolonged delays increase the failure rate.

Failure of the cultured cells to divide can be caused by a very small sample size, an extremely high white blood cell count, a hemodilute specimen, or improper storage or transport. Small sample size can lead to an inadequate number of metaphase cells for analysis, and specimens with extremely high white blood cell counts are likely to fail because the majority of cells are incapable of division, and their presence inhibits those that can divide. It is often recommended to include a peripheral blood specimen at the same time as the marrow to be set up as a back-up culture, which can be particularly useful if there are greater than 15% peripheral blasts.

THE ROLE OF CONVENTIONAL CYTOGENETIC STUDIES AND FLUORESCENCE IN SITU HYBRIDIZATION

Cytogenetic abnormalities detected at clinical presentation are one of the main predictors of outcome in AML.[2,6,7] Conventional cytogenetic (CC) studies have defined certain chromosomal rearrangements as favorable risk, standard risk, and high risk (**Table 1**).[8–14] Allied to this, these studies play an essential role in contemporary AML diagnosis and classification. Although most of the disease-defining aberrations are detected by CC studies, fluorescence in situ hybridization (FISH) and sometimes also reverse-transcription polymerase chain reaction (RT-PCR) may also play a central role at diagnosis.

Table 1
AML risk stratification by cytogenetic abnormalities at diagnosis

	Adult		Pediatric	
	Cytogenetic Abnormality	Incidence	Cytogenetic Abnormality	Incidence
Favorable risk[a]	t(15;17)(q24;q21)	5%–13%	t(15;17)(q24;q21)	8%–11%
	t(8;21)(q22;q22)	5%–7%	t(8;21)(q22;q22)	11%–13%
	inv(16)(p13.1q22)/ t(16;16)(p13.1;q22)	5%–8%	inv(16)(p13.1q22)/ t(16;16)(p13.1;q22)	3%–6%
			t(1;11)(q21;q23)	3%
Intermediate risk	t(9;11)(p21;q23)	2%	t(9;11)(p21;q23)	10%
	normal karyotype	40%–45%	t(1;22)(p13;q13)	2%–3%
	−Y	3%	normal karyotype	20%–25%
	+8	10%	<3 abnormalities	6%–7%
Adverse risk[b]	inv(3)(q21q26)/t(3;3)(q21;q26)	1%–2%	inv(3)(q21q26)/t(3;3)(q21;q26)	1%–2%
	−5/ del(5q)/ add(5q)	4%–12%	−5/ del(5q)/ add(5q)	5%–6%
	−7/ del(7q)/ add(7q)	8%	−7/ del(7q)/ add(7q)	1%–2%
	t(8;16)(p11;p13)	<1%	t(11q23) [excluding t(9;11)]	18%–22%
	t(11q23) [excluding t(9;11)]	3%–4%	t(6;9)(p23;q34)	1%
	t(6;9)(p23;q34)	1%–2%	t(9;22)(q34;q11.2)	1%
	t(9;22)(q34;q11.2)	1%	−17/ abn(17p)	2%
	−17/ abn(17p)	5%	Complex (≥3 unrelated abnormalities)	10%
	Complex (≥3 unrelated abnormalities)	6%–14%		

[a] Irrespective of additional cytogenetic abnormalities.
[b] Excluding favorable cytogenetic abnormalities.

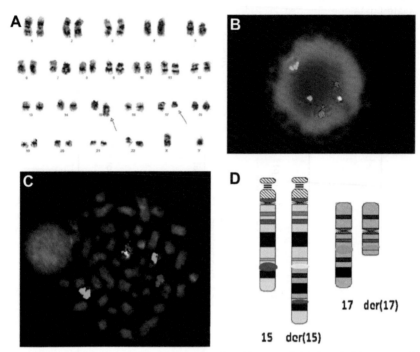

Fig. 1. Variant *PML-RARA* rearrangement elucidated by FISH. (*A*) G-banded karyotype from the bone marrow of a patient with a diagnosis of acute promyelocytic leukemia showing an atypical rearrangement involving chromosomes 15 and 17. (*B*) FISH for the *PML-RARA* rearrangement in an interphase nucleus from the same specimen with a single yellow fusion signal, 2 red (*PML*) signals, and 2 green (*RARA*) signals, confirming an atypical rearrangement involving *PML* and *RARA*. (*C*) Metaphase FISH shows the normal chromosome 15 (large red signal), the derivative chromosome 15 (yellow signal, red signal), the normal chromosome 17 (green signal), and the derivative chromosome 17 with the fusion (smaller green signal). This changes the karyotype to 46,XY,ins(15;17)(q24;q21q25). (*D*) Ideogram of the rearrangement, showing the localization of the *PML* and *RARA* probe signals. ([*D*] *From* Hiller B, Bradtke J, Balz H, et al. CyDAS: a cytogenetic data analysis system. Bioinformatics 2005;21:1282–3; with permission.)

When FISH is performed at diagnosis, it is usually considered to be either an adjunct to conventional cytogenetic studies to unravel the components of complex translocations or a way to identify underlying abnormalities that are cytogenetically cryptic (**Fig. 1**). Thus, FISH is often useful at diagnosis to identify subtle abnormalities or to define breakpoints. Often, metaphase spreads from diagnostic marrows for AML can have poor morphology that can render certain rearrangements equivocal, such as some *MLL* translocations and deletions of 17p13. In such cases, FISH can be helpful in discerning questionable rearrangements that might alter classification and treatment options. For example, some cases of t(15;17) might be missed by CC studies, and only detected by FISH (or RT-PCR). Furthermore, there is also some evidence that FISH can have predictive value at diagnosis in AML. For example, *TP53* deletions identified by FISH portend a poor response to chemotherapy.[15]

In general, interphase FISH correlates extremely well with abnormalities detected by CC. There is some evidence from a large prospective study in a series of older AML patients that some common rearrangements [inv(16), *MLL* rearrangements] in AML are missed by CC studies but readily identified by FISH.[16] The Eastern Collaborative

Oncology Group compared CC studies and FISH in 237 AML specimens and found that a probe panel to detect monosomy 5/deletion 5q, monosomy 7/deletion 7q, trisomy 8, t(8;21), t(9;22), *MLL* rearrangements with various partners, t(15;17), and inv(16)/t(16;16), had a concordance between 98% and 100%.[17] In cases without sufficient metaphase cells for evaluation or metaphase cells with poor morphology or those with nonevaluable chromosomes, FISH studies can be extremely helpful in defining specific entities and the determination of cytogenetic risk groups.

Spectral Karyotyping, Multicolor FISH, and Combined Binary Ratio FISH

Spectral karyotyping (SKY), multicolor FISH (M-FISH), and combined binary ratio FISH (COBRA FISH) are molecular cytogenetic techniques that permit simultaneous visualization of all chromosomes in a different color by combinatorial chromosome painting, using slightly different methodologies.[18] This group of techniques is useful in the detection of translocations, unbalanced rearrangements, and complex karyotypes, in which the resolution of G-banding may be too poor to detect all the rearrangements present. Because these are performed on a background of metaphase chromosomes, they allow the visualization of chromosomal rearrangements, including changes in copy number and location. However, none of these is currently used in most diagnostic laboratories.

Multiplex PCR

The combination of cytogenetic and molecular methods for detection of translocations in AML has multiple benefits and should be considered at diagnosis to detect common rearrangements. Numerous platforms are available that target the common recurrent cytogenetic abnormalities seen in AML, with the benefit of detection of cryptic rearrangements.[19] The technique of multiplex RT-PCR for translocation detection has the advantage of shorter turnaround time and no requirement for dividing cells in the diagnosis of AML, both of which are essential for conventional cytogenetics.

AML WITH RECURRENT GENETIC ABNORMALITIES

There are currently 7 chromosome rearrangements that fall under the category of AML with recurrent genetic abnormalities. They are typically balanced translocations or inversions and are identified in 20% to 30% of all cases of AML. Often these aberrations seemingly occur as the sole cytogenetic abnormality, but they can be seen in the background of complex abnormalities or molecularly detected mutations, which, in some cases, alter risk stratification. In the 2001 edition of the WHO Classification of Tumours of Haematopoietic and Lymphoid Tissues, four such translocations were formally integrated into the diagnosis of AML, and in 2008 edition they were modified and increased to seven (**Table 2**). These balanced rearrangements usually lead to fusion genes and chimeric protein expression and are considered necessary but not sufficient for development of AML.[20]

t(8;21)(q22;q22.3)

The t(8;21) involves *RUNX1T1* on 8q22 and *RUNX1* on 21q22 (**Fig. 2**A) (formerly *ETO* and *AML1/CBFA2*, respectively), and this type of AML is associated with a favorable prognosis in children and adults.[2,21] There is some correlation with the previously designated FAB type of M2 (myeloblastic with maturation), especially those with characteristic blastic morphology (delicate Auer rods, salmon-pink granules) and coexpression of a number of B-cell antigens. The t(8;21) is seen in

Table 2
AML with recurrent chromosomal abnormalities: consequences of genetic disruptions

Abnormality	Critical Chromosome	Involved Genes	Effect of Translocation
t(8;21)(q22;q22)	der(8)	RUNX1-RUNX1T1	Chimeric transcription factor, repression of CBF-regulated genes
inv(16)(p13.1q22)/ t(16;16)(p13.1; q22)	16p	CBFB-MYH11	Chimeric transcription factor, repression of CBF-regulated genes
t(15;17)(q24;q21)	der(15)	PML-RARA	Chimeric transcription factor, resistant to normal RARA activation
t(9;11)(p21;q23)	der(11)	MLLT3-MLL	Dysregulated transcriptional activation
t(6;9)(p22;q34)	der(6)	DEK-NUP214	Increased global gene expression (increased translation?)
inv(3)(q21q26)/ t(3;3)(q21;q26)	3q26 moves to the 3q21 locus	RPN1-EVI1	EVI1 overexpression
t(1;22)(p13;q13)	der(22)	RBM15-MKL1	Transcriptional deregulation

approximately 5% to 7% of de novo AML in adults. Of note, cases with a t(8;21)(q22;q22) are considered to be AML regardless of the percentage of blasts in the bone marrow (ie, it is acceptable to diagnose AML with <20% blasts). Although this is an easy translocation to identify cytogenetically, recognition can be complicated by a complex karyotype or a cryptic insertion. In approximately 3% to 4% of t(8;21)-positive cases, the translocation is complex, involving 8q22, 21q22, and another chromosome[22,23] with evidence indicating that the derivative chromosome 8 is the chromosome harboring the critical abnormal fusion. Secondary abnormalities include sex chromosome loss (X in females, Y in males) and deletions of the long arm of chromosome 9. There appears to be no significant difference in overall survival in patients with a deletion of 9q or loss of an X chromosome; however, loss of the Y chromosome is associated with better overall survival.[2] Individuals with t(8;21) AML have a complete remission rate of 97% and a 10-year overall survival rate of 61%.

RUNX1 encodes the core binding factor subunit alpha 2, with the fusion gene leading to the transcriptional repression of genes that are normally physiologically activated by RUNX1, preventing granulocytic differentiation through dominant-negative inhibition.[24] Although the t(8;21) appears to be necessary for AML development, it is not sufficient, in that additional mutations are necessary for development of this form of AML. This is not unique to t(8;21) AML and is operative in other AMLs; however, this phenomenon is perhaps best studied in this context. This has been demonstrated in a number of ways, including the identification of the t(8;21) in utero followed by a latency of up to 10 years before the development of AML.[25] There is also evidence that the RUNX1T1-RUNX1 transcript persists in patients in long-term, sometimes decades-long, remission,[26,27] although these patients are more likely to relapse than those in whom the transcript is undetectable molecularly.[28] Interestingly, even after relapse, t(8;21)-positive leukemias maintain their good prognosis and can respond well to bone marrow transplantation.

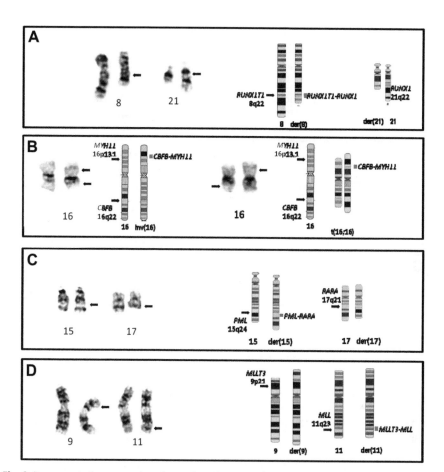

Fig. 2 Representative examples of translocations seen in AML with recurrent genetic abnormalities. Shown are G-banded translocation partner pairs of the WHO group of AML with recurrent genetic changes, with chromosome images (*arrows* indicate the breakpoints on the abnormal homologue) and ideograms to demonstrate the rearranged regions. The blue square represents the critical location for the gene fusion. (*A*) t(8;21)(q22;q22). (*B*) inv(16)(p13.1q22), left, and t(16;16)(p13.1;q22), right. (*C*) t(15;17)(q24;q21). (*D*) t(9;11)(p21; q23). (*E*) inv(3)(q21q26), left, and t(3;3)(q21;q26), right. (*F*) t(6;9)(p22;q34). (*G*) t(1;22)(p13; q13). ([*F*] *Courtesy of* Drs Jinglan Liu and Shashikant Kulkarni, Washington University School of Medicine; [*G*] *Courtesy of* Dr Susana Raimondi, St. Jude Children's Research Hospital.)

Several factors alter the favorable prognosis of t(8;21) AML. Recently, identification of a more potent form of *RUNX1T1-RUNX1* was identified, which shows enhanced leukemogenic potential caused by alternative splicing of exon 9a of the fusion transcript.[28] Although the exon 9 splice variant was seen in patients with *RUNX1-RUNX1T1* rearrangements, the patients who remained in complete remission were found to have a faster disappearance of the *RUNX1-RUNX1T1* exon 9a splice variant compared with patients bound to relapse. Mutations in the *KIT* gene, a receptor tyrosine kinase, have been identified in a subset of patients with t(8;21). Several studies have associated the presence of *KIT*-activating mutations (most commonly affecting an aspartate residue at codon 816) with poorer prognosis in adult patients

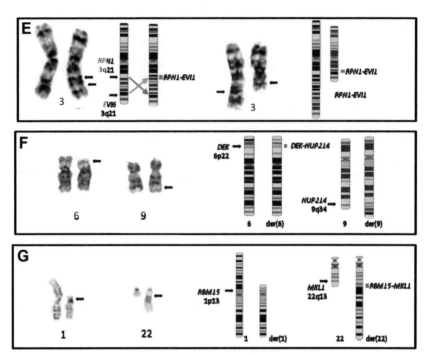

Fig. 2 (continued).

with this translocation.[29,30] However, these mutations appear not to be prognostically relevant in pediatric patients.[31]

inv(16)(p13.1q22) or t(16;16)(p13.1;q22)

These molecularly identical events involve *CBFB* on 16q22 and *MYH11* on 16p13.1 (formerly *PEBP2B* and *SMMHC/SMHC*, respectively), and this form of AML is usually, but not invariably, associated with acute myelomonocytic leukemia with abnormal eosinophils harboring basophilic granules (previously designated FAB M4Eo). Such rearrangements of chromosome 16 are seen in approximately 5% to 8% of all cases of adult AML, with the inversion much more common (95%) (see **Fig. 2**B, left) than the translocation (5%) (see **Fig. 2**B, right).[3] As with the t(8;21)(q22;q22) above, it is possible to diagnose AML when this translocation/inversion is present, regardless of the percentage of blasts.

The inv(16)/t(16;16) is the sole abnormality in 70% of cases. The most frequent secondary changes, trisomy 22, trisomy 8, deletion 7q, and trisomy 21 do not alter the favorable prognosis of this rearrangement; indeed, there is evidence that +22 improves overall outcome.[2] Approximately 20% of cases harbor *KIT* mutations in exons 8 and 17, and this is associated with a less-favorable outcome.[32,33] *RAS* mutations occur in approximately 36% of cases, with *NRAS* more commonly mutated than *KRAS* (32% vs 6%); however, these are not currently considered prognostically significant.[34] Individuals harboring inv(16)/t(16;16) have a complete remission rate of 92% and a 10-year overall survival rate of 55%.[2]

Physiologically, the RUNX1 protein, genetically disrupted in the t(8;21), and CBFB, genetically disrupted here, associate to form core binding factor (CBF), which is a key transcription factor central to the regulation of normal hematopoiesis, via its ability to positively control the expression of a variety of hematopoietically important genes.[20,35] Like *RUNX1-RUNX1T1*, the *CBFB-MYH11* fusion gene product acts in a dominant-negative fashion by preventing normal heterodimer formation[36] leading to a differentiation block. Thus, *CBFB-MYH11* and *RUNX1T1-RUNX1* AMLs can be considered together as CBF-AMLs; interestingly, they have similarly good outcomes.

t(15;17)(q24;q21)

The t(15;17) is essentially synonymous with the diagnosis of acute promyelocytic leukemia (APL), which is equivalent to the entity designated by FAB as AML M3 (see **Fig. 2C**). The translocation was one of the first balanced translocations described in acute leukemia.[37] The breakpoint on chromosome 15 has recently been modified from 15q22 to 15q24.1 (UCSC Human Genome Browser, February 2009, hg19).[38]

It is important to recognize this translocation quite rapidly because of the need to begin (targeted and specific) treatment due to the high rate of the development of disseminated intravascular coagulation in APL. t(15;17) AML comprises about 5% to 13% of all cases of AML and is seen as the sole abnormality in approximately 75% of cases. As above for the 2 CBF AMLs, it is possible to diagnose AML (specifically APL) if this translocation is present, even if there are less than 20% blasts/leukemic promyelocytes. The most common additional abnormalities include trisomy 8, deletion 7q, deletion 9q, and an isochromosome of the derivative 17q from the t(15;17). However, these additional chromosome rearrangements, including those that would typically be considered adverse (eg, abnormalities of 17p and complex abnormalities), do not alter the excellent prognosis of APL.[2] Individuals with a t(15;17) AML have a 93% complete remission rate and a 10-year overall survival rate of 81%.[2]

The translocation involves *PML* on chromosome 15 and *RARA* on chromosome 17, resulting in a chimeric protein, fusing *PML*, and *RARA* on the derivative chromosome 15. The normal PML protein is involved in a variety of cellular processes, whereas RARA encodes a transcription factor for retinoic acid response genes, important in myeloid differentiation. The PML-RARA gene product is exquisitely sensitive to pharmacologic doses of all-trans retinoic acid (ATRA), and APL is thus the hallmark genetic defect-targeted therapy form of AML. Per the 2008 WHO classification of AML with recurrent genetic abnormalities [3], only the presence of t(15;17) is associated with this entity. However, *RARA* is rather promiscuous and can rearrange with several other genes in APL although at a much lower frequency. The t(5;17)(q35;q21) results in its fusion with *NPM1*, the t(11;17)(q13;q21) results in its fusion with *NUMA1*, the t(11;17)(q23;q21) leads to its fusion with *ZBTB16*, the t(4;17) leads to its fusion with *FIP1L1*, and an interstitial deletion of 17(q11.2q21) results in its fusion with *STAT5B*. One rationale for refining this WHO entity in 2008[3] (restricting it to cases with t(15;17) only, and removing these variant translocations that were included in WHO 2001) is that some variants, such as the most common t(11;17)(q23;q21), do not respond to ATRA.

FLT3 mutations in APL are seen in 40% of cases and are associated with higher white blood cell count and the morphologic hypogranular variant. However, these mutations have not been shown to have a significant impact on treatment sensitivity, remission status, or overall outcome in APL.[39]

t(9;11)(p22;q23)

This translocation involves *MMLT3* on 9p22 and *MLL* on 11q23 and is associated with AML with monocytic features (see **Fig. 2D**). The t(9;11) constitutes one-third of all *MLL* rearrangements in AML.[40] It is more common in pediatric AML (10%)[41] than in adult

AML (2%). Trisomy 8 is the most common secondary abnormality (20% of cases), with trisomy 6, 19, and 20 also seen with t(9;11), but none appear to affect the association of this translocation with an intermediate prognosis. This form of AML is considered to have a better prognosis than AML with other translocations involving *MLL* (and for this reason it was separated out in WHO 2008) and has an overall 10-year survival rate of approximately 39%.[2]

inv(3)(q21q26)/t(3;3)(q21;q26)

These 3q rearrangements are seen in 1% to 2% of cases of AML. Unlike the aforementioned translocations that result in fusion genes and chimeric proteins, the consequence of this genetic event is dysregulated (over)expression of *EVI1*. Multi-lineage dysplasia and megakaryocytic differentiation are common features, and the prognosis is typically poor. The inversion (see **Fig. 2E**, left) is at least twice as common as the translocation (see **Fig. 2E**, right), and rare cryptic rearrangements have been identified. The most common secondary abnormality is monosomy 7 (approximately 50% of cases), and this worsens the already dismal poor prognosis associated with this rearrangement.[42] This is not unexpected, because this combination meets criteria for a monosomal karyotype (see later discussion). Deletions of 5q, trisomy 8, and complex karyotypes can also be seen with these 3q rearrangements. However, these additional abnormalities do not influence the extremely poor outcome of these patients who have a 10-year overall survival rate of 3%.[2]

t(6;9)(p22;q34)

This translocation (see **Fig. 2F**) is seen in 1% to 2% of cases of AML, which often have a basophilic component. These cases have a poor prognosis; this is particularly dismal in pediatric patients, with some reports of 0% overall survival rate at 4 years,[43] whereas the 10-year overall survival rate in adults is 27%.[2] The genes involved are *DEK* at 6p22 and *NUP214 (CAN)* at 9q34 and are the sole abnormality in approximately 80% of cases.[44] When additional abnormalities are seen, trisomy 8, del(12p), and trisomy 13 are the most common; however, their effect on outcome is unclear. More than 70% of cases with a t(6;9) also contain the *FLT3* internal tandem duplication, with the combination associated with a high white blood cell count and an even poorer prognosis.[44,45]

t(1;22)(p13;q13)

This translocation fuses *RBM15* (formerly *OTT*) at 1p13 with *MKL* (formerly *MAL*) at 22q13 (see **Fig. 2G**)[46] and is seen in less than 1% of AML.[2] The translocation is most often seen in infants or young children, with most cases being observed in the first 6 months of life. The t(1;22) is associated with acute megakaryoblastic leukemia (AMKL) and is the most common abnormality seen in pediatric AMKL in the first year of life. Although the prognosis of AMKL is poor, infants with the t(1;22) fare better than those lacking the translocation.[3] The t(1;22) has been associated with an intermediate outcome, with a 3-year event-free survival rate of approximately 50%. This is the sole abnormality in 60% of cases (mostly those under 6 months of age), with older children more likely to have a hyperdiploid karyotype [2, +19, +der(1)t(1;22), +6, +21]. These additional changes are reported to have no effect on outcome. The presence of supernumerary der(22)t(1;22) and the retention of the der(22) as the sole abnormality in some cases suggest that the critical event lies on the der(22), leading to the fusion gene *RBM15-MKL*.

Table 3
AML with myelodysplasia-related changes: cytogenetic features and genetic correlates

Cytogenetic Abnormality	Frequency	Genetic Consequence[a]
Monosomy 5/del5q	1%–11%	*EGR1, CSF1R, RPS14, CTNNA1*
Monosomy 7/del 7q	1%–7%	Unknown
iso(17q)/del(17p)	0.5%–1.5%	*TP53*
del (11q)	0.6%–5%	*MLL*
t(11;16)(q23;p13.3)	<0.2%	*MLL-CBP*
t(3;21)(q26.2;q22)	<0.5%	*RUNX1-RPL22L1, RUNX1-MDS1-EVI1*
t(2;11)(p21;q23)	<0.5%	Unknown-*MLL*
t(5;12)(q33;p12)	<0.5%	*ETV6-PDGFRB*
t(5;7)(q33;q11.2)	<0.5%	*HIP1-PDGFRB*
t(5;17)(q33;p13)	<0.5%	*RABEP1-PDGFRB*
t(5;10)(q33;q21)	<0.5%	*H4(D10S170)-PDGFRB*
t(3;5)(q25;q34)	<0.5%	*NPM1-MLF1*
Complex karyotypes ≥ 3 abnormalities	10%–15%	Not applicable

[a] In all except for the numerical abnormalities in the first 4 rows (which are assumed to lead to haploinsufficiency of the noted genes), the effects are mostly a consequence of fusion genes that typically, but not always, lead to chimeric proteins.

AML WITH MYELODYSPLASIA-RELATED CHANGES

This WHO AML category can be diagnosed when there are greater than 20% blasts and 1 criterion of 3 is met: (1) a history of a myelodysplastic syndrome (MDS) or MDS/myeloproliferative neoplasm (MPN), (2) an MDS-related genetic abnormality (**Table 3**), or (3) morphologic evidence of multilineage dysplasia. Important exclusionary criteria are a history of prior chemotherapy or radiotherapy (described below) and an absence of a recurring cytogenetic abnormality (described in AML with recurrent genetic changes above). This category, AML with myelodysplasia-related changes (AML-MRC) may account for between one-fourth and one-third of all cases of adult AML.[47] AML-MRC has a poor prognosis with low rates of achieving complete remission and is more common in the elderly, being rarely seen in the pediatric population.

Of the 3 criteria that allow for the diagnosis of AML-MRC, it appears that it is the presence (or absence) of associated genetic abnormalities that best defines this category and dictates prognosis. For example, there are a number of cases with a preceding MDS or MDS/MPN with a normal karyotype. In general, such cases are associated with a better prognosis than those with MDS-related cytogenetic abnormalities. Some cases of AML with multilineage dysplasia have been found to have mutations in *NPM1*, *FLT3*, or *CEBPA* (described in later discussion). In the background of a normal karyotype, these are considered to be important prognostic markers, but here MDS-related cytogenetic abnormalities assume diagnostic precedence[47]; however, this may not be the case in AML-MRC defined by multilineage dysplasia.[48] Chromosome abnormalities identified within this group are most commonly unbalanced rearrangements, including monosomy 5/5q−, monosomy 7/deletion 7q, abnormalities of 3q26 [including inv(3)(q21q26), t(3;3)(q21;q26), and ins(3;3)(q21;q26)], as well as complex cytogenetics with ≥ 3 abnormalities.

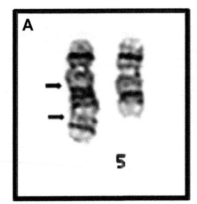 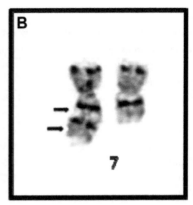

Fig. 3. Representative examples of deletions seen in AML with myelodysplasia-related changes. Shown are G-banded deletion partner pairs of the WHO group of AML with myelodysplasia-related changes (*arrows* indicate the proximal and distal breakpoints on the normal homologue). (*A*) Deletion 5q13-q31. (*B*) Deletion 7q22-q34.

Deletion 5q/monosomy 5

Monosomy 5 and deletion 5q are seen in approximately 6% of all cases of AML (**Fig. 3**A). Although these are often lumped together, monosomy 5 is rarely seen as the sole abnormality and is often seen with trisomy 8, monosomy 7, and trisomy 21. Loss of chromosome 5 in the context of structural abnormalities or other chromosome loss is considered to be a poor predictor of outcome, fitting the definition of a monosomal karyotype (see later discussion).

Deletion of the long arm of chromosome 5 can be seen as the sole change or in the context of additional abnormalities. When deletions occur in the context of more complex karyotypes, the prognosis is poor. The molecular consequence of the deletion is almost certainly the loss of tumor suppressor genes, rather than creation of a fusion gene, because there are many different proximal and distal breakpoints described. The majority of the deletions are interstitial and usually inclusive of bands 5q31 to q33. Numerous candidate genes have been identified, including *CTNNA1*, *EGR1*, and *RPS14*,[49,50] as well as microRNAs *miR-145* and *miR-146a*.[51] Abnormalities of chromosome 5 are also seen in therapy-related AML (see later discussion).

Deletion 7q/monosomy 7

Monosomy 7 is the second most common numerical chromosome abnormality seen in AML (trisomy 8 is more common; see later discussion) and is seen in approximately 10% of cases, as the sole abnormality in approximately 5%, and as a secondary abnormality in approximately 5%.[52] Deletions of the long arm of chromosome 7q are also common in AML (see **Fig. 3**B), typically involve bands within 7q22 to q34, and are usually inclusive of 7q31.1, but this deletion is frequently seen in the context of additional abnormalities as compared with monosomy 7. There are multiple breakpoints on 7q, and although numerous groups have performed mapping studies, the identification of a putative tumor suppressor gene remains elusive.[53]

Both monosomy 7 and deletion 7q are common secondary abnormalities that can be associated with specific translocations. For example, and as noted above, monosomy 7 is seen as a secondary abnormality in 50% of cases of inv(3)(q21q26)/ t(3;3)(q21q26). Monosomy 7 and deletion 7q, as with monosomy 5 and deletion 5q, are commonly seen in the context of prior exposure to alkylating agents and radiotherapy (see later discussion).

THERAPY-RELATED AML

Therapy-related acute leukemia (t-AML) is a complication of cytotoxic therapy used for primary cancer treatment and accounts for 10% to 20% of myeloid neoplasms. These forms of AML are incorporated under the WHO group of therapy-related myeloid neoplasms, which also includes MDS and MDS/MPN. WHO does not separate out these otherwise distinct and typically morphologically and hematologically defined categories when a myeloid neoplasm arises in the context of prior therapy,[54] because they all seem to involve similar genetic pathogeneses and have a uniformly dismal prognosis. Further, although 2 distinct groups of therapy-related AML have been well recognized (arising with topoisomerase II inhibitors or alkylating agents/radiation therapy), they are now considered together, because many polychemotherapeutic regimens often include drugs from both classes. Nevertheless, it is worth highlighting some distinguishing differences (**Table 4**).

Abnormalities associated with prior treatment with topoisomerase II inhibitors typically involve gene rearrangements leading to gene fusions, classically involving 11q23/*MLL*. These patients typically do not have an intervening MDS phase, there is usually a relatively short latency period (<5 years), and morphologically there is often a monocytic component. Although approximately two-thirds of such AMLs associated with topoisomerase II inhibitors harbor 11q23 translocations, the remaining one-third do not. The latter include some translocations that had previously been construed of as classical de novo AMLs [those with t(15;17), t(8;21), inv(16)/t(16;16), as well as 11p15 rearrangements, involving *NUP98*]. Patients with these structural abnormalities often present in a similar manner to the de novo AMLs. However, there is some evidence that these apparently identical translocations do not have the same favorable outcome when occurring in the setting of cytotoxic therapy.[55]

Abnormalities associated with alkylating agents (such as melphalan and chlorambucil) typically involve chromosomal deletions and monosomies. The 2 abnormalities most commonly associated with alkylating agents are monosomy 7/deletion 7q, and monosomy 5/deletion 5q.[56] These abnormalities are typically seen 5 to 10 years after treatment, after an MDS phase, and may be associated with a complex karyotype. Patients with these abnormalities have a poor therapeutic response.

AML IN CHILDREN WITH DOWN SYNDROME

Early in infancy, up to 10% of children with Down syndrome can present with transient abnormal myelopoiesis (TAM),[57] a typically reversible phenomenon associated with acquired *GATA1* mutations but that can mimic AML morphologically. There are no clonal cytogenetic abnormalities in TAM, but cytogenetic studies should be performed, primarily to exclude bona fide AML. The appearance of such chromosomal abnormalities can be a harbinger of acute transformation. In the majority (70% to 80%) of cases, TAM resolves without treatment over a period of several weeks to months. However, in 20% to 30% of cases, it can evolve into AML, typically AMKL, albeit without the t(1;22) seen in AMKL in children without Down syndrome.

OTHER COMMON AND RELEVANT CYTOGENETIC ABNORMALITIES THAT DO NOT CURRENTLY DEFINE SPECIFIC TYPES OF AML CURRENTLY DESIGNATED BY WHO

Monosomal Karyotype

The poor outcome of individuals with complex karyotypes, defined as 3 or more abnormalities, has long been recognized (**Fig. 4**). Reanalysis of patients with complex

Table 4
Therapy-Related AML: Associations with different therapeutic agents

Therapy	Abnormality	Frequency	MDS Phase	Approximate Time from Exposure
Alkylating agents—70% (for example, melphalan, cyclophosphamide, chlorambucil) Ionizing radiation therapy	5q deletion/ monosomy 5[a] 7q deletion/ monosomy 7[a]	70%[b]	Common	Long latency (5–10 y)
Topoisomerase inhibitors—30% (for example, etoposide, daunorubicin, mitoxantrone)	*MLL* rearrangements *RUNX1* rearrangements t(15;17) inv(16)/t(16;16) Others	3%–32% 2.5%–4.5% 2% 2% 15%–20%	Rare	Short latency (1–5 y)

[a] Often associated with additional cytogenetic abnormalities [del(13q), del(20q), del(11q), del(3p), −17, −18, −21, +8].
[b] Of abnormalities of chromosome 5, 7, or both.

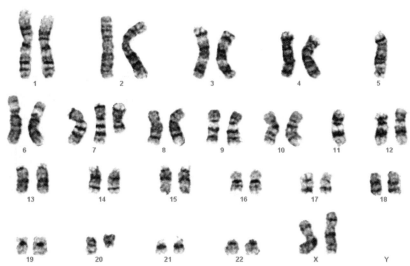

Fig. 4. Monosomal karyotype. G-banded karyogram from a woman with AML with a karyotype of 44,XX,–5,+del(7)(q22),–11,del(20)(q11.2), with numerical and structural abnormalities present.

karyotypes (including numerical aberrations, structural abnormalities, and marker chromosomes) identified a unique subset of individuals with an extremely poor outcome, designated the monosomal karyotype (MK).[58] MK is defined as 2 or more monosomies or a single monosomy in the presence of structural abnormalities. A large study by SWOG[59] showed that MK is more frequent in elderly AML patients. In this group, the 4-year overall survival rate of patients with unfavorable cytogenetics was only 3%, compared with 13% without MK. MK in AML is quite common (approximately 10% of all AML and up to 20% in older populations) and its recognition is paramount, so that alternative therapies can be used to potentially modify the associated dismal prognosis.[60]

Trisomy 8

The most common numerical abnormality observed in AML is trisomy 8, which is seen in approximately 10% to 20% of AMLs, either as the sole abnormality (in one-third of cases) or as an additional abnormality in the remainder.[52] The molecular genetic consequences of acquired trisomy 8 are unclear.

Trisomy 8 is not associated with a particular morphology or immunophenotype and is considered in some studies to be an intermediate prognostic marker. It does not alter a favorable prognosis when seen as a secondary abnormality with t(8;21), inv(16)/t(16;16), or t(15;17).

11q23 Rearrangements Other Than the t(9;11)

In addition to the t(9;11)(p22;q23) described above, there are numerous other rearrangements involving the *MLL* gene on 11q23, which are found in 3% to 10% of cases of both de novo and therapy-related AML (**Fig. 5**A, B). The der(11) harbors the fusion oncogene, with the N-terminus of *MLL* joined in-frame with the various partner genes. The *MLL* rearrangement is the sole chromosome abnormality in 60% of cases,

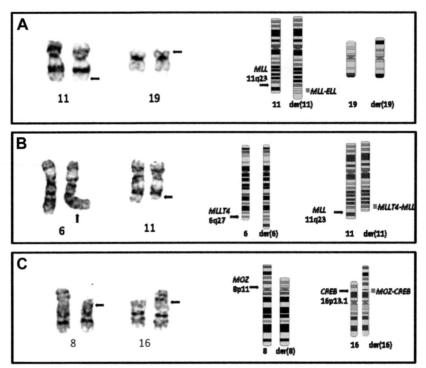

Fig. 5. Representative examples of recurrent translocations seen in AML that do not currently define specific types of AML. (*A*) t(11;19)(q23;p13.1). (*B*) t(6;11)(q27;q23). (*C*) t(8;16)(p11;p13.1).

and the most common rearrangement is a translocation, but many variants have been identified, including insertions, inversions, and partial tandem duplications.[53] The MLL protein has histone methyltransferase activity and thus affects chromatin remodeling. *MLL* is promiscuous, with greater than 80 different partners in AML, more than 45 of which have been cloned. *MLL* rearrangements are also seen in acute lymphoblastic leukemia. Although there is some partner specificity for *MLL* rearrangements (in acute lymphoblastic leukemia vs AML), there is also overlap.

Like t(9;11), these other *MLL* translocations are most often seen in AML with monocytic differentiation; unlike the t(9;11), however, they are associated with a poor prognosis. As noted above, *MLL* translocations may occur (apparently) de novo and in therapy-related contexts. Curiously, these different *MLL* rearrangements often have different breakpoints, with the de novo cases more likely to have a 5' breakpoint and the therapy-related cases a 3' breakpoint.[61]

Two *MLL* rearrangements, t(6;11)(q27;q23) (see **Fig. 5**B) and t(10;11)(p12;q23) involving the *MLLT4* and *MLLT10* genes predict a particularly poor prognosis, with a median survival of 9 months and a 10-year overall survival rate of approximately 10%.[2,62] By contrast, the t(1;11)(21;23), involving *MLLT11*, is associated with a good prognosis in pediatric AML.[63]

t(8;16)(p11;p13)

AML with t(8;16) is rare (0.2% of cases of AML) and is often associated with acute monocytic/monoblastic leukemias that display erythrophagocytosis (see **Fig. 5**C).

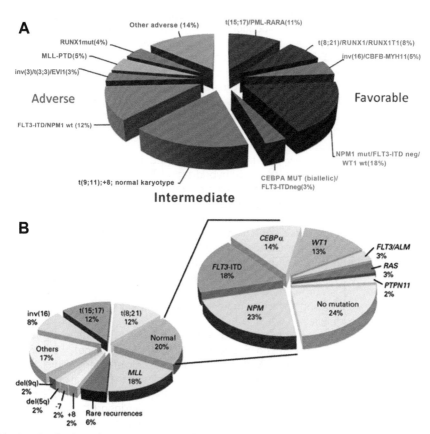

Fig. 6. Distribution of recurrent genetic abnormalities in AML. (*A*) Cytogenetic and molecular genetic abnormalities to refine risk groups in adult AML. (*B*) In pediatric AML, approximately 80% of patients have chromosome rearrangements, and the majority of those with a normal karyotype have single gene mutations.[66,67] (*Adapted from* Smith ML, Hills RK, Grimwade D. Independent prognostic variables in acute myeloid leukaemia. Blood Rev 2011;25:39–51; *with permission.*)

This translocation involves *MYST3* (formerly *MOZ*) on 8p11.2 and *CREB* (formerly *CBP*) on 16p13.1, leading to an in-frame fusion. AML associated with *MYST3* rearrangements are associated with a poor prognosis, with median overall survival of 4.7 months.[64]

MOLECULOCENTRIC APPROACHES TO AML CLASSIFICATION

Although the typically grossly detectable translocations and numeric abnormalities discussed above are central to the diagnosis and classification of AML, it has become increasingly clear that multiple other submicroscopic lesions are also germane to the pathogenesis and prognosis of these genetically complex neoplasms (**Fig. 6A, B**).[65] Although these cannot be detected by CC or FISH, technologies that are the focus of this review, they are nevertheless worth highlighting given their significant relevance, at many levels, in AML (**Table 5**). Detection of some of these mutations in diagnostic specimens of AML is essential, regardless of karyotype. Although many are enriched

Table 5
Gene mutations in AML: Contextual frequency, biologic consequences, and prognostic significance

Gene	Typical (cyto)genetic context		Mutations	Consequence	Prognostic Significance
	Normal Karyotype	Associated Cytogenetic Abnormality			
NPM1	50%–60%	14%–15%	~50 variants. Mutation A (TCTG tetra-nucleotide duplication) commonest (70%–80%)	Cytoplasmic mislocalization, p14/ARF dysregulation	Favorable (with normal karyotype, in the absence of FLT3-ITD)
CEBPA	10%–15%	9q deletions (40%)	Out-of-frame insertions and deletions in the N-terminal region; In-frame insertions and deletions in the C-terminal region	Transcriptional repression	Favorable (when biallelic, with normal karyotype, in the absence of FLT3-ITD)
FLT3	25%–30%	t(6;9) (70%) t(15;17) (40%)	ITD (75%–80%) TKD (20%–25%)	Increase signal transduction, decreased apoptosis	Poor (when there is aUPD)
KIT	2%–8%	t(8;21) (16%–45%) inv(16)/t(16;16) (29%) trisomy 4	TKD D816 TKD N822	Gain of function, increase signal transduction	Poor
RUNX1	5%–33%, MLL-PTD (20%) FLT3 (16%) NRAS (9%)	trisomy13 (90%)	Missense, nonsense, frameshift mutations	Decrease transcription of CBF target genes	Poor
MLL	5%–11%, FLT3	trisomy 11 (25%–45%)	PTD	Transcriptional activation of MLL target genes, histone hyper-methylation	Unclear (? poor)
WT1	1%–2% FLT3-ITD (8%)	?	Insertions and deletions within exons 7 and 9	? transcriptional repression	Unclear (? poor with FLT3-ITD)

continued on next page

Table 5
(Continued)

Gene	Typical (cyto)genetic context		Mutations	Consequence	Prognostic Significance
	Normal Karyotype	Associated Cytogenetic Abnormality			
NRAS	10%–13%	inv(16)/t(16;16) (37%) t(8;21) (7%) inv(3)/ t(3;3) (23%)	Missense, codons 12, 13, and 61	Activating mutations, increased signal transduction	Unclear
KRAS	2.5%	inv(16)/t(16;16) inv(3)/ t(3;3) (24%)	Missense, codons 12, 13	Activating mutations, increased signal transduction	Unclear
TP53	1%–11%	Complex karyotype with or without 17p deletion (66%–88%)	Missense (most common), nonsense, splice site, deletions, insertions	Loss of tumor suppressor activity	Poor
IDH1	7%–8%	Monosomy 8	Missense (R132)	Oncometabolite leading to DNA hypermethylation	Unclear (? poor)
IDH2	8%–9%	Unclear	Missense (R140, R172)	Oncometabolite leading to DNA hypermethylation	Unclear (? poor)
DNMT3A	22%	Unclear	Missense	Genome-wide hypomethylation	Poor
ASXL1	8%–25%	9%, including favorable [eg, t(8; 21)) and poor (eg, −7, i(17q)]	Exon 12	Chromatin modification	Unknown
TET2	12%–17%	Unknown	Deletion, frameshift nonsense	Epigenetic regulation	?poor
CBL	2%–4%	CBP-AML (3%–5%)	Missense	E3 ubiquitin ligase, gain of function	Unknown

Abbreviations: PTD, partial tandem duplication; TKD, tyrosine kinase domain; ?, currently unknown or questionable.

in cases with normal cytogenetics, some are associated with recurrent cytogenetic abnormalities, often modifying the prognosis. Hence, incorporation of these data with cytogenetic results can provide critical clinically applicable information.[68,69] Of note, provisional status has been given by the 2008 WHO classification to AMLs with mutations in *NPM1* and *CEBPA*.[3]

NPM1

The gene encoding nucleophosmin (*NPM1*) is located at 5q35 and is the most frequent molecular target in AML, seen in about 25% to 30% of de novo AML,[70] but overrepresented in patients with a normal karyotype (50% to 60%). The most common mutations involve an insertion of 4 to 11 base pairs in the terminal exon (causing a frame shift) and leads to the cytoplasmic distribution of the NPM1 protein, which is physiologically housed in the nucleus. NPM1 is associated with many pathways, including ribosome biogenesis, chromatin remodeling, DNA repair, replication, and transcription. More than 50 mutations have been identified in *NPM1* and are typically heterozygous.[70] *NPM1* mutation status has been associated with a favorable prognosis when seen in the background of a normal karyotype and without the presence of a *FLT3-ITD* mutation.[71]

CEBPA

The gene for CCAAT/enhancer-binding protein-α (CEBPA) is located at 19q13 and the protein is a transcription factor involved in myeloid differentiation. Mutations in *CEBPA* differ somewhat from the other gene mutations seen in AML in that the mutations are only prognostically relevant when biallelic.[72] As such, they are associated with a favorable prognosis. *CEBPA* mutations are seen in approximately 10% to 15% of AML, with a slight overrepresentation in the presence of a normal karyotype (15% to 18%).[3,73] Concurrent *FLT3* and *NPM1* mutations are rarely seen with *CEBPA* mutations.[72]

FLT3

FLT3 located at 13q12 codes for a receptor tyrosine kinase expressed on the cell surface of hematopoietic progenitor cells. Mutations leading to constitutive activation of the FLT3 receptor are seen in approximately 25% to 30% of cases of cytogenetically normal AML (and approximately 15% of all cases). In-frame internal tandem duplications (ITD) of the juxtamembrane domain are the most common mutations, representing approximately three-fourths of *FLT3* mutations. Mutations within the tyrosine kinase 2 domain account for the remaining one-fourth, most commonly at position D835.[74] Although these mutations lead to autophosphorylation and constitutive activation of the tyrosine kinase activity, only those with the ITD are clearly prognostically relevant. This adverse prognosis is especially evident in the absence of wild-type *FLT3*, typically occurring as a consequence of acquired uniparental disomy.

Although *FLT3* mutations are most often seen in AML with normal karyotype, there are 2 translocations with which it is seen in a high percentage of cases. Approximately 70% of cases of AML with t(6;9) have this mutation, and it is seen in 40% to 45% of cases of t(15;17)-positive APL,[75] particularly in the microgranular morphologic variant and with the 'short' (*PML* bcr3) *PML-RARA* isoform.

KIT

KIT is a receptor tyrosine kinase that is structurally related to FLT3. Mutations of *KIT*, located at 4q11.2, occur in 2% to 8% of all cases of AML with gain of function mutations leading to intermolecular autophosphorylation and increased signal transduction.[76] The mutations in *KIT* are variable; those in exon 8 lead to dimerization, whereas those in exon 17 affect the activation loop. *KIT* mutations are enriched in CBP-AMLs [t(8;21) and inv(16)/t(16;16)], seen in 16% to 46% of cases. In adults with CBP-AMLs, *KIT* mutations have been associated with a poor prognosis, but this does not seem to be the case in pediatric AML.

A variety of other single gene mutations have been described, with the advent of high throughput sequencing yielding many new discoveries, and it is challenging to keep abreast of these. Some are detailed in **Table 5**[77,78]; no doubt others will have been described subsequent to this review being written, and more after it has been read.

NASCENT AND EMERGING GENETIC TECHNOLOGIES

A number of newer technologies, some of which are being applied clinically while others still remain in the research realm, have led to fundamental discoveries in AML and are very briefly reviewed here.

DNA Copy Number/Single Nucleotide Polymorphism Microarrays

Array comparative genomic hybridization (aCGH) is a cytogenomic technique that allows genome-wide detection of chromosomal gains and losses. Approaches include the use of bacterial artificial chromosomes in standard aCGH and single nucleotide polymorphisms (SNP) in SNP arrays. A clear advantage of SNP arrays is the ability to detect acquired uniparental disomy (aUPD)/copy number neutral loss of heterozygosity.[79] For example it has recently been shown that aUPD of the *TP53* locus, seen in approximately 11% of cases, is an independent negative prognosticator, portending an extremely short survival.[80] Multiple studies have shown that aCGH leads to better global identification of copy number changes, greatly increasing the resolution obtained by both conventional cytogenetics and FISH.[80–82]

Gene Expression Profiling

Gene-expression profiling is a technique by which RNA expression patterns are identified and clustered into subgroups according to parameters of interest, including chromosomal rearrangement and mutation status or clinical outcomes. A number of studies have evaluated genomic signatures in AML. Initial studies found that AMLs defined by recurrent cytogenetic abnormalities had distinctive expression profiles, which validated their classification as AML entities. Novel subgroups have also emerged in an attempt to discern different genetic signatures in cytogenetically normal AML.[83–85]

Genome-wide Methylation Analysis

There are multiple epigenetic mechanisms that have been shown to alter gene expression in AML (reviewed in Chen and coworkers[86]). These mechanisms include methylation of DNA (for example, on cytosine residues in promoter regions) as well as a variety of histone modifications. Analysis of genome-wide promoter methylation patterns appears to provide important additional information regarding risk and outcome, and prognostic subgroups based on DNA methylation profiles have been identified.[82] The DNA methyltransferase, DNMT3A, plays a central role in epigenetic regulation; *DNMT3A* is mutated in approximately 20% of cases of acute myelomonocytic leukemia,[87] leading to differential methylation and gene expression profiles and a poor prognosis.[88]

miRNA Profiling

miRNAs are short RNA molecules that are transcribed, but not translated, and are involved in the posttranscriptional regulation of gene expression through gene silencing. They regulate many developmental processes, including hematopoiesis. Prognostically significant aberrant miRNA profiles have been identified in AML.[89,90] These abnormal patterns can be detected by RT-PCR or miRNA arrays.

Whole Genome, Transcriptome, and Exome Sequencing

The human diploid genome is approximately 6 Gb. Although unthinkable only a decade ago, advances in next-generation massively parallel sequencing technologies are bringing about the day when the entire genomic sequence of a patient or a patient's malignancy will be readily attainable.[91] The first AML genome from a cytogenetically normal case has been sequenced, identifying many submicroscopic changes.[91]

Alternatively, to sequence the transcriptome (the set of all RNA molecules produced in a population of cells), is a smaller project, consisting of about 10% of the genome. Transcriptome sequence comparison of a diagnostic and remission marrow of a patient with AML identified mutations in genes associated with leukemogenesis.[92] The exome (expressed RNAs) is only about 1% to 1.5% of the genome, about 30 to 45 Mb in size.[93] This is currently a more manageable fraction of the genome to sequence and is more amenable to bioinformatics models related to understanding the functional relevance of SNPs and common insertion/deletions (indels). For example, exome sequencing identified mutations in DMNT3A alluded to above.[88] However, these sequencing technologies are potentially hindered by the presence of constitutional DNA sequence variants, and each individual has been estimated to have as many as 4 million variants. Hence, when determining whether a variant is significant in AML, a normal tissue control must be used for assessing whether the variation is acquired or constitutional.

SUMMARY

It is a truism to state that the diagnosis of AML is multifaceted, harnessing such laboratory-based parameters as morphology, immunophenotype, and genetics. The requirement for integration also applies and indeed expands within genetic testing, in that the extremely important findings from conventional karyotyping (aided and abetted by FISH and RT-PCR) now need to be synthesized with an explosion of new data emerging at the molecular level. This is especially (but not exclusively) and fortuitously (not only from the viewpoint of the dissection of the pathophysiology) evident in the approximately one-half of AMLs that are karyotypically normal. Thus, those from this group with isolated NPM1 mutations or biallelic CEPBA mutations are now elevated from intermediate or standard prognosis to a category of good prognosis, in which stem cell transplantation is now no longer a front-line therapeutic consideration. Conversely, AMLs with a normal karyotype and a FLT3 ITD mutation (with loss of wild type) have a poor outcome, requiring alternative, and perhaps more targeted, therapies. The unraveling of the genetic basis of AML at the molecular level, which is already altering diagnostic, prognostic, and therapeutic algorithms, is likely to continue with the application of other technologic modalities of interrogating not only DNA (or exomes) by high throughput sequencing and RNA by targeted arrays or multiplex RT-PCR, but also at the epigenomic level, such as through methylation and miRNA profiling. This is likely to become even more exciting (but daunting and complicated), by analyses of the patient's constitutional genome, to ascertain specific drug sensitivity.

REFERENCES

1. Jemal A, Siegel R, Ward E, et al. Cancer statistics, 2008. CA Cancer J Clin 2008;58: 71–96.
2. Grimwade D, Hills RK, Moorman AV, et al.National Cancer Research Institute Adult Leukaemia Working Group. Refinement of cytogenetic classification in acute myeloid leukemia: determination of prognostic significance of rare recurring chromosomal abnormalities among 5876 younger adult patients treated in the United Kingdom Medical Research Council trials. Blood 2010;116:354–65.
3. Arber DA, Brunning RD, Le Beau MM, et al. Acute myeloid leukaemia with recurrent genetic abnormalities. In: Swerdlow SH, Campo E, Harris NL, et al, editors. World Health Organization Classification of Tumours of Haematopoietic and Lymphoid Tissues. Lyon: IARC; 2008. p.110–23.
4. Gilliland DG. Hematologic malignancies. Curr Opin Hematol 2001;8:189–91.
5. Reilly JT. Pathogenesis of acute myeloid leukaemia and inv(16)(p13;q22): a paradigm for understanding leukaemogenesis? Br J Haematol 2005;128:18–34.
6. Betts DR, Ammann RA, Hirt A, et al. The prognostic significance of cytogenetic aberrations in childhood acute myeloid leukaemia: a study of the Swiss Paediatric Oncology Group (SPOG) Eur J Haematol 2007;78:468–76.
7. von Neuhoff C, Reinhardt D, Sander A, et al. Prognostic impact of specific chromosomal aberrations in a large group of pediatric patients with acute myeloid leukemia treated uniformly according to trial AML-BFM 98. J Clin Oncol 2010;28;2682–9.
8. Berger R, Bernheim A, Ochoa-Noguera ME, et al. Prognostic significance of chromosomal abnormalities in acute nonlymphocytic leukemia: a study of 343 patients. Cancer Genet Cytogenet 987;28:293–9.
9. Samuels BL, Larson RA, Le Beau MM, et al. Specific chromosomal abnormalities in acute nonlymphocytic leukemia correlate with drug susceptibility in vivo. Leukemia 1988;2:79–83.
10. Keating MJ, Smith TL, Kantarjian H, et al. Cytogenetic pattern in acute myelogenous leukemia: a major reproducible determinant of outcome. Leukemia 1988;2:403–12.
11. Fenaux P, Preudhomme C, Lai JL, et al. Cytogenetics and their prognostic significance in acute myeloid leukaemia: a report on 283 cases. Br J Haematol 1989;73: 61–7.
12. Marosi C, Köller U, Koller-Weber E, et al. Prognostic impact of karyotype and immunologic phenotype in 125 adult patients with de novo AML. Cancer Genet Cytogenet 1992;61:14–25.
13. Dastugue N, Payen C, Lafage-Pochitaloff M, et al. Prognostic significance of karyotype in de novo adult myeloid leukemia. Leukemia 1995;9:1491–8.
14. Damm F, Heuser M, Morgan M, et al. Integrative prognostic risk score in acute myeloid leukemia with normal karyotype. Blood 2011. [Epub ahead of print].
15. Tavor S, Rothman R, Golan T, et al. Predictive value of TP53 fluorescence in situ hybridization in cytogenetic subgroups of acute myeloid leukemia. Leuk Lymphoma 2011;52:642–7.
16. Fröhling S, Kayser S, Mayer C, et al. AML Study Group Ulm. Diagnostic value of fluorescence in situ hybridization for the detection of genomic aberrations in older patients with acute myeloid leukemia. Haematologica 2005;90:194–9.
17. Vance GH, Kim H, Hicks GA, et al. Utility of interphase FISH to stratify patients into cytogenetic risk categories at diagnosis of AML in an Eastern Cooperative Oncology Group (ECOG) clinical trial (E1900). Leuk Res 2007;31:605–9.

18. Volpi EV, Bridger JM. FISH glossary: an overview of the fluorescence in situ hybridization technique. Biotechniques 2008;45:385–6.
19. King RL, Naghashpour M, Watt CD, et al. A comparative analysis of molecular genetic and conventional cytogenetic detection of diagnostically important translocations in over 400 cases of acute leukemia, highlighting the frequency of false negative conventional cytogenetics. Am J Clinic Path 2011;135:921–8.
20. Speck NA, Gilliland DG. Core-binding factors in haematopoiesis and leukaemia. Nat Rev Cancer 2002;2:502–13.
21. Harrison CJ, Hills RK, Moorman AV, et al. Cytogenetics of childhood acute myeloid leukemia: United Kingdom Medical Research Council Treatment trials AML 10 and 12. J Clin Oncol 2010;28:2674–81.
22. Groupe Francais de Cytogenetique Hematologique. Acute myelogenous leukemia with an 8;21 translocation; a report on 148 cases from the Groupe Francais de Cytogenetique Hematologique. Cancer Genet Cytogenet 1990;44:169–79.
23. Huang L, Abruzzo LV, Valbuena JR, et al. Acute myeloid leukemia associated with variant t(8;21) detected by conventional cytogenetic and molecular studies: a report of four cases and review of the literature. Am J Clin Pathol 2006;125:267–72.
24. Elagib KE, Goldfarb AN. Oncogenic pathways of AML1-ETO in acute myeloid leukemia: multifaceted manipulation of marrow maturation. Cancer Lett 2007;251: 179–86.
25. Wiemels JL, Xiao Z, Buffler PA, et al. In utero origin of t(8;21) AML1-ETO translocations in childhood acute myeloid leukemia. Blood 2002;99:3801–5.
26. Jurlander J, Caligiuri MA, Ruutu T, et al. Persistence of the AML1/ETO fusion transcript in patients treated with allogeneic bone marrow transplantation for t(8;21) leukemia. Blood 1996;88:2183–91.
27. Miyamoto T, Nagafuji K, Akashi K, et al. Persistence of multipotent progenitors expressing AML1/ETO transcripts in long-term remission patients with t(8;21) acute myelogenous leukemia. Blood 1996;87:4789–96.
28. Ommen HB, Ostergaard M, Yan M, et al. Persistent altered fusion transcript splicing identifies RUNX1-RUNX1T1+ AML patients likely to relapse. Eur J Haematol 2010; 84:128–32.
29. Paschka P, Marcucci G, Ruppert AS, et al. Adverse prognostic significance of KIT mutations in adult acute myeloid leukemia with inv(16) and t(8;21): a Cancer and Leukemia Group B Study. J Clin Oncol 2006;24:3904–11.
30. Schnittger S, Kohl TM, Haferlach T, et al. KIT-D816 mutations in AML1-ETO-positive AML are associated with impaired event-free and overall survival. Blood 2006;107: 1791–9.
31. Pollard JA, Alonzo TA, Gerbing RB, et al. Prevalence and prognostic significance of KIT mutations in pediatric patients with core binding factor AML enrolled on serial pediatric cooperative trials for de novo AML. Blood 2010;115:2372–9.
32. Care RS, Valk PJ, Goodeve AC, et al. Incidence and prognosis of c-KIT and FLT3 mutations in core binding factor (CBF) acute myeloid leukaemias. Br J Haematol 2003;121:775–7.
33. Paschka P, Marcucci G, Ruppert AS, et al,Cancer and Leukemia Group B. Adverse prognostic significance of KIT mutations in adult acute myeloid leukemia with inv(16) and t(8;21): a Cancer and Leukemia Group B Study. J Clin Oncol 2006;24:3904–11.
34. Boissel N, Leroy H, Brethon B, et al. Incidence and prognostic impact of c-Kit, FLT3, and Ras gene mutations in core binding factor acute myeloid leukemia (CBF-AML). Leukemia 2006;20:965–70.
35. Paschka P. Core binding factor acute myeloid leukemia. Semin Oncol 2008;35: 410–7.

36. Huang G, Shigesada K, Wee HJ, et al. Molecular basis for a dominant inactivation of RUNX1/AML1 by the leukemogenic inversion 16 chimera. Blood 2004;103:3200-7.
37. Rowley JD. Identification of a translocation with quinacrine fluorescence in a patient with acute leukaemia. Ann. Genet 1973;16:109-12.
38. Kent WJ, Sugnet CW, Furey TS, et al. The human genome browser at UCSC. Genome Res 2002;12:996-1006. Available at: http://genome.ucsc.edu/cgi-bin/hgTracks?hgHubConnect.destUrl=..%2Fcgi-%09bin%2FhgTracks&clade=mammal&org=Human&db=hg19&position=chr15%3A74287014-%0974340153&hgt.suggest=PML&hgt.suggestTrack=knownGene&Submit=submit&hgsid=21192596%095&hgt.newJQuery=1&knownGene=pack. Accessed August 15, 2011.
39. Beitinjaneh A, Jang S, Roukoz H, et al. Prognostic significance of FLT3 internal tandem duplication and tyrosine kinase domain mutations in acute promyelocytic leukemia: a systematic review. Leuk Res 2010;34:831-6.
40. Krauter J, Wagner K, Schäfer I, et al. Prognostic factors in adult patients up to 60 years old with acute myeloid leukemia and translocations of chromosome band 11q23: individual patient data-based meta-analysis of the German Acute Myeloid Leukemia Intergroup. J Clin Oncol 2009;27:3000-6.
41. Raimondi SC, Chang MN, Ravindranath Y, et al. Chromosomal abnormalities in 478 children with acute myeloid leukemia: clinical characteristics and treatment outcome in a cooperative pediatric oncology group study-POG 8821. Blood 1999; 94:3707-16.
42. Lugthart S, Gröschel S, Beverloo HB, et al. Clinical, molecular, and prognostic significance of WHO type inv(3)(q21q26.2)/t(3;3)(q21;q26.2) and various other 3q abnormalities in acute myeloid leukemia. J Clin Oncol 2010;28:3890-8.
43. Stark B, Jeison M, Gabay LG, et al Classical and molecular cytogenetic abnormalities and outcome of childhood acute myeloid leukaemia: report from a referral centre in Israel. Br J Haematol 2004;126:320-37.
44. Slovak ML, Gundacker H, Bloomfield CD, et al. A retrospective study of 69 patients with t(6;9)(p23;q34) AML emphasizes the need for a prospective, multicenter initiative for rare 'poor prognosis' myeloid malignancies. Leukemia 2006;20:1295-7.
45. Thiede C, Steudel C, Mohr B, et al. Analysis of FLT3-activating mutations in 979 patients with acute myelogenous leukemia: association with FAB subtypes and identification of subgroups with poor prognosis. Blood 2002;12:4326-35.
46. Dastugue N, Lafage-Pochitaloff M, Pagès MP, et al. Cytogenetic profile of childhood and adult megakaryoblastic leukemia (M7): a study of the Groupe Français de Cytogénétique Hématologique (GFCH). Blood 2002;100:618-26.
47. Arber DA, Brunning RD, Le Beau MM, et al. Acute myeloid leukaemia with myelodysplasia-related changes. In: Swerdlow SH, Campo E, Harris NL, et al, editors. World Health Organization Classification of Tumours of Haematopoietic and Lymphoid Tissues. Lyon: IARC; 2008. p. 124-6.
48. Falini B, Macijewski K, Weiss T, et al. Multilineage dysplasia has no impact on biologic, clinicopathologic, and prognostic features of AML with mutated nucleophosmin (NPM1). Blood 2010;115:3776-86.
49. Ebert BL. Genetic deletions in AML and MDS. Best Pract Res Clin Haematol 2010;23:457-61.
50. Gondek LP, Tiu R, O'Keefe CL et al. Chromosomal lesions and uniparental disomy detected by SNP arrays in MDS, MDS/MPD, and MDS-derived AML. Blood 2008; 111:1534-42.
51. Starczynowski DT, Kuchenbauer F, Argiropoulos B. et al. Identification of miR-145 and miR-146a as mediators of the 5q- syndrome phenotype. Nat Med 2009;16: 49-58.

52. Johansson B, Harrison CJ. Acute myeloid leukemia. In: Heim S, Mitelman F, editors. Cancer cytogenetics, chromosomal and molecular genetic aberrations in tumor cells. Hoboken (NJ): John Wiley & Sons; p. 45–139.

53. Curtiss NP, Bonifas JM, Lauchle JO, et al. Isolation and analysis of candidate myeloid tumor suppressor genes from a commonly deleted segment of 7q22. Genomics 2005;85:600–7.

54. Vardiman JW, Arber DA, Brunning RD, et al. Acute myeloid leukaemia with recurrent genetic abnormalities. In: Swerdlow SH, Campo E, Harris NL, et al, editors. World Health Organization Classification of Tumours of Haematopoietic and Lymphoid Tissues. Lyon: IARC; 2008. p.127–9.

55. Gustafson SA, Lin P, Chen SS, et al. Therapy-related acute myeloid leukemia with t(8;21) (q22;q22) shares many features with de novo acute myeloid leukemia with t(8;21)(q22;q22) but does not have a favorable outcome. Am J Clin Pathol 2009;131: 647–55.

56. Qian Z, Joslin JM, Tennant TR, et al. Cytogenetic and genetic pathways in therapy-related acute myeloid leukemia. Chem Biol Interact 2010;184:50–7.

57. Baumann I, Niemeyer CM, Brunning RD, et al. Myeloid proliferations related to Down syndrome. In: Swerdlow SH, Campo E, Harris NL, et al, editors. World Health Organization Classification of Tumours of Haematopoietic and Lymphoid Tissues. Lyon: IARC; 2008. p.124–6.

58. Breems DA, Van Putten WL, De Greef GE, et al. Monosomal karyotype in acute myeloid leukemia: a better indicator of poor prognosis than a complex karyotype. J Clin Oncol 2008;26:4791–7.

59. Medeiros BC, Othus M, Fang M, et al. Prognostic impact of monosomal karyotype in young adult and elderly acute myeloid leukemia: the Southwest Oncology Group (SWOG) experience. Blood 2010;116:2224–8.

60. Breems DA, Löwenberg B. Acute myeloid leukemia with monosomal karyotype at the far end of the unfavorable prognostic spectrum. Haematologica 2011;96:491–3.

61. Broeker PL, Super HG, Thirman MJ, et al. Distribution of 11q23 breakpoints within the MLL breakpoint cluster region in de novo acute leukemia and in treatment-related acute myeloid leukemia: correlation with scaffold attachment regions and topoisomerase II consensus binding sites. Blood 1996;87:1912–22.

62. Schoch C, Schnittger S, Klaus M, et al. AML with 11q23/MLL abnormalities as defined by the WHO classification: incidence, partner chromosomes, FAB subtype, age distribution, and prognostic impact in an unselected series of 1897 cytogenetically analyzed AML cases. Blood 2003;102:2395–402.

63. Balgobind BV, Raimondi SC, Harbott J, et al. Novel prognostic subgroups in childhood 11q23/MLL-rearranged acute myeloid leukemia: results of an international retrospective study. Blood. 2009;114:2489–96.

64. Haferlach T, Kohlmann A, Klein HU, et al. AML with translocation t(8;16)(p11;p13) demonstrates unique cytomorphological, cytogenetic, molecular and prognostic features. Leukemia 2009;23:934–43.

65. Smith ML, Hills RK, Grimwade D. Independent prognostic variables in acute myeloid leukaemia. Blood Rev 2011;25:39–51.

66. Reaman GH, Smith FO. Childhood leukemia: a practical handbook. Heidelberg (Germany): Springer Verlag; 2011.

67. Pui CH, Carroll WL, Meshinchi S, et al. Biology, risk stratification, and therapy of pediatric acute leukemias: an update. J Clin Oncol 2011;29:551–65.

68. Watt CD, Bagg A. Molecular diagnosis of acute myeloid leukemia. Expert Rev Mol Diagn 2010;10:993–1012.

69. Marcucci G, Haferlach T, Döhner H. Molecular genetics of adult acute myeloid leukemia: prognostic and therapeutic implications. J Clin Oncol 2011;29:475–86.
70. Falini B, Martelli MP, Bolli N, Acute myeloid leukemia with mutated nucleophosmin (NPM1): is it a distinct entity? Blood 2011;117:1109–20.
71. Wertheim G, Bagg A. Nucleophosmin (NPM1) mutations in acute myeloid leukemia: an ongoing (cytoplasmic) tale of dueling mutations and duality of molecular genetic testing methodologies. J Mol Diagn 2008;10:198–202.
72. Taskesen E, Bullinger L, Corbacioglu A. Prognostic impact, concurrent genetic mutations, and gene expression features of AML with CEBPA mutations in a cohort of 1182 cytogenetically normal AML patients: further evidence for CEBPA double mutant AML as a distinctive disease entity. Blood 2011;117:2469–75.
73. Döhner K, Schlenk RF, Habdank M, et al Mutant nucleophosmin (NPM1) predicts favorable prognosis in younger adults with acute myeloid leukemia and normal cytogenetics: interaction with other gene mutations. Blood 2005;106:3740–6.
74. Breitenbuecher F, Schnittger S, Grundler R. Identification of a novel type of ITD mutations located in nonjuxtamembrane domains of the FLT3 tyrosine kinase receptor. Blood 2009;113:4074–7.
75. Gale RE, Hills R, Pizzey AR, et al., Relationship between FLT3 mutation status, biologic characteristics, and response to targeted therapy in acute promyelocytic leukemia, Blood 2005;106:3768–776.
76. Schnittger S, Kohl TM, Haferlach T, et al. KIT-D816 mutations in AML1-ETO-positive AML are associated with impaired event-free and overall survival. Blood 2006;107:1791–9.
77. Basecke J, Whelan JT, Griesinger F, et al. The MLL partial tandem duplication in acute myeloid leukaemia. Br J Haematol 2006;135:438–49.
78. Chandra P, Luthra R, Zuo Z, et al. Acute myeloid leukemia with t(9;11)(p21-22;q23): common properties of dysregulated ras pathway signaling and genomic progression characterize de novo and therapy-related cases. Am J Clin Pathol 2010;133:686–93.
79. Raghavan M, Smith LL, Lillington DM, et al. Segmental uniparental disomy is a commonly acquired genetic event in relapsed acute myeloid leukemia. Blood 2008;112:814–21.
80. Parkin B, Erba H, Ouillette P, et al. Acquired genomic copy number aberrations and survival in adult acute myelogenous leukemia. Blood 2010;116:4958–67.
81. Tiu RV, Gondek LP, O'Keefe CL, et al. New lesions detected by single nucleotide polymorphism array-based chromosomal analysis have important clinical impact in acute myeloid leukemia. J Clin Oncol 2009;27:5219–26.
82. Bullinger L, Kronke J, Schon C, et al. Identification of acquired copy number alterations and uniparental disomies in cytogenetically normal acute myeloid leukemia using high-resolution single nucleotide polymorphism analysis. Leukemia 2010;24:438–49.
83. Bullinger L, Rücker FG, Kurz S, et al. Gene-expression profiling identifies distinct subclasses of core binding factor acute myeloid leukemia. Blood 2007;110:1291–300.
84. Metzeler KH, Hummel M, Bloomfield CD, et al.Cancer and Leukemia Group B; German AML Cooperative Group. An 86-probe-set gene-expression signature predicts survival in cytogenetically normal acute myeloid leukemia. Blood 2008;112:4193–201.
85. Radmacher MD, Marcucci G, Ruppert AS, et al. Independent confirmation of a prognostic gene-expression signature in adult acute myeloid leukemia with a normal karyotype: a Cancer and Leukemia Group B study. Blood 2006;108:1677–83.

86. Chen J, Odenike O, Rowley JD. Leukaemogenesis: more than mutant genes. Nat Rev Cancer 2008;10:23–36.
87. Ley TJ, Ding L, Walter MJ, et al. DNMT3A mutations in acute myeloid leukemia. N Engl J Med 2010; 363:2424–33.
88. Yan XJ, Xu J, Gu ZH, et al. Exome sequencing identifies somatic mutations of DNA methyltransferase gene DNMT3A in acute monocytic leukemia [Epub ahead of print]. Nat Genet 2011.
89. Garzon R, Volinia S, Liu CG, et al. MicroRNA signatures associated with cytogenetics and prognosis in acute myeloid leukaemia. Blood 2008;111:3183–9.
90. Marcucci G, Mrózek K, Radmacher MD, et al. The prognostic and functional role of microRNAs in acute myeloid leukemia. Blood 2011;117:1121–9.
91. Ley TJ, Mardis ER, Ding L, et al. DNA sequencing of a cytogenetically normal acute myeloid leukaemia genome. Nature 2008;456:66–72.
92. Greif PA, Eck SH, Konstandin NP, et al. Identification of recurring tumor-specific somatic mutations in acute myeloid leukemia by transcriptome sequencing [Epub ahead of print]. Leukemia 2011.
93. Ng SB, Turner EH, Robertson PD, et al. Targeted capture and massively parallel sequencing of 12 human exomes. Nature 2009;461:272–6.

Chronic Myeloid Leukemia: Current Perspectives

Yanming Zhang, MD[a,b,*], Janet D. Rowley, MD[c]

KEYWORDS

• CML • Cytogenetics • FISH • t(9;22) • *BCR* • *ABL1*

CLINICAL AND PATHOLOGIC FEATURES OF CML

Chronic myeloid leukemia (CML) is a rare type of leukemia (1–2 per 100,000 people) but is the most common chronic myeloproliferative neoplasm with the proliferation of multiple myeloid lineages. It occurs commonly in older patients with a median age of about 65, although it also affects some pediatric patients.[1] Clinically, CML typically has a high white blood count, a massively enlarged spleen (splenomegaly) owing to extramedullary hematopoietic proliferation, and symptoms of chronic fatigue, weight loss, bleeding, and fever.[2] Typically, CML consists of 3 clinical phases: chronic, accelerated and blast phases. Before the era of imatinib mesylate (first named as STI571, and then Gleevec) and other tyrosine kinase (TK) inhibitors, the chronic phase usually lasted for 3–5 years, and then eventually evolved to the accelerated and blast phases, when patients presented with a worsening of overall performance status, fever, sweats, weight loss, bone pain, progressive splenomegaly and lymphoadenopathy, and loss of response to therapy.

Leukocytosis, ranging from 20 to 500 $\times$ 10^9/L with a mean of approximately 100 $\times$ 10^9/L, mostly with neutrophilic elements at all stages of maturation and absolute basophilia in the peripheral blood, is one of the striking features of CML in the chronic phase.[2] Bone marrow examination shows a typical picture of a granulocytic expansion with increased basophilic and eosinophilic cells, and megakaryocytic proliferation with small hypolobated (dwarf) megakaryocytes in clusters. When CML evolves,

Disclosure: Supported partly by the Leukemia and Lymphoma Society Translational Research Grant (to JDR), and the Spastic Paralysis Foundation of Illinois, Eastern Iowa Brand of Kiwanis International (to JDR).

[a] Department of Pathology, Feinberg School of Medicine, Northwestern University, 303 East Chicago Avenue, Tarry Building 7-729, Chicago, IL 60611, USA
[b] Cytogenetics Laboratory, Northwestern Memorial Hospital, Northwestern University, Chicago, IL
[c] Department of Medicine, Molecular Genetics & Cell Biology, and Human Genetics, Section of Hematology/Oncology, The University of Chicago, 900 East 57th Street, KCBD Building, Office 7-132, MC 2115, Chicago, IL 60637, USA
* Corresponding author. Department of Pathology, Feinberg School of Medicine, Northwestern University, 303 East Chicago Avenue, Tarry Building 7-729, Chicago, IL 60611.
E-mail address: yanming-zhang@northwestern.edu

Clin Lab Med 31 (2011) 687–698
doi:10.1016/j.cll.2011.08.012
0272-2712/11/$ – see front matter © 2011 Elsevier Inc. All rights reserved.

peripheral blood and bone marrow analysis shows a further increase in leukocytosis, a high percentage of blasts, and dysplastic features in myeloid lineages and myelofibrosis.

Historical Review of the Philadelphia Chromosome and the t(9;22) in CML and Its Model in Cancer Biology

CML is a hematopoietic stem cell disease always observed with t(9;22) that results in a novel fusion of the BCR (22q11.2) and ABL1 (9q34) genes. The chimeric BCR–ABL1 protein is a constitutively activated TK, and leads to autophosphorylation of the oncoprotein (ABL1) that can activate downstream signaling pathways including RAS, RAF, JNK, MYC, JAK/STAT, and nuclear factor-κB during cell proliferation, differentiation and survival.[1]

CML serves as the best model for our understanding of the mechanisms of genetic abnormalities in leukemogenesis.[3] CML was the first cancer to be associated with a recurring chromosome abnormality. In 1960, Nowell and Hungerford[4] identified a consistently small G-group chromosome in leukemia cells in CML, later called the Philadelphia (Ph) chromosome after the place where it was discovered.[4] Using novel chromosome banding techniques, Rowley[5] demonstrated in 1973 that the Ph chromosome was actually a translocation between chromosomes 9 and 22, i.e., t(9;22), which was the second recurring chromosome translocation identified in cancer shortly after the t(8;21) was discovered in acute myeloid leukemia, also by Rowley in the same year.[5] CML was also the first disease in which a molecular rearrangement was recognized as resulting in a novel fusion gene and a chimeric protein that was fundamental to leukemogenesis. In 1982, de Klein[6] elucidated that the ABL1 gene at 9q34 was relocated to the Philadelphia chromosome in the t(9;22). In 1984 and 1985, Heisterkamp and associates[7] and Groffen and colleagues[8] identified the "breakpoint cluster region" (BCR) on the derivative chromosome 22, and later Shtivelman and co-workers[9] and Grosveld and colleagues[10] revealed that the BCR and ABL1 genes were fused together to give rise to a novel chimeric mRNA and protein in CML with t(9;22). Furthermore, CML serves as the first cancer with a rationally designed drug treatment that directly targets the molecular consequence responsible for the pathogenesis of the disease. By 1996, Druker and colleagues[11] were able to identify a TK inhibitor Imatinib that specifically bound to the fusion BCR/ABL1 protein and inhibited the constitutively active ABL1 gene function. Since then, many other novel chromosome abnormalities in leukemia, lymphoma, sarcoma, and recently in epithelial cancer have been discovered, and other genes and protein-specific drugs are used in patient treatment and clinical trials. Therefore, CML is a valid research model in cancer stem cell biology, normal and abnormal hematopoiesis and lineage commitment, disease progression, and in targeted drug development and therapy.[3]

CYTOGENETIC TESTS IN THE DIAGNOSIS AND DIFFERENTIAL DIAGNOSIS OF CML
The t(9;22) in CML: Standard and Variants

The standard t(9;22) can be detected by conventional cytogenetic analysis in bone marrow or peripheral blood samples in more than 90% of CML patients. Presumably occurring in a stem cell, the t(9;22) is detectable in all myeloid lineage cells, including granulocytes, monocytes, erythroid precursors, megakaryocytes, and in all B and some T lymphocytes. At the time of diagnosis, the t(9;22) is usually seen in all metaphase cells analyzed from 24- or 48-hour cultures, indicative of a high mitotic index. In the remaining 2% to 10% of patients with CML, a variant of the t(9;22), involving a third (or more) chromosome can be observed. Either the chromosome 9 or

22 may not exhibit the usual abnormal banding pattern; rather, they may show a 3-way inter-chromosome translocation involving 9q34 (*ABL1*) and 22q11.2 (*BCR*), and a third chromosome. Certain chromosome bands are commonly involved in variant t(9;22), such as 1p36.1, 3p21, 11q13, 12p13, and 17q25, although all chromosomes have been observed in variant translocations.[12] Careful analysis will enable the identification of a 3- or 4-way translocation involving both chromosomes 9 and 22.

In a few cases, the t(9;22) is cryptic such that conventional cytogenetic analysis does not reveal any apparent chromosomal changes at 9q34 or 22q11.2. Instead, insertion of the *BCR* gene into the *ABL1* gene or vice versa has been identified. FISH analysis or polymerase chain reaction (PCR) studies would be needed to detect the *BCR/ABL1* fusion. However, in all patients, the BCR-ABL1 fusion, owing to the t(9;22), is the hallmark of CML as recognized by the 2008 World Health Organization classification of hematopoietic and lymphoid neoplasms.[2] The t(9;22) is also one of the recurring chromosome abnormalities in acute lymphoblastic leukemia (ALL), in particular in adult patients; the consequence of the t(9;22) is the chimeric mRNA and protein with the fusion between the 3' end of the first exon of the *BCR* gene and the 5' terminus of the second exon of the *ABL1* gene on the derivative chromosome 22 (Ph chromosome).[13] The breakpoints in *ABL1* are always proximal to the second exon in both CML and ALL, whereas the breakpoints in *BCR* are variably different between CML and ALL. In CML, the breakpoints in *BCR* are more telomeric in the major breakpoint cluster region (M-bcr, between exons 12 and 15) or micro-bcr region (between exons 19 and 21), giving rise to the P210 and P230 fusions, respectively. In contrast, the breakpoints in the *BCR* gene in ALL are far more proximal to exon 2 in a minor breakpoint cluster region (m-bcr), producing the P190 fusion. The location of the breakpoints and the amount of the *BCR* gene that is included in the *BCR/ABL1* fusion determines whether the leukemia will be CML or ALL, both showing a similar but not identical BCR/ABL1 fusion protein.[13]

Secondary Chromosome Aberrations in CML at Diagnosis

The t(9;22) or its variants are detectable as a single cytogenetic abnormality in up to 90% of CML patients in the chronic phase at the time of diagnosis. In some patients, other chromosome aberrations are observed in addition to the t(9;22). The most common ones are loss of the Y chromosome, gain of chromosome 8, and a second Philadelphia chromosome, and isochromosome 17, that is, i(17q). Loss of the Y chromosome is generally related to increasing age (>70 years), and seems to have no effect on the disease course or phenotypic features. Notably, the remaining additional chromosome aberrations, namely, +8, +Ph, and i(17q), are also frequent in CML during the accelerated and blast phases. Thus, it is reasonable that these patients with t(9;22) and additional chromosome aberrations do poorly in comparison with those with t(9;22) as the sole abnormality. In fact, it has been demonstrated that such additional abnormalities indeed are associated with poor survival, and a higher risk of relapse.[14] Particularly, the i(17q) is a predictor for poor cytogenetic and clinical response. It remains to be seen if the negative association of additional chromosome aberrations with poor prognosis in CML can be overcome by imatinib treatment.

Cytogenetic Evolution in CML During the Accelerated and Blast Phases

The chronic phase of CML usually lasts about 3 to 5 years, and then evolves to an advanced stage. The disease evolution is accompanied in more than 60% of patients with additional chromosome aberrations, which can be reliably identified by cytogenetic analysis in many cases.[12] The most common additions are gain of chromosome

8 (33%), followed by an additional Ph chromosome (30%), i(17q) (20%), and +19 (12%); loss of the Y chromosome (8% in males), trisomy 21 (7%) and loss of chromosome 7 (5%). They may occur individually or in combination. In certain situations, the appearance of additional abnormalities, such as +8 and i(17q), is a strong indicator of an occult disease progression, often several months earlier than morphologic evidence on bone marrow examination or clinical symptoms.

The blast phase is about two thirds in myeloid and one third in lymphoid lineages. In addition to those common karyotypic evolutions described above, additional chromosome aberrations, specific for acute myeloid leukemia, can be observed such as t(8;21), and inv(16) in CML in myeloid blasts with abnormal eosinophilia, or even t(15;17) in CML with acute promyelocytic blasts. The t(3;21) and inv(3q)/t(3;3) that result in the overexpression of the *EVI1* gene at 3q26.2 are also one of the recurring abnormalities in CML in transformation.

Fluorescence in Situ Hybridization Detection of the BCR/ABL1 Fusion Gene

Fluorescence in situ hybridization (FISH) technique is a molecular cytogenetic tool that complements conventional chromosome analysis. Because of its high sensitivity and easy use in both metaphase and interphase cells, FISH can be used to rapidly confirm the *BCR/ABL1* fusion in diagnosis and in disease follow-up and in monitoring treatment response. FISH is also very helpful in clarifying a variant, cryptic, or complex karyotype in CML patients. At the time of diagnosis of CML, FISH can be used in parallel with cytogenetic analysis to confirm the t(9;22) and determine fusion signal patterns in bone marrow or peripheral blood samples. It is particularly important if the sample was suboptimal, or there were only few dividing cells in the cultured cells. FISH is also a very sensitive tool in monitoring treatment response and disease course by comparing the percentages of the *BCR/ABL1* fusion positive leukemia cells because 200 or more interphase cells are examined as compared with 20 metaphase cells in conventional cytogenetic analysis.

FISH Probe Strategy Selection

There are several commercial FISH probes available from various vendors. A dual fusion probe set is preferred with large genomic bacterial artificial chromosome probes covering the entire or a part of the genomic breakpoint regions of the *BCR* and *ABL1* genes labeled in different colors. It has a very low cutoff value (around 0%–1%) for a positive result and, thus, is particularly useful in monitoring the treatment response. In certain situations, a *BCR-ABL1* fusion probe with an extra signal pattern is helpful in distinguishing the major and minor breakpoints in the *BCR* gene. Another probe strategy is to use an internal control probe on chromosome 9q34 to detect a partial deletion of the *ABL1-BCR* reciprocal fusion on the derivative chromosome 9 (see below).

Interpretation of FISH Results in Combination With Cytogenetic Analysis

A combined conventional cytogenetics and FISH analysis is important in CML for diagnosis. Although it is at a low-resolution level, chromosome analysis provides a complete picture of all metaphase chromosome changes. It is particularly helpful to identify a variant of t(9;22) and clonal evolution, which is informative of disease status. FISH not only confirms the t(9;22) but it establishes a reference FISH signal pattern as well for monitoring disease status and treatment response. FISH on metaphase cells helps to identify complex karyotypes and clarify unusual chromosome aberrations, such as 3-way translocations of the t(9;22), a cryptic translocation, or a partial deletion of the genomic fusion on the derivative chromosome 9. In most patients, the percentages of leukemia cells with t(9;22) is comparable in both tests, with a little bit lower percentage seen in the FISH analysis.[15,16] Once the FISH pattern has been identified at diagnosis, FISH can be used to monitor treatment response in bone marrow or peripheral blood samples at appropriate intervals, without the need to perform standard cytogenetic analysis. However, before the patient enters hematologic and cytogenetic remission, karyotyping should be done every 3 to 6 months to avoid missing additional chromosome aberrations associated with blast crisis.

MONITORING DISEASE PROGRESSION AND RESPONSE TO TK INHIBITOR TREATMENT USING CYTOGENETICS AND FISH

Ideally, a bone marrow aspirate should be studied for CML at diagnosis, although peripheral blood is usually suitable for chromosome analysis as well. However, a peripheral blood sample commonly results in a low mitotic index, and the chromosome banding morphology is inferior to that from bone marrow cells. In various clinical trials, conventional cytogenetic analysis is performed every 3 to 6 months before achieving a complete cytogenetic response as a reliable tool to monitor the cytogenetic response in CML patients receiving imatinib and other TK inhibitor treatment. One criterion of treatment efficiency in many clinical trials on imatinib and other TK inhibitors in CML is to measure the percentage of residual metaphase cells with t(9;22) at various time periods, such as at 6, 12, and 18 months after initiation of imatinib treatment.[17] A major cytogenetic response has less than 35% of the Ph-positive cells based on the analysis of at least 20 metaphase cells, whereas a minor cytogenetic response shows fewer than 65%. A complete cytogenetic response or a major reduction of the Ph-chromosome–positive metaphase cells in a short period of time is strongly associated with improved disease-free and overall survival in CML.[17,18]

FISH analysis is extremely useful in monitoring the treatment response using peripheral blood samples in CML patients. Several studies have showed that the percentage of cells with the BCR/ABL1 fusion in peripheral blood and bone marrow samples is comparable.[15,16] Thus, FISH is a reliable monitoring tool on peripheral blood samples, and cytogenetic analysis can be performed on bone marrow cells as an alternative in close monitoring of the disease course. It is now known that imatinib and other TK inhibitors cannot eradicate all CML stem cells with t(9;22); thus, repeating cytogenetic and/or FISH analysis in CML patients on imatinib and other TK inhibitor treatment is necessary. About one fourth of CML patients became resistant to imatinib in a 5-year follow up study.[18] Point mutations in the ABL1 protein-binding pocket in the BCR/ABL1 gene are the most common mechanism, in particular in secondary resistance. Other resistance is owing to genomic amplification or the development of alternative pathways that escape from imatinib targeting.[19] Early detection of suboptimal responses by cytogenetic and/or FISH analysis permits prompt treatment modification.

CORRELATION OF CYTOGENETICS AND FISH ANALYSIS WITH HEMATOPATHOLOGY AND OTHER LABORATORY TESTS

Per the World Health Organization 2008 classification of hematopoietic and lymphoid tissue, all patients diagnosed with CML must have the t(9;22) or the BCR/ABL1 fusion confirmed by cytogenetic, FISH or PCR analysis. The detection of t(9;22) is not only critical for the diagnosis, but important for the treatment choice using imatinib and other TK inhibitors as well. The differential diagnosis between CML and other myeloproliferative neoplasms, such as chronic neutrophilic leukemia and chronic myelomonocytic leukemia, may be challenging because they share many morphologic features on bone marrow biopsy and in the clinical findings. Regarding CML in the lymphoid blast phase, it may be impossible to separate it from de novo ALL with t(9;22) if there was no previous clinical indication of leukemia and any background pictures of CML on bone marrow examination.

From our experience, bone marrow samples may show a picture with no clear-cut diagnostic evidence of residual CML when patients with CML are under treatment with imatinib or other TK inhibitors. However, cytogenetic and FISH analysis often reveals a small, and sometimes even a large, population of metaphase cells with t(9;22) and interphase cells with the BCR/ABL1 fusion. This can be confirmed with qualitative PCR analysis. Therefore, either cytogenetic, FISH, or PCR analysis should be performed to confirm the disease status to guide the treatment course.

GENOMIC IMBALANCES IN CML AND ITS TRANSFORMATION

The t(9;22) is the hallmark of CML and is required for establishing the diagnosis of CML. The causative evidence of the BCR/ABL1 fusion in leukemogenesis are from mouse animal studies; mice transplanted with bone marrow retrovirally transduced with the BCR/ABL1 fusion developed a myeloproliferative syndrome that recapitulated the CML features.[20] However, the BCR/ABL1 fusion alone may not lead to the progression of CML. It is also assumed that additional cooperative genetic events interact with the BCR/ABL1 fusion in initiating CML.[1,3]

Single nucleotide polymorphism (SNP) microarray or array comparative genomic hybridization techniques provide much higher resolution than conventional cytogenetic analysis in detecting genomic and chromosomal abnormalities, leading to copy number alterations in hematologic neoplasms.[21] SNP arrays can detect genomic imbalances such as loss or gain of gene copy numbers, and copy-neutral loss of heterozygosity, so-called acquired uniparental disomy, owing to incomplete chromosome segregation or to mitotic recombination.

In a recent study of 118 CML patients in chronic phase, SNP array analysis identified 39 clonal copy number alternations in 25 (21%) of the patients, ranging from 0.1 to 52 Mb, including 35 genomic losses, 2 gains, and 2 copy neutral loss of heterozygosity.[22] Twelve and 15 losses existed in 9q34 or 22q11.2, respectively, among the ABL1 and BCR gene regions, and 8 additional losses occurred in 2q, 7q, 8q, 11q, 13q, and 16p. Two gains were defined in 8p and 9p, whereas 2 copy-neutral loss of heterozygosity were detected in 9p/JAK2 and 1p. Thus, the most common genomic aberrations in CML in chronic phase are deletions at 9q34 and 22q11.2, at or around the ABL1 and BCR regions. As noted below, partial deletions of the derivative chromosome 9 containing either or both ABL1 and BCR genomic sequences have been identified by FISH using specific bacterial artificial chromosome and other genomic probes. Large, but not small, deletions—in particular those involving both ABL1 and BCR—indicated a shorter survival time. Interestingly, copy-neutral loss of heterozygosity in CML are extremely rare in comparison with other leukemias.

Using array comparative genomic hybridization with 2600 bacterial artificial chromosome probes on 54 samples from 44 patients in chronic phase, 11 in myeloid and 1 in lymphoid blast phase together with 12 CML cell lines, Brazma and colleagues[23] found that disease progression is accompanied by a spectrum of recurrent genome imbalances, including losses at 1p36, 5q21, 9p21 and 9q34, and gains at 1q, 8q24, 9q34, 16p, and 22q11. These genome imbalances were detected in clinically manifested or suspected accelerated/blast phase alike, but not seen in chronic phase samples, and some of these imbalances were seen in the CD34-positive stem cells only. Oligo-comparative genomic hybridization array analysis of 78 CML in lymphoid blast phase found a unique signature of genome deletions within the immunoglobulin heavy chain and T-cell receptor regions, frequently accompanied by concomitant loss of sequences within the short arm regions of chromosomes 7 and 9, including the *IKZF1, HOXA7, CDKN2A/2B, MLLT3, IFNA/B, RNF38, PAX5, JMJD2C,* and *PDCD1LG2* genes, indicating that their presence is essential for the development of a malignant clone with a lymphoid phenotype.[24]

Thus, genomic microarray analysis has provided information of additional genomic imbalances in CML in chronic phase and its transformation to the myeloid and lymphoid blast phases. Importantly, genomic imbalances or breakpoints identified by high-resolution microarray analysis may pinpoint important genes that are also implicated in the pathogenesis of CML.[25,26]

A PARTIAL DELETION OF THE DERIVATIVE CHROMOSOME 9 IN CML AND IIS SIGNIFICANCE TO DISEASE PROGNOSIS

It is well known that apparently balanced chromosome translocations detected by cytogenetic analysis may not be balanced at the genomic level, with a variable size of microdeletions and duplications at the genomic translocation breakpoint regions.[27] In about 10% to 16% of CML patients, FISH analysis reveals a cryptic partial deletion of the *ABL1/BCR* fusion on the derivative chromosome 9. FISH analysis using multiple genomic probes along the long arms of chromosomes 9 and 22 show that the deletion sizes are quite variable ranging from 0.5 to greater than 10 Mb, and involve either or both the *ABL1* and *BCR* genes and their surrounding areas.[28–30] However, FISH analysis using large genomic probes might have underestimated the incidence of del(9q) in CML owing to its low-resolution and nonobjective evaluation, in particular in cases with small (<200 kb) deletions. Applying genomic SNP microarray enables a genome wide search for genomic imbalances and a more precise deletion mapping in der(9q) in CML.[22,25] Three small common deletion regions near the *BCR* and *ABL1* genes were identified, with one of 162 kb involving 9q34, and 2 of 138 kb, and 102 kb on 22q only. However, more than half of patients have a deletion involving both *BCR* and *ABL1* regions. Thus, genomic microarray analysis also confirmed these 3 scenarios, that is, deletions involving the proximal segment, the distal part of *BCR* or *ABL1*, and the *ABL1/BCR* fusion. It seems that a partial deletion of the *ABL1/BCR* fusion on the derivative chromosome 9 occurs as part of the same process as the formation of the *BCR-ABL1* translocation.[31]

The significance of a deletion of the der(9q) is controversial in terms of its effect on the prognosis of CML, partly owing to using various treatment protocols. Most studies were based on the results of the treatment with interferon-α and conventional chemotherapy before the imatinib era. Few analyses involved patients with CML in a late phase or after the treatment with imatinib. In several studies, a deletion of the der(9q) is associated with a poor prognosis, in particular short survival due to a rapid disease progression, whereas others were not able to confirm the association and found that the del(9q) is not correlated with clinical features, laboratory findings or disease phases.[32–35] In a recent study of a large series of 521 Italian CML patients, including 60 patient with the del(9q) in the early chronic phase on imatinib treatment, the cumulative incidence of complete cytogenetic response and major molecular response and the overall survival are comparable in 5 years follow-up between CML patients with and without the del(9q).[36] Thus, the del(9q) does not seem to influence the response and outcome of CML in the early chronic phase on imatinib treatment.[29] Molecular mapping analysis provided some consistent observation that only those with a deletion involving the *ABL1/BCR* fusion region are associated with a relatively poor prognosis.[32,33] However, it is not clear if the reciprocal *ABL1/BCR* fusion or other genes near the fusion on the derivative chromosome 9 may contribute to it. Notably, the reciprocal *ABL1/BCR* fusion is not expressed in about one of third of CML patients. In addition, all CML patients with del(9q) lost the *ABL1/BCR* expression, whereas only about a half of CML with no del(9q) have no *ABL1/BCR* expression.[28,36,37] It was assumed that the effect of del(9q) on a poor prognosis was due to the loss of a yet-identified tumor suppression gene around the *ABL1* and/or *BCR* genes. Thus, it is possible that the del(9q) may have some negative impact only on those patients with a large deletion or one involving both *BCR* and *ABL1* sequences, which can be partially overcome with treatment using Imatinib and other TK inhibitors.[29]

APPEARANCE OF PHILADELPHIA-CHROMOSOME–NEGATIVE CLONES AND THEIR SIGNIFICANCE IN MYELOID PROLIFERATION IN CML

The treatment of CML has been evolving over the past decades from the interferon-α era to bone marrow transplantation and the availability of many TK inhibitors, such as imatinib, dasatinib, and nilotinib. During the treatment course, patients respond to the TK inhibitors well by showing dramatically decreasing percentages of cells with t(9;22) detected cytogenetically.[11] After a period of 1 to 2 years, most patients enter clinical, hematologic, and cytogenetic remission. However, a small Ph-negative abnormal clone may appear in about 5% to 10% of CML patients in remission. The latency from the cytogenetic remission to the appearance of a Ph-negative abnormal clone is variable, but usually occurs after more than 1 year. Most common abnormal clones have a gain of chromosome 8 and deletion of the long arm of chromosome 7 or loss of chromosome 7, followed by loss of chromosome 5 and deletion of 20q.[38,39] Remarkably, all these chromosome aberrations are also recurring abnormalities in acute myeloid leukemia, MDS, and chronic myeloproliferative neoplasms, although none of these are specifically associated with any subtype of leukemia or myelodysplasia. The significance of the occurrence of these Ph-negative clones in CML is not clear because many patients perform well on imatinib treatment and remain in continuous remission; there is frequently no evidence of abnormal morphologic changes of the myeloid lineage in the bone marrow at the time of the appearance of Ph-negative clones. It is evident that the occurrence of these Ph-negative clones in patients with CML in remission is not indicative of CML progression, because these clones may disappear when CML relapses. In a recent study of 10 CML patients with del(20q) in remission, no morphologic evidence of dysplasia was observed at the time of the occurrence of the del(20q) and no MDS developed after a follow-up time of more than 4 years.[40] Nevertheless, the development of MDS and/or acute myeloid leukemia has been reported in a few patients with a Ph-negative clone, in particular −7 or +8; this is confirmed by our own clinical observations. Thus, it is likely that the appearance of Ph-negative clones in CML remission after TK inhibitor treatment is a reflection of an early malignant myeloid change at least in some patients; repeating cytogenetic analysis, not just FISH tests, at regular intervals (annually) is warranted to monitor CML patients in remission.

The mechanism of the occurrence of Ph-negative clones in CML patients in remission after TK inhibitor treatment is poorly understood. One possibility is that such occurrences of Ph-negative clones are probably a result of therapy-related myeloid disease owing to some unknown side effect of TK inhibitors on the *ABL1* gene that participates in the DNA damage and repair system. Another, more likely thought is that the appearance of Ph-negative clones is due to the disappearance of the Ph-positive CML clone after imatinib treatment, which leads to the proliferation and release of the previously suppressed and minor antecedent clone with +8, −7, or other chromosomal aberrations.[39]

CML IN THE ERA OF IMATINIB AND OTHER TK INHIBITORS TREATMENT

CML is a disease model for understanding leukemogenesis and cancer biology. Use of imatinib and other TK inhibitors as the front-line drugs has revolutionized the treatment of CML, and has significantly improved the outcome of patients with CML, with a superior outcome of 97% of complete hematologic response and 87% of complete cytogenetic remission in a 5-year follow-up study.[18] The natural course of CML before the era of imatinib has completely been changed because no CML patients with complete cytogenetics remission and an excellent molecular response with more than a 3-log reduction of the BCR/ABL1 fusion evolved to the accelerated or blast phase during 5 years of imatinib treatment.[18]

Many questions remain about the initiation and progression of CML. The genomic instabilities that lead to the formation of the BCR/ABL1 fusion are not fully understood. It is important to search for those genes that are involved in regulating the signaling pathway in the evolution of CML; what drives the CML chronic phase to the accelerated and blast phases and what genes are responsible for arresting the differentiation of the leukemic stem cells. The significance of the partial deletion of the derivative chromosome 9 related to disease prognosis in patients with CML remains controversial. Genomic SNP array analysis can discover subtle genomic lesions that are cooperating with the BCR/ABL1 fusion in disease initiation and evolution, and enable us to define the deletion size and location on the der(9q) more precisely, and classify the relationship of the deletions and clinical and pathological features.[41] Expression microarray studies will provide important information as to what genes are differentially expressed at the various phases of the disease, and may distinguish an early and late chronic phase stage.[42] Studying microRNAs that are usually targeting multiple genes will help us to understand the network of gene interaction and epigenetic regulation in cancer evolvement. Indeed, miR-219-2 and miR-199b are located near to the ABL1 gene and are deleted in CML patients with del(9q).[43] It is clear that, with continuing research, we will better understand the molecular basis of the generation of the BCR/ABL1 fusion and its effect in producing CML.

However, chromosome analysis and FISH tests will likely remain as the gold standard in helping make the diagnosis and in monitoring the treatment response and disease evolution in CML. The diagnosis of CML requires the presence of t(9;22) and or the BCR/ABL1 fusion by conventional cytogenetics, FISH, or PCR. In a clinical cytogenetics laboratory, either or both cytogenetic and FISH analysis should be routinely performed at the time of diagnosis of CML, and during the treatment course. Although it is relatively straightforward to confirm t(9;22) and the BCR/ABL1 fusion, there may be some unique situations or challenges needing extensive analysis with various techniques in CML. It is critical to understand the advantages and disadvantages of each test in terms of their correlation with hematopathologic observation and clinical changes. Repeat analysis is warranted in monitoring treatment response and disease progression, and in detecting Ph-negative clones in CML remission.

REFERENCES

1. Sawyers CL. Chronic myeloid leukemia. N Engl J Med 1999;340:1330–40.
2. Swerdlow SH, Campo E, Harris N, et al. WHO classification of tumors of hematopoietic and lymphoid tissue. 4th edition. Lyon (France): IARC Press; 2008.

3. Melo JV. The molecular biology of chronic myeloid leukemia. Leukemia 1996;10: 751–6.

4. Nowell PC, Hungerford DA. A minute chromosome in human chronic granulocytic leukemia. Science 1960;132:1497–9.

5. Rowley JD. A new consistent abnormality in chronic myelogenous leukaemia identified by quinacrine fluorescence and Giemsa staining. Nature 1973;243: 290–3.

6. de Klein A, van Kessel AG, Grosveld G, et al. A cellular oncogene is translocated to the Philadelphia chromosome in chronic myelocytic leukaemia. Nature 1982;300:765–7.

7. Heisterkamp N, Stam K, Groffen J, et al. Structural organization of the BCR gene and its role in the Ph' translocation. Nature 1985;315:758–61.

8. Groffen J, Stephenson JR, Heisterkamp N, et al. Philadelphia chromosomal breakpoints are clustered within a limited region, bcr, on chromosome 22. Cell 1984;36:93–9.

9. Shtivelman E, Lifshitz B, Gale RP, et al. Fused transcript of ABL1 and BCR genes in chronic myelogenous leukaemia. Nature 1985;315:550–4.

10. Grosveld G, Verwoerd T, van Agthoven T, et al. The chronic myelocytic cell line K562 contains a breakpoint in *bcr* and produces a chimeric bcr/c-ABL1 transcript. Mol Cell Biol 1986;6:607–16.

11. Druker BJ, Tamura S, Buchdunger E, et al. Effects of a selective inhibitor of the ABL1 tyrosine kinase on the growth of BCR-ABL1 position cells. Nat Med 1996;2:561–6.

12. Johansson B, Fioretos T, Mitelman F. Cytogenetic and molecular genetic evolution of chronic myeloid leukemia. Acta Haematol 2002;107:76–94.

13. Deininger MW, Goldman JM, Melo JV. The molecular biology of chronic myeloid leukemia. Blood 2000;96:3343–56.

14. Sokal JE, Gomez GA, Baccarani M, et al. Prognostic significance of additional cytogenetic abnormalities at diagnosis of Philadelphia chromosome-positive chronic granulocytic leukemia. Blood 1988;72:294–8.

15. Lima L, Bernal-Mizrachi L, Saxe D, et al. Peripheral blood monitoring of chronic myeloid leukemia during treatment with Imatinib, second-line agents, and beyond. Cancer 2011;117:1245–52.

16. Landstrom AP, Ketterling RP, Knudson RA, et al. Utility of peripheral blood dual color, double fusion fluorescent in situ hybridization for BCR/ABL1 fusion to assess cytogenetic remission status in chronic myeloid leukemia. Leuk Lymphoma 2006;47: 2055–61.

17. Baccarani M, Saglio G, Goldman J, et al. Evolving concepts in the management of chronic myeloid leukemia: recommendations from an expert panel on behalf of the European LeukemiaNet. Blood 2006;108:1809–20.

18. Drucker BJ, Guilhot F, O'Brien SG, et al. Five-year follow-up of patients receiving in Imatinib for chronic myeloid leukemia. N Engl J Med 2006;355:2408–17.

19. La Rosée P, Hochhaus A. Molecular pathogenesis of tyrosine kinase resistance in chronic myeloid leukemia. Curr Opin Hematol 2010;17:91–6.

20. Daley GO, van Etten RA, Baltimore D. Induction of chronic myelogenous leukemia in mice by the P210 bcr/ABL1 gene of the Philadelphia chromosome. Science 1990; 247:824–30.

21. Maciejewaski JP, Mufti GJ. Whole genome scanning as a cytogenetic tool in hematological malignancies. Blood 2008;112:965–74.

22. Huh J, Jung CW, Kim JW, et al. Genome-wide high density single-nucleotide polymorphism array-based karyotyping improves detection of clonal aberrations including der(9) deletion, but does not predict treatment outcomes after Imatinib therapy in chronic myeloid leukemia. Ann Hematol 2011;90(11):1255–64.

23. Brazma D, Grace C, Howard J, et al. Genomic profile of chronic myelogenous leukemia: imbalances associated with disease progression. Gene Chrom Cancer 2007;46:1039–50.

24. Nacheva EP, Brazma D, Virgili A, et al. Deletions of immunoglobulin heavy chain and T cell receptor gene regions are uniquely associated with lymphoid blast transformation of chronic myeloid leukemia. BMC Genomics. 2010;11:41–52.

25. Gondek LP, Dunbar AJ, Szpurka H, et al. SNP array karyotyping allows for the detection of uniparental disomy and cryptic chromosomal abnormalities in MDS/MPD-U and MPD. PLOS One 2007;2:e1225.

26. Hosoya N, Sanada M, Nannya Y, et al. Genome-wide screening of DNA copy number changes in chronic myelogenous leukemia with the use of high-resolution array-based comparative genomic hybridization. Gene Chrom Cancer 2006;45:482–94.

27. Zhang Y, Rowley JD. Chromatin structural elements and chromosomal translocations in leukemia. DNA Repair 2006;5:1282–97.

28. Huntly BJ, Bench AJ, Delabesse E, et al. Derivative chromosome 9 deletions in chronic myeloid leukemia: poor prognosis is not associated with loss of ABL1-BCR expression, elevated BCR-ABL1 levels, or karyotypic instability. Blood 2002;99:4547–53.

29. Castagnetti F, Testoni N, Luatti S, et al. Deletions of the derivative chromosome 9 do not influence the response and the outcome of chronic myeloid leukemia in early chronic phase treated with Imatinib mesylate: GIMEMA CML Working Party analysis. J Clin Oncol 2010;28:2748–54.

30. Sinclair PB, Nacheva EP, Leversha M, et al. Large deletions at the t(9;22) breakpoint are common and may identify a poor-prognosis subgroup of patients with chronic myeloid leukemia. Blood 2000;95:738–43.

31. Huntly BJ, Reid AG, Bench AJ, et al. Deletions of the derivative chromosome 9 occur at the time of the Philadelphia translocation and provide a powerful and independent prognostic indicator in chronic myeloid leukemia. Blood 2001;98:1732–8.

32. Kreil S, Pfirrmann M, Haferlach C, et al. Heterogeneous prognostic impact of derivative chromosome 9 deletions in chronic myelogenous leukemia. Blood 2007;110: 1283–90.

33. Huntly BJ, Bench A, Green AR. Double jeopardy from a single translocation: deletions of the derivative chromosome 9 in chronic myeloid leukemia. Blood 2003;102:1160–8.

34. Huntly BJ, Guilhot F, Reid AG, et al. Imatinib improves but may not fully reverse the poor prognosis of patients with CML with derivative chromosome 9 deletions. Blood 2003;102:2205–12.

35. Fourouclas N, Campbell PJ, Bench AJ, et al. Size matters: the prognostic implications of large and small deletions of the derivative 9 chromosome in chronic myeloid leukaemia. Haematologica 2006;91:952–5.

36. de la Fuente J, Merx K, Steer EJ, et al. ABL1-BCR expression does not correlate with deletions on the derivative chromosome 9 or survival in chronic myeloid leukemia. Blood 2001;98:2879–80.

37. Melo JV, Gordon DE, Cross NC, et al. The ABL1-BCR fusion gene is expressed in chronic myeloid leukemia. Blood 1993;81:158–65.

38. Bumm T, Muller C, Al-Ali HK, et al. Emergence of clonal cytogenetic abnormalities in Ph–cells in some CML patients in cytogenetic remission to Imatinib but restoration of polyclonal hematopoiesis in the majority. Blood 2003;101:1941–9.

39. Jabbour E, Kantarjian HM, Abruzzo LV, et al. Chromosomal abnormalities in Philadelphia chromosome negative metaphases appearing during Imatinib mesylate therapy in patients with newly diagnosed chronic myeloid leukemia in chronic phase. Blood 2007;110:2991–5.

40. Sun J, Yin C, Cui W, et al. Chromosome 20q deletion. A recurrent cytogenetic abnormality in patients with chronic myelogenous leukemia in remission. Hematopathol 2011;135:391–7.

41. Storlazzi C, Specchia G, Anelli L, et al. Break-point characterization of der(9) deletions in chronic myeloid leukemia patients. Gene Chrom Cancer 2002;35:271–6.

42. Oehler VG, Yeung KY, Choi YE, et al. The derivation of diagnostic markers of chronic myeloid leukemia progression from microarray data. Blood 2009;114:3292–8.

43. Chaubey A, Karanti S, Rai D, et al. microRNAs and deletion of the derivative chromosome 9 in chronic myeloid leukemia. Leukemia 2009;23:186–8.

Multiple Myeloma: Current Perspectives

Marilyn L. Slovak, PhD

KEYWORDS

- Multiple myeloma • Cytogenetics
- Fluorescence in situ hybridization • Monoclonal gammopathy
- Plasma cell dyscrasia • Microarray

INTRODUCTION

Multiple myeloma (MM) is a rarely curable malignancy defined by a proliferation of monoclonal plasma cells (PCs) in the bone marrow (BM), often with an elevated serum or urine paraprotein (M protein, or monoclonal protein). It is the second most common hematologic cancer in the United States and Europe, with an incidence of 20,000 or more cases per year,[1,2] representing 1% of all cancers and 2% of all cancer deaths. MM is primarily a disease of the elderly (median age at diagnosis, 67 years) with only approximately 3% of patients diagnosed before the age of 40. The cause of MM remains unknown, but associated risk factors include obesity and a family history of lymphoid hematopoietic cancers. The disease is more prevalent in men than in women and is highest in blacks and lowest in Asians.[3]

MM is heterogeneous at many levels, including clinical presentation, pathogenetic characteristics, response to treatment, and outcome. MM emerges through a multistep transformation from one or two asymptomatic, premalignant phases—monoclonal gammopathy of undetermined significance (MGUS) and smoldering MM (SMM).[4,5] Patients with symptomatic MM present with one or more features of CRAB, an acronym for hypercalcemia, renal insufficiency, anemia, and bone lesions.[6] The International Myeloma Working Group laboratory criteria for the different stages of MM are shown in **Table 1**.[6]

MGUS, with a reported incidence of about 3% per year in people aged older than 60 years, and the more advanced premalignant stage of SMM share the same primary genetic aberrations detected in MM. They are not treated, however, because of the low likelihood of progression and the unknown effects of early intervention. The risk of progression to MM is about 1% per year for MGUS patients and about 10% per year for the first 5 years for SMM patients. Many patients remain under observation for years before transformation occurs.[7,8] There is also no supporting evidence that early intervention in asymptomatic disease will improve overall survival (OS) or quality

The author has nothing to disclose.
Quest Diagnostics Nichols Institute, 14225 Newbrook Drive, Chantilly, VA 20151, USA
E-mail address: marilyn.l.slovak@questdiagnostics.com

Clin Lab Med 31 (2011) 699–724
doi:10.1016/j.cll.2011.08.009
0272-2712/11/$ – see front matter © 2011 Elsevier Inc. All rights reserved.

Table 1
Multiple myeloma categories proposed by the International Myeloma Working Group

Category	Criteria	Treatment	Risk of MM Progression per Year	Comments
MGUS	Serum M protein[a] <3 g/dL Clonal bone marrow plasma cells <10% No evidence of related organ or tissue impairment (CRAB[b])	None Observation and close follow-up are recommended	~1%	Progresses to MM in ~20% of patients
SMM	Serum M protein ≥3 g/dL or clonal bone marrow plasma cells ≥10% or both No evidence of related organ or tissue impairment (CRAB)	Treatment (within clinical trials only) Bisphosphonates given for bone loss	~10%	
MM	≥10% clonal bone marrow plasma cells Serum or urine M protein (except in nonsecretory MM[c]) Related organ or tissue impairment (CRAB)	Immediate treatment Clinical trials Bisphosphonates for patient with bone lesions		Aggressive relapses occur in some genetic subtypes[d]

[a] M protein, or monoclonal protein, is the abnormal immunoglobulin produced by myeloma cells.
[b] CRAB is an acronym for the major clinical features of myeloma— hypercalcemia (serum Ca ≥11.5 mg/dL), renal insufficiency (serum creatinine >2 mg/dL), anemia (>2 g/dL below normal), and bone lesions.
[c] Nonsecretory myeloma requires ≥10% clonal plasma cells; no M protein is detectable by serum/urine electrophoresis or elevated κ or λ light chains by the free light chain assay; 1% to ~2% of patients present with nonsecretory MM.
[d] Aggressive relapse is characterized by acute renal failure, circulating plasma cells, deep cytopenias, extramedullary plasmacytomas (malignant plasma cells that localize to bone or soft tissue), and resistance to conventional anti-MM therapies.

of life, lead to unexpected complications such as secondary myeloid neoplasia, or result in an earlier onset or more aggressive disease.[8] MM, in contrast, with destruction of bone and suppression of bone marrow function, among other symptoms, requires immediate treatment.

The critical event in MM pathogenesis is thought to be the transformation of a proliferative "plasmablastic" cell located in the lymphoid germinal centers.[9,10] The progeny of this "stem cell" migrate to the bone marrow where they mature to terminally differentiated antibody-secreting PCs. Acquired cytogenetic and molecular alterations associated with malignant transformation of PCs dysregulate the normal developmental pathway, leading to altered cell behavior. Based on the premise that hyperdiploidy or an aberrant *IGH* gene rearrangement leading to cyclin D dysregulation is an early, disease-defining event in the transformation process,[9,11,12] Gonzalez and colleagues[9] compared serial samples collected from patients in transition from MGUS to MM or at relapse and found no intraclonal diversity. These data suggest that from the precursor states of MGUS and SMM to MM, the abnormal plasma cell clone carries the same primary chromosomal aberration (*IGH* translocations or hyperdiploidy) and secretes the same paraprotein for the duration of the disease.[8,9] Fulminant MM and its progression are typically associated with the presence of additional karyotypic aberrations, shorter therapeutic responses, and shortened OS.

Heterogeneity of disease course and outcome shows a striking relationship with the genetic alterations of the malignant PCs. Traditionally, MM has been associated with a poor prognosis and an OS of 3 to 7 years from diagnosis, although the range has varied from less than 1 year in patients with aggressive disease to greater than 10 years in patients with indolent disease. But the management of patients with MM has changed dramatically over the past decade. Emerging new therapies, such as thalidomide, lenalidomide, and bortezomib, have increased the median OS to 4 to 5 years and a 20% chance of surviving to greater than 10 years.[13–15] Despite these achievements, MM is usually considered incurable. Refinement of the current genetically defined risk groups is needed to identify high-risk patients who may benefit from novel treatments from patients with predictable clinical courses who benefit from existing treatments. To address this need, the International Myeloma Working Group recently proposed consensus guidelines for the workup of patients with suspected MM using standardized diagnostic, prognostic, and response criteria.[6,16–18] Currently, patient stratification is based on the known pathogenetic factors of age; tumor burden; renal function; serum levels of lactic dehydrogenase (LDH); β_2-microglobulin (Sβ_2M); and albumin, plasma cell labeling index, functional status, and cytogenetics (**Table 2**). This stratification model will soon be strengthened with the incorporation of oncogenomic diagnostic techniques including analysis of DNA copy number alteration by array comparative genomic hybridization (aCGH), single nucleotide polymorphism (SNP) microarrays, and gene expression profiling (GEP).[18–20] This article reviews the conventional cytogenetics (CC), molecular cytogenetics, and genomic diagnostics of MM and highlights a few recent clinical trials that demonstrate the impact of genetic risk stratification on the treatment of this plasma cell malignancy.

HISTORICAL PERSPECTIVE OF CYTOGENETICS IN MM

Dewald and colleagues were the first to describe the clinical utility of chromosome studies in MM.[21] In their seminal paper, they showed that compared with patients with karyotypically normal bone marrow cells, patients with karyotypically abnormal

Table 2
International Myeloma Working Group risk stratification guidelines for multiple myeloma

Minimal recommendations for risk stratification	Additional studies suggested for optimal risk stratification
Serum albumin and β_2-microglobulin assays	Conventional (metaphase) cytogenetics
Bone marrow examination with FISH to detect t(4;14), t(14;16), and del(17p) in PCs[a,b]	Labeling index
Lactic acid dehydrogenase levels	MRI/PET imaging
Immunoglobulin type	Microarrays (CGH/SNP) to determine DNA copy number alterations
Histology to determine plasmablastic disease	Gene expression profiling

[a] Identified by plasma cell specific FISH protocols.
[b] Genetic testing in MM clinical trials may also include: (1) FISH testing for deletion 1p and 1q gains, (2) DNA copy number alterations by CGH/SNP microarrays, or (3) gene expression profiling, or a combination of these.

bone marrow cells had reduced OS, underscoring the relevance of the plasma cell genome to disease outcome. Normal PCs are terminally differentiated cells with low proliferative activity. The presence of karyotypically normal bone marrow studies in MM patients provides clear evidence of active, normal hematopoiesis, whereas patients with abnormal karyotypes show a higher proliferative, less differentiated PC neoplasm indicative of active disease and higher tumor burden. Over the following 15 years, conventional cytogenetic studies reported an incidence of abnormal PC karyotypes in 30% to approximately 40% of newly diagnosed and 35% to approximately 60% of previously treated MM patients.[22–27] Despite the relatively low abnormality rate, the data exposed two clinically significant findings: (1) conventional cytogenetic studies are a surrogate for the plasma cell proliferative index assay, with either test capable of indicating active proliferating disease in the bone marrow; and (2) prognostic differences are associated with ploidy level and with specific recurring cytogenetic aberrations (**Fig. 1**).

Because the low proliferative potential of terminally differentiated PCs limits detection of chromosomal aberrations by CC, which requires metaphases, interphase fluorescence in situ hybridization (I-FISH) has become an attractive technique to interrogate MM-specific chromosomal aberrations. All patients with abnormal karyotypes show known abnormalities by I-FISH, but the two assays provide slightly different information. I-FISH detects specific prognostically significant cytogenetic markers in malignant PCs, in particular, high-risk *IGH* translocations such as t(4;14)/*IGH/FGFR3* and t(14;16)/*IGH/MAF* that are not obvious by CC because they are cryptic or hidden in complex karyotypes.[28] However, I-FISH detects only its intended target and provides no information about additional abnormalities that may be present or may signal disease progression. Metaphase cytogenetics, however, is an excellent tool for detecting the wide range of karyotypic alterations observed in MM and, as mentioned previously, serves as a surrogate index for active proliferative disease. Thus, I-FISH is not a substitute for CC; it has clear clinical utility when CC is either noninformative or not interpretable and is a necessary adjunct to metaphase cytogenetics for detecting subtle *IGH* translocations. In addition, both interphase and metaphase

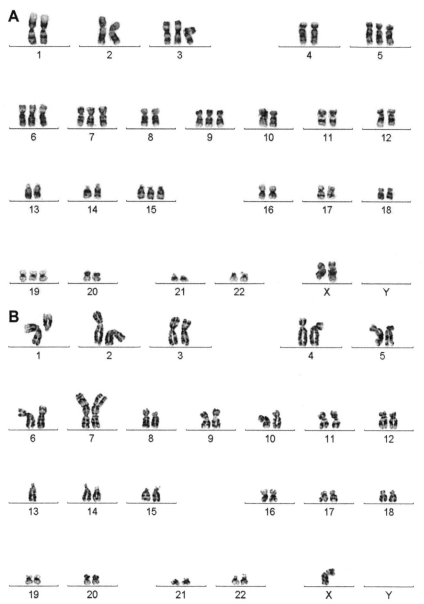

Fig. 1. Representative abnormal karyotypes found in MM. (*A*) Hyperdiploid karyotype (53 chromosomes) showing gain of the typical "odd number" chromosomes. (*B*) Hypodiploid karyotype (44 chromosomes) showing loss of chromosome Y, monosomy 13, gain of 1q by unbalanced rearrangements involving chromosome 7, and deletion of 8p and 11q. A "cryptic" *IGH* gene rearrangement was also detected by FISH (not shown).

FISH studies extend the advantage that the residual cell pellet from metaphase studies or the G-banded slides can be used to refine data gleaned from the CC study. Together, CC and FISH (both metaphase and interphase) play important and independent roles in MM stratification by providing timely and prognostically relevant information for newly diagnosed patients and by defining secondary aberrations associated with clonal evolution.

CC Methods

The tissue of choice for the study of MM is BM collected at presentation. A small aliquot of a BM aspirate is cultured for 24 to approximately 72 hours and a minimum of 20 metaphase cells from two or more cultures is analyzed. Some laboratories report a higher yield of metaphase cells if they add B-cell cytokines or growth factors such as interleukin-4 (IL4) or IL6 to the medium.

A comprehensive analysis includes G-banded karyotyping and metaphase FISH, when applicable. With metaphase cytogenetics alone, a laboratory can expect informative results in approximately 40% of cases, but metaphase FISH is required to show cryptic or hidden *IGH* fusions and deletions in approximately 10% of cases.[28] Periodic follow-up cytogenetic studies should be recommended to detect clonal evolution of disease or evolving therapy-related myeloid neoplasms.

FISH Studies

Dewald and colleagues[28] reported that bone marrow aspirates from 54% of newly diagnosed MM patients with normal CC showed clonal anomalies by I-FISH. However, when BM samples contained 20% or more PCs, the percentage of detected anomalies by I-FISH rose to approximately 85%. A Mayo Clinic/Eastern Cooperative Oncology Group (ECOG) study using a FISH assay combined with an immunoglobulin (cIg) assay that stains PC cytoplasmic Ig light chains detected 60% *IGH* translocations compared with 11% detected by karyotyping, with all 11% showing t(11; 14)(q13;q32) (**Fig. 2**).[29] Based on those findings, the International Myeloma Working Group discourages the use of FISH on unselected BM cells and recommends the use of plasma cell–specific FISH.[6] Using CC and PC FISH, laboratories can expect to find a PC clone in more than 90% of newly diagnosed MM patients.[19,28]

Identifying PCs for FISH analysis may be accomplished in any of three ways: (1) magnetic-activated cell sorting using anti-CD138 microbeads (purity approximately 90%)[19,30–35]; (2) cIg-FISH[36]; or (3) morphology using sequential May–Grünwald Giemsa staining to identify malignant PCs by their characteristic morphology, followed by FISH (**Fig. 3A–J**).[37] The last technique has the advantage of correlating cytogenetic aberrations with cell lineage. Correlating discrepant CC results with cell morphology allows for the detection of myeloid neoplasms coexisting with MM (see **Fig. 3K,L**).

The Mayo Clinic and the International Myeloma Working Group recommend the following FISH probes for risk stratification: –13/del(13q), del(17p)/TP53, and the two *IGH* high-risk translocations that are not clearly visible by CC, t(4;14)(p16;q32) and t(14;16)(q32;q23) (**Fig. 4**; see **Table 2**).[15,18] Because hyperdiploidy and t(11;14)(q13; q32) are the most common aberrations observed in MM and define the standard risk group, many clinical laboratories test for them routinely.

Other Molecular Assays

Information on copy number alterations in bone marrow samples can be detected with array comparative genomic hybridization (aCGH) or high-resolution single nucleotide polymorphism (SNP) arrays. These DNA-based arrays are highly effective in determining the chromosomal site, size, and genetic content of copy number alterations and defining the minimal region of gain or loss. Together with GEP, mutation analysis, and methylation studies, these genomic tools have the potential to

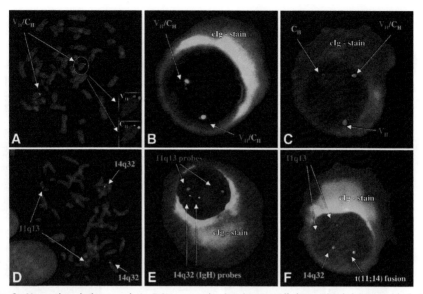

Fig. 2. Normal and abnormal cIg FISH examples in plasma cell dyscrasia. (*A*) Normal hybridization pattern of the variable heavy chain (V$_H$) and constant heavy chain (C$_H$) probes of the immunoglobulin heavy chain (*IGH*) gene localize to their locus on chromosome 14 at band 14q32 on a normal male metaphase cell. (*B*) Normal *IGH* pattern with the V$_H$C$_H$ probes closely paired. Note the intense blue fluorescence of the cytoplasmic light chain (cIg). (*C*) 14q32/*IGH* translocation detected by separation of one V$_H$C$_H$ pair using a break-apart probe set. (*D*) A normal hybridization pattern using the t(11;14)(q13;q32) or *IGH/CCND1* probe set on a normal male metaphase cell. No fusions are seen. Probes localized to their normal sites. (*E*) Normal hybridization pattern for t(11;14) probe set in a plasma cell. No fusions are present. (*F*) A fusion is present in this plasma cell indicating the presence of a t(11;14) or *CCND1/IGH* gene rearrangement. (*Reprinted from* Hayman SR, Bailey RJ, Jalal SM, et al. Translocations involving the immunoglobulin heavy-chain locus are possible early genetic events in patients with primary systemic amyloidosis. Blood 98:2266–8, 2001 [**Fig. 1**]; with permission.)

identify candidate genes important in myeloma pathogenesis and to establish a new molecular risk stratification model. As with PC-FISH, these molecular assays yield the best results when purified PCs are used.[18,30–35,38,39]

CLINICAL SIGNIFICANCE OF CYTOGENETIC ABERRATIONS

The first broad classification of MM is based on ploidy. Hyperdiploidy and non-hyperdiploidy represent the two major pathways for MGUS progression to MM (**Table 3**; see **Fig. 1**).[7,11,24,29,40–45] The hyperdiploid subgroup comprises approximately 60% of MM patients and demonstrates better OS than the non-hyperdiploid subgroup. Key findings in the hyperdiploid subgroup include karyotypes with 48 to 74 chromosomes, frequent gains of odd-numbered chromosomes (especially 3, 5, 7, 9, 11, 15, 19, or 21), and compared with the non-hyperdiploid subgroup, less frequent structural aberrations and less frequent *IGH* translocations (~10%–20%). Using high-resolution SNP arrays, the rank order of frequency of whole chromosomes gained in hyperdiploid MM is 15 > 9 > 5 > 19 > 3 > 11 > 7 > 21.[33] In the non-hyperdiploid subtype, in contrast, the 40% of MM patients with generally poor OS share chromosome counts of 47 or less or 75 or greater and numerous structural

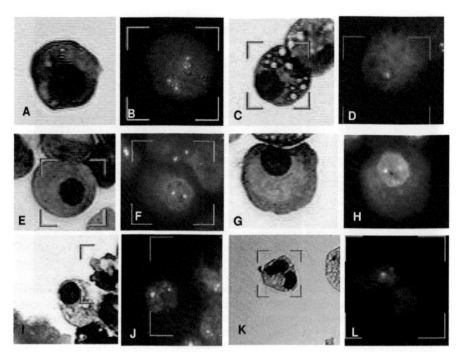

Fig. 3. Examples of a sequential morphology/FISH technique using May–Grünwald Giemsa to identify PCs by their characteristic morphology followed by FISH to detected specific MM aberrations. The plasma cell in (*A*) shows gain of chromosomes 5, 9, and 15 (hyperdiploid) in frame (*B*). The plasma cell in (*C*) shows a monosomy 13 hybridization pattern in (*D*). The plasma cell in (*E*) shows an *IGH* gene rearrangement using a breakapart probe set (*F*). The plasma cell in (*G*) shows a fusion in (*H*) indicating the presence of the derivative chromosome 4 using a t(4;14) probe set. The red and green signals in this plasma cell denote the normal chromosomes 4 and 14; the derivative chromosome 14 is not present in this PC. The plasma cell in (*I*) shows a normal chromosome 13 hybridization in (*J*); however, a myeloid cell (segmented neutrophil) in (*K*) from the same patient sample shows a hybridization pattern consistent with deletion 13q, indicating the presence of a coexisting myelodysplastic disorder. (*Modified from* Slovak ML, Bedell V, Pagel K, et al. Targeting plasma cells improves detection of cytogenetic aberrations in multiple myeloma: phenotype/genotype fluorescence in situ hybridization. Cancer Genet Cytogenet 2005;158:99–109; with permission).

aberrations, including frequent *IGH* translocations (~70%).[11,29,43–47] Chromosomes 13, 14, 16, and 22 are frequently lost in hypodiploid (defined as less than 45 chromosomes) MM. Near-tetraploid karyotypes are included in the non-hyperdiploid group because they appear to be doubling products of pseudodiploid or hypodiploid karyotypes.[24,29,43,48]

IGH Translocations Are Primary Aberrations in MM

IGH translocations targeting the *IGH* class switching region are reported in approximately 65% of patients with MM.[29,42,49] Because *IGH* translocations are detected in MGUS and SMM, they are considered the primary "immortalizing" events, yet alone they are not sufficient for transformation.[11] At the molecular level, these translocations juxtapose oncogenes into the proximity of the *IGH*

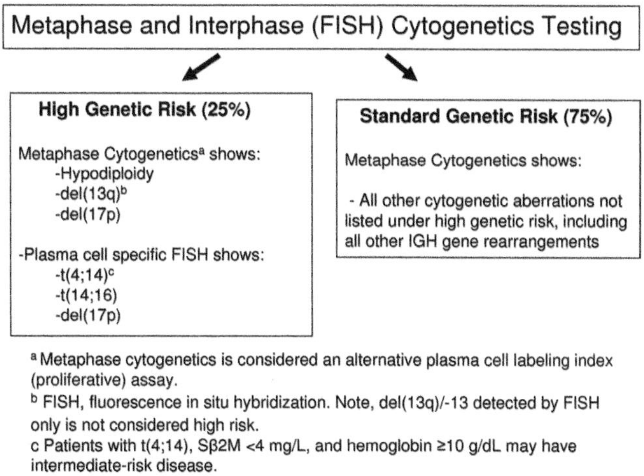

| Metaphase and Interphase (FISH) Cytogenetics Testing |

High Genetic Risk (25%)

Metaphase Cytogenetics[a] shows:
-Hypodiploidy
-del(13q)[b]
-del(17p)

-Plasma cell specific FISH shows:
-t(4;14)[c]
-t(14;16)
-del(17p)

Standard Genetic Risk (75%)

Metaphase Cytogenetics shows:

- All other cytogenetic aberrations not listed under high genetic risk, including all other IGH gene rearrangements

[a] Metaphase cytogenetics is considered an alternative plasma cell labeling index (proliferative) assay.
[b] FISH, fluorescence in situ hybridization. Note, del(13q)/-13 detected by FISH only is not considered high risk.
[c] Patients with t(4;14), Sβ2M <4 mg/L, and hemoglobin ≥10 g/dL may have intermediate-risk disease.

Fig. 4. Genetic testing in newly diagnosed multiple myeloma for risk stratification. (*Adapted from* **Fig. 1** from Kumar SK, Mikhael JR, Buadi FK, et al. Management of newly diagnosed symptomatic multiple myeloma: updated Mayo Stratification of Myeloma and Risk-Adapted Therapy [mSMART] consensus guidelines. Mayo Clin Proc 2009;84:1095–110; with permission.)

enhancers, driving abnormal expression of the translocated oncogenes. Each translocation subgroup is associated with dysregulation of one of three cyclin D genes—*CCND1*, *CCND2*, or *CCND3*. *CCND1* and *CCND3* are directly overexpressed as the result of t(11;14) and t(6;14), respectively, while *CCND2* is indirectly upregulated in the t(4;14) and MAF translocation group [7] (see **Table 2**). An additional approximately 20% of MM patients harbor *IGH* translocations involving other partner genes.[29] The frequency of *IGH* translocations increases from MGUS to MM, suggesting some *IGH* translocations occur as secondary events in patients who present with hyperdiploid MM.[29] In the absence of an *IGH* translocation, a diagnosis of κ and λ light chain immunoglobulin gene translocations, which have reported frequencies of up to 20% in MM, should be considered.[11] The most common *IGH* translocation partners—4p16 (*FGFR3* and *MMSET*), 11q13 (*CCND1*), 6p21 (*CCND3*), 16q23 (*MAF*), and 20q12 (*MAFB*)—are discussed in more detail in the text that follows, along with associated therapy and outcomes (see **Table 3**; **Table 4**). For a comprehensive discussion of the role of immunoglobulin gene rearrangements in antibody diversity and the pathogenesis of MM, see the review by Gonzalez and colleagues.[9]

t(4;14)(p16;q32)

t(4;14)(p16;q32) occurs in approximately 15% of MM patients and results in the direct dysregulation of both the fibroblast growth factor receptor 3 gene (*FGFR3*) and a histone methyltransferase gene referred to as the MM SET domain gene (*MMSET*). *MMSET* is also known as *WHSC1*, or the Wolf-Hirschhorn syndrome candidate gene. Derivative 14 expresses *FGFR3*, an oncogenic tyrosine kinase receptor, and *MMSET* is overexpressed as a result of the der(4) fusion.[45,49] Approximately 20% of t(4;14)-positive tumors lack *FGFR3* expression, a finding that correlates with loss of der(14).[50,51] The translocation results in the exchange of two subtelomeric light staining G-bands, so the best methods for detecting this

Table 3
Most common cytogenetic abnormalities in MM

Abnormality	% Frequency	Other associations	Survival characteristics
Ploidy status			
Hyperdiploidy	~60	48 to 74 chromosomes Gain of the odd chromosomes, esp. 5, 9, & 15; Less likely to show del(13q) or −13	Best OS among the abnormal ploidy subgroups
Non-hyperdiploid	~40	<48 or >74 chromosomes Usually (70%~90%) associated with *IGH* translocations	Less favorable than hyperdiploid karyotypes
Hypodiploid	~30	≤44 chromosomes Frequent (88%) *IGH* translocations with ≥50% showing t(4;14)	
Pseudodiploid	~18	45 to 47 chromosomes	
Tetraploid	~1~2	≥75 chromosomes Usually coexist near 2n and 4n clones; Frequent (~90%) *IGH* translocations	
Primary IGH aberrations			
t(4;14)(p16;q32)	~15	~90% have concurrent del(13q) Indirectly dysregulates *CCND2*	Poor Short remission (21 to ~30 months) after high dose-chemotherapy and SCT
t(6;14)(p21;q32)	~4	~66% have concurrent del(13q) Directly dysregulates *CCND3* Indirectly dysregulates *CCND2* Variant translocation involves *IGL/22q11*	Similar to MM with t(11;14)
t(11;14)(q13;q32)	~20	~50% have concurrent del(13q) Directly up-regulates *CCND1* Associated with CD20 expression, lymphoplasmacytic morphology, hyposecretory disease, and λ light chains in serum	Variable (heterogeneous group): poor if presenting with PC leukemia *RAS* mutations may predict disease progression

(continued on next page)

Table 3
(continued)

Abnormality	% Frequency	Other associations	Survival characteristics
t(14;16)(q32;q23)	~3	Up-regulates *MAF* and indirectly up-regulates *CCND2* Frequent del(13q) and IgA isotype	Suggests high-risk clinical course
t(14;20)(q32;q12)	~1	Up-regulates *MAFB* Observed in non-hyperdiploid karyotypes (>80%), del(13q) (~75%), and gain of 1q (>50%)	Trend suggests poor risk—similar to t(14;16)
Other IGH translocations	~20	Concurrent del(13q) (~45%)	Little data available—neutral prognosis
Common aberrations—reported as primary or secondary			
Deletion of 1p	~30	Non-specific	Reflects disease progression; determinant of high-risk disease
Gain of 1q21	~35	Non-specific	Reflects disease progression; determinant of high-risk disease
t(8;14)(q24;q32) or MYC variants	2 to ~4	Deregulates *MYC*	Reflects disease progression
Deletion of 12p	~10	Cryptic deletions at or near *CD27*	Short EFS and OS
del(13q) or −13*	~45*	Monosomy 13 (~85%) vs del(13q) (15%); reported in ~75% non-hyperdiploid vs ~35% hyperdiploid MM; concurrent with high-risk *IGH* translocations	Does not appear to affect prognosis in hyperdiploid cases; A marker for clonal expansion in t(4;14) and t(14;16) MM
Deletion of 17p	8~14	Uncommon in MGUS Present in ~10% newly dx cases; MM with ≥60% have ultra-high-risk disease and the poorest prognosis	Rapid disease progression

Table 4
Correlation between MM therapy and cytogenetics

Abnormality	Relationship with Treatment	References
Deletion 1p	Associated with short remission and survival in patients undergoing high-dose therapy and a single autologous transplant.	Qazilbash et al[75]
Deletion of 1p21 or 17p	Adversely affects outcome for lenalidomide- plus dexamethasone-treated patients with relapsed or refractory MM. Co-presence of t(4;14) does not appear to be an adverse risk factor for PFS or OS.	Reece et al[102]
Amplification of 1q	Thalidomide improved 5 year EFS in patient lacking amp(1q21) but not in patients with amp(1q21) and did not improve OS in either group.	Hanamura et al[74]
del(17p13) or gain of 1q21	Associated with a dismal OS when treated with lenalidomide and dexamethasone.	Klein et al[104]
Absence of metaphase chromosome 13 aberrations and hypodiploidy	Favorable prognostic factor in tandem autologous SCTs.	Shaughnessy et al[117]
t(4;14) and low *TP53* expression	Bortezomib may overcome poor prognosis significance of t(4;14) but cannot overcome the adverse outcome of low *TP53* expression or the high-risk 17-gene MM model.	Barlogie et al[118]
Low *TP53* gene expression and del(17p13)	Deletion is an independent adverse prognostic marker in newly diagnosed MM treated with autologous SCT.	Xiong et al[32]
TP53 deletion	Patients with del17p/*TP53* show an extremely poor outcome with VRD (lenalidomide, dexamethasone [RD] and bortezomib) combination.	Dimopoulos[103]

IGH rearrangement are PC FISH and reverse transcription polymerase chain reaction (RT-PCR) for the hybrid *IGH/MMSET* transcript.[29,52] The translocation has been reported in both asymptomatic and symptomatic disease.[45,52] When observed in asymptomatic disease (MGUS and SMM), approximately 25% of cases progress to symptomatic MM in less than a year from diagnosis,[53] and associated features include frequent IgA isotype (~50%), concurrent 13q deletion (~90%), high $S\beta_2M$ concentration (usually $\geq$2.3 mg/L), up-regulation of *CCND2*, and infrequent presentation with bone lesions.[7,41,50,52–55] Although the overall initial therapy response rate for this subgroup is good, median progression-free survival is approximately 12 months, and more than one-third of patients experience rapid, aggressive, and drug-resistant relapses.[53] High-dose chemotherapy with stem cell transplantation offers better rates of overall response and progression-free survival.[53,55] In addition, emerging data using proteasome inhibitors (bortezomib) show promise for this poor-risk subgroup (see **Table 4**).[53,56]

CCND1 and CCND3 Translocations

The t(11;14)(q13;q32) translocation occurs in approximately 20% of MM patients and results in a CCND1/IGH rearrangement with concomitant up-regulation of cyclin D1 (CCND1). This translocation has been associated with frequent expression of CD20, lymphoplasmacytic morphology, IgM myeloma, hyposecretory disease, λ light-chain serum monoclonal protein of less than 10 g/L, and a lower plasma cell labeling index: it may be seen in hyperdiploid karyotypes.[29,57–59] The prognostic significance of this translocation in plasma cell dyscrasias is unclear. Although reported in MGUS that has been stable for more than 10 years, patients presenting with t(11;14)-positive plasma cell leukemia show an aggressive course and poor OS.[7,42,57–59] Other genetic alterations, such as RAS mutations, appear to be an important factor associated with disease progression in t(11;14) MM.[60,61] These data are consistent with the two distinct t(11;14) subgroups emerging from the microarray based studies (see "Molecular Classification of MM" section).[19,30]

CCND3 translocations are less frequent and are found in only approximately 4% of MM patients. The more common t(6;14)(p21;q32) results in CCND3/IGH rearrangement, and the less common variant t(6;22)(p21;q11) results in a CCND3/IGL rearrangement.[62] In general, the prognosis of patients with CCND1 and CCND3 translocation positive MM is considered neutral.[63]

MAF Translocations

MAF translocations t(14;16)(q32;q23) and t(14;20)(q32;q12) occur in approximately 5% of MM patients and confer a poor prognosis,[64,65] but the Intergroupe Francophone du Myeloma has questioned that poor prognostic designation for t(14;16) on the basis of small sample cohorts.[66] The prognosis appears to be linked to MAF and CCND2 up-regulation, which results in apoptosis resistance.[67,68] Non-hyperdiploid karyotypes are frequently associated with t(14;16), as are a higher prevalence in IgA myeloma,[65] a higher frequency of leukemic presentation, and frequent concurrent 13q deletions (78%).[66] Although the translocation has been detected in MGUS,[12] it confers an aggressive phenotype in MM. The 16q23 breakpoint occurs within the WWOX gene, which spans the FRA16D fragile site, raising suspicion that WWOX plays a tumor suppressor role in both t(14;16)-positive and del(16q)-positive MM.[11,69,70] Of interest, a novel MEK (mitogen-activated or extracellular signal-regulated protein kinase) inhibitor, U0126, selectively induces apoptosis of MAF-expressing myelomas, justifying clinical trials of MEK inhibitors for those cases.[20]

Like t(14;16)(q32;q23), t(14;20)(q32;q12) is strongly associated with del(13q) (76%), non-hyperdiploidy (83%), and gain of 1q (58%).[65] The translocation has been reported in approximately 1.0% of patients with MM and in 5% with MGUS. Patients with t(14;20)-positive MGUS or SMM may have stable disease for years before progressing.[65]

Secondary Aberrations in MM

Secondary aberrations are in keeping with the multistep progression of MGUS or SMM to MM.[4,5] These genetic events are not disease defining but may have important implications for prognosis, response to therapy, and potential therapeutic targets. Neither the events nor their sequence within translocation subtypes is well defined. The most common secondary aberrations are described in the following subsections.

Chromosome 1

Chromosome 1 aberrations occur in about one third of patients and are often observed as gain of the long arm with or without deletion of the short arm.[33,71–79]

Deletions involving chromosome 1 span the entire short arm but most lie within the 1p13p32 region.[33,75–78,80] The minimal regions of deletion were identified as 1p31p32 in an aCGH study [80] and as 1p21 in a SNP study.[78] Deletion of 1p is strongly associated with 1q gains and less strongly with 17p deletions[76,78] and with an overall poor outcome.[75,76,78] In a study of 203 MM cases, patients with 1p21 deletions showed shorter progression-free and OS than patients without such deletions. After adjusting for del(13q), del(17p)/*TP53*, t(4;14), and 1q21 gains, multivariate analysis indicated that del(1)(p21) was an independent poor prognostic factor associated with disease progression.[78] When present with del(17p), del(1)(p21) appears to adversely affect the outcome of patients with relapsed or refractory MM treated with lenalidomide and dexamethasone.[79]

Gains of 1q, observed as tandem duplications, isochromosomes, whole arm translocations, jumping translocations, or segmental duplications of the 1q12q32 region, are thought to result from instability of the 1q pericentromeric heterochromatin.[71,73,74] Jumping and unbalanced 1q translocations show receptor preference, usually targeting 6q, 8p, 16q, 19q, or 17p.[71–73] The frequency of 1q gain is approximately 40% in newly diagnosed MM, increasing to approximately 70% in relapsed disease.[41] The minimal critical region of gain within band 1q21[31] contains many candidate genes, including *PDZK1, IL6R, BCL9, CSK1B, PSMD4,* and *ANP32E.* [31,34,81–83] A second 1q region where gain or amplification is reported to be prognostically significant is 1q23.3.[19]

Defined as greater than 2 copies of 1q21 by FISH,[74] amp(1q21) is associated with disease progression and poor OS.[33,41,74,79,84] Using aCGH on DNA isolated from PCs from SMM patients, Rosinol and colleagues[84] showed that the risk of conversion to overt disease was linked to gains of 1q21 and loss of chromosome 13. Similarly, using I-FISH, Hanamura and colleagues[74] showed that 1q21 gain was associated with a higher risk of transition from SMM to MM. When seen concurrently with t(14;16) and t(4;14), it confers a poorer survival, especially if the 1q copy number increases at relapse. Amp 1q21 has also been associated with adverse prognosis and disease progression in MM patients treated with autologous stem cell transplantation (SCT) and in patients with relapsed or refractory disease treated with bortezomib (see **Table 4**).[74,78,79,82,85,86] These data support the contention that 1q21 houses genes that trigger disease progression and a more aggressive clinical course.

Chromosome 8

MYC/8q24 rearrangements are thought to be late disease-progression events because of their similar frequency in hyperdiploid and non-hyperdiploid MM [46]; however, a single report suggests a frequency in primary MM as high as 15%.[87] MYC/8q24 duplications and translocations are generally seen in complex karyotypes and are associated with 1q gains.[46,73,87,88] The 8q region appears to play a complex role in MM. Using high-resolution aCGH, Carrasco and coworkers[31] defined minimal regions of gains within 8q24.12–q24.13 and 8q24.2–8q24.3, and GEP studies suggest that within the 8q21q24 region, *FABP5, YWHAZ, EXOSC4,* and *EIFC2* contribute to high-risk disease.[34]

Chromosome 12

DNA-based microarrays show 12p deletions of variable size in approximately 12% of patients with a minimal deletion region near *CD27* at band 12p13.31.[19,42] Several studies have linked del(12p) to low expression of *CD27*, leading to high-risk disease and a poor prognosis.[19,89–91]

Chromosome 13

Chromosome 13 aberrations are subdivided into monosomy 13 (85%) and deletion 13q (15%) with no known difference in prognosis. They are common to hyperdiploid and non-hyperdiploid MM. By I-FISH, the incidence of chromosome 13 abnormalities is 50%, but only 15% of newly diagnosed patients showed chromosome 13 aberrations by CC.[31,42,52,92,93] The timing of detection and the method of detection is of prognostic significance. Chromosome 13 aberrations are not a high-risk feature when detected only by FISH[18] but are when detected by CC because cells detected by CC are proliferating, and proliferating PCs denote active disease and poor OS.[28,94] Actually, chromosome 13 aberrations seem to garner prognostic significance based on the company they keep. They are highly correlated with high-risk *IGH* translocations (see **Table 3**),[42,65,94] and one detailed study reported chromosome 13 aberrations in 57% of patients studied, of whom approximately 40% also showed t(4;14), t(14;16), and/or del(17p).[28] In relapsed refractory disease, −13 or del(13q) was observed concurrently with both t(4;14) and del(17p).[79] Finally, the low prevalence of chromosome 13 aberrations in MGUS and SMM, especially the absence in *IGH* translocation-positive MGUS and SMM, provides compelling evidence that chromosome 13 aberrations are secondary. Their presumed role is related to disease progression perhaps by activation of cyclin D overexpression in *IGH* translocation-specific MM. [42,94]

In GEP studies involving 13q14, *TRIM13* (also known as *RFP2*) exhibited copy number and expression differences in MM and was linked to poor survival,[31] although it is not listed in the 17-gene model proposed to define high-risk MM (see "Molecular Classification of MM" section).[34] *TRIM14* is a candidate tumor-suppressor gene in B cell chronic lymphocytic leukemia (B-CLL) with significant homology to *BRCA1*.[95]

Chromosome 17

Del(17p) was first reported to confer an adverse prognosis in 1998[96] and is now considered the most prognostically significant chromosome aberration in MM. The short arm of chromosome 17 houses the tumor suppressor gene *TP53*, a transcriptional regulator that influences cellular response to DNA damage. *TP53* deletions are detected by FISH in approximately 10% (range, 9%–34%) of newly diagnosed MM cases,[33,96–98] but most occur as secondary events marking disease progression.[32,98,99] When observed at diagnosis, patients with del(17p) are more likely to have an aggressive clinical course, drug-resistant disease, short survival, plasmacytomas (extramedullary disease), and other high-risk features.[33,42,79,96,100,101] Most (90%) *TP53* deletions in MM are monoallelic; mutations of the *TP53* gene are rare and exclusively found in relapsed MM samples.[32]

In a comprehensive investigation, Xiong and colleagues[32] reported that low *TP53* expression correlates highly with *TP53* loss; their results also confirmed that *TP53* loss is a significant and independent adverse prognostic factor in newly diagnosed MM. It is associated with shorter event-free and OS, even in the setting of other high-risk disease features, such as high levels of LDH, a high number of bone lesions, an increased incidence of chromosome 13 deletion, amplification of 1q21, and high-risk translocations. Deletion of 17p predicts short survival regardless of therapeutic approach (see **Table 4**).[96,97,102–104]

Ultra-High-Risk MM

The definition of ultra-high-risk myeloma varies, but in general it is given as myeloma that is likely to lead to death within 24 months. It is diagnosed in 15% to 20% of MM patients and correlates with International Staging System stage 3, a high plasma cell

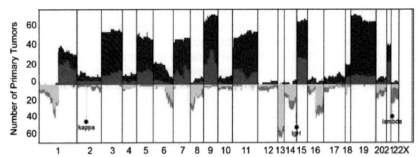

Fig. 5. Composite histogram summarizing the copy number alterations detected by aCGH in samples from 67 newly diagnosed MM patients. The recurring copy number aberrations for each chromosome (x-axis) is plotted against the number of primary tumors (y-axis) showing the aberration. Dark red and green bars indicate the number of samples with gain or loss of chromosome material and bright red or green bars represent the number of samples showing amplification or deletion. Asterisks show focal deletions of the *IGK* (2p12), *IGH* (14q32), and *IGL* (22q11). (*Reprinted from* Carrasco DR, Tonon G, Huang Y, et al. High-resolution genomic profiles define distinct clinico-pathogenetic subgroups of multiple myeloma patients. Cancer Cell 2006;9:313–25; with permission.)

proliferative rate, and del(17p).[101] A recent report suggests that del(17p) should be considered ultra high risk when seen in 60% or more of bone marrow PCs.[56] Patients who present with plasma cell leukemia or show poor-risk gene expression profiles (see "Molecular Classification of MM" section) may also be included in this subgroup. Because the t(4;14) subgroup has shown promising responses with proteasome inhibitors, it is considered high risk rather than ultra high risk.[56,104]

COEXISTENCE OF MYELOID NEOPLASMS AND MM

Therapy-related myelodysplastic syndromes (t-MDS) and acute myeloid leukemia (t-MN) are known complications in MM patients treated with intensive chemotherapy.[37,105–108] MDS-defined clones may be isolated or mixed among abnormal MM karyotypes. In a single-institution study of 3000 MM patients who received autologous stem cell transplants, approximately 5% showed cytogenetic evidence of MDS.[108] The most common reported t-MN aberrations among MM patients are der(1;7)(q10;p10), del(20q), del(5q), -7/del(7q), +8, del(11q), and del(13q). The presence of del(13q) as a sole aberration should suggest to cytogeneticists the possibility of an underlying t-MN (**Fig. 3**k,l).[37,105–108]

MOLECULAR CLASSIFICATION OF MM

High-resolution copy number (aCGH and SNP) microarrays and gene expression profiling are refining the genetic characterization of MM and its prognostic significance.[19,30–35] I discuss here how comparing molecular genetic data with patient outcomes after current therapeutic approaches will advance the molecular prognostic classification of MM.

Using high-resolution aCGH, Carrasco and colleagues [31] identified 87 discrete minimal common regions of recurrent copy number alterations (CNAs) in 67 newly diagnosed MM patients (**Fig. 5**). Of those, 14 CNAs, including TP53 deletions, were found to be associated with poor survival. Using unsupervised clustering, hyperdiploid MM was segregated into two groups, one exhibiting gain of odd-number chromosomes and another exhibiting gain of 1q and 7, deletion of 13q, and absence of trisomy 11. The study also identified two non-hyperdiploid subtypes, one characterized by high-level amplification of 1q21q22, deletion of 1p, and chromosome 13 aberrations and another characterized by absence of chromosome 1 abnormalities with deletions of chromosomes 8 and 13. In a study using high-density SNP arrays in 192 newly diagnosed MM cases, Avet-Loiseau and colleagues[19] proposed two prognosis subgroups—an adverse prognosis group associated with 1q gain or amplification and deletions involving 1p, 12p, 14q, 16q, or 22q, and a more favorable prognosis group associated with hyperdiploidy (gain of chromosomes 5, 9, 11, 15, or 19). Multivariate analysis with confirmation by an independent series resulted in the identification of del(12)(p13.31) as an independent adverse marker and amp(5q31.1) with low Sβ_2M as a favorable prognostic marker. Generally speaking, these data concur with the known MM cytogenetic data and refine the alterations down to the specific cytogenetic band.

In a combined high-density SNP and GEP investigation of 258 samples from the Medical Research Council Myeloma IX study, Walker and colleagues [33] reported frequent deletions of 1p (30%), 6q (33%), 8p (25%), 12p (15%), 13q (59%), 14q (39%), 16q (35%), 17p (7%), 20 (12%), and 22 (18%) and observed acquired isodisomy or copy number-neutral loss of heterozygosity (CN-LOH) for 1q (8%), 16q (9%), or X (20%). This study and another[31] confirmed the following: (1) direct associations between *IGH* translocations and del(13q), 1q gain and del(13q), and t(4;14) and del(13q); (2) inverse associations between 1q gain or del(13q) and trisomy 11, and t(4;14) with del(16q); (3) two hyperdiploid subgroups based on the presence of trisomy 11 with or without 1q gain and del(13q); and (4) a clinical disadvantage in hyperdiploid MM with concurrent 1q gain with or without del(13q), when compared with hyperdiploid cases with disomy 1q.

In a large SNP and GEP investigation of the significance of 16q deletions in MM, Jenner and colleagues[70] delineated two subgroups—those with del(16q) and those with LOH 16q23, which included all t(14;16) cases. The minimal region of deletion in the del(16q) subgroup pinpointed band 16q12, the normal locus for *CYLD*, a negative regulator of the NF-κB pathway, whereas the LOH 16q23 subgroup showed reduced *WWOX* expression. When either group was observed in combination with del(17p), OS was poor.

Three large GEP studies have refined the classification of MM at the transcriptional level.[30,34,109] Zhan and colleagues[30] identified seven distinct molecular subclasses associated with *CCND* gene expression, the recurrent *IGH* translocations, and hyperdiploidy: HY, MF, MS, CD1, CD2, LB, and PR. The hyperdiploid (HY) group overexpressed many genes that mapped to chromosomes 3, 5, 7, 9, 11, 15, and 19. The MF group comprised cases with ectopic expression of *MAF* genes, which included t(14;16)(q32;q23) and t(14;20)(q32;q11), which led to dysregulation of their common downstream targets. The t(4;14)(p16;q32) cases clustered within the MS group, which highly overexpressed *FGFR3* and *WHSC1/MMSET*. Cases clustered within CD-1 and CD-2 were defined by overexpression of the cyclin D genes. CD-1 included the t(11;14) cases and overexpressed *CCND1*. CD-2 samples included the t(6;14) cases and overexpressed *CCND3, PAX5, CD20*, and several genes localized to 1p. The LB (low bone disease) group showed low *DKK-1* expression. The PR (proliferation) subgroup was characterized by high expression of numerous cell cycle and proliferation-related genes (eg, *CCNB2, CCNB1, MCM2, CDCA2, BUB1, CDC2*, and *TYMS*) and cancer/testis antigen genes (eg, *MAGEA6, MAGEA3, GAGE1*, and *GAGE4*). The PR group showed a strong association with highly complex karyotypes. Approximately 27% of the MM cases studied showed a myeloid/normal plasma cell gene expression signature (MY), a finding that may reflect a copurification of myeloid and PCs or aberrant expression of myeloid genes in malignant PCs.

Within those seven groups, overexpression of genes localized to 1q was highest in the poor-risk PR and MS groups. HY, CD-1, CD-2, and LB subgroups were associated with superior event-free and OS after high-dose therapy and stem cell transplantation whereas the PR and MF groups were associated with poorer outcomes. Using Kaplan–Meier plots, the CD-1, CD-2, LB, and HY groups were associated with low-risk MM and the MF, MS, and PR cases were associated with high-risk MM, with 48-month estimates of event free survival of 68% versus 31% ($P<.001$) and OS of 79% versus 51% ($P<.001$), respectively. By multivariate analysis, these genetic groups, along with abnormal cytogenetics and elevation of $S\beta_2M$ and LDH, were significant independent predictors of OS. The HOVON group [35] independently confirmed the existence of these seven subgroups and added three novel subgroups—the NF-κB cluster based on the overexpression of positive regulator genes in the NF-κB pathway, the CTA cluster overexpressing a number of cancer testis antigens and the PRL-3 cluster overexpressing *PTP4A3*, *PTPRZ1*, and *SOC3*. Activation of the NF-κB pathway either by deletion of NF-κB inhibitors (such as *TRAF3* or *CYLD*) or by activation of NF-κB activators (such as *NIK* or *CD40*) has been reported in approximately 20% of MM patients.[70,110–113]

To improve the molecular classification of high-risk MM, Shaughnessy and colleagues[34] developed a 70-gene model based on GEP of which 21 genes (30%) mapped to chromosome 1. Of those, 12 up-regulated genes mapped to 1q and 9 down-regulated genes mapped to 1p. This model carved out approximately 13% of MM patients with shorter complete remissions and event-free and OS. The marked increase in the frequency of high-risk designation from 13% at diagnosis to 76% at relapse provides molecular evidence of disease evolution influencing post-relapse outcome. Multivariate discriminant analysis was used to redesign the 70-gene model to a more manageable 17-gene model for the detection of high-risk disease in a clinical setting. Predictably, 9 (53%) of the 17 genes mapped to chromosome 1, supporting the contention that chromosome 1 aberrations concomitant with altered transcriptional regulation of the affected genes play a role in disease progression.[33,71,73–78,80]

The Intergroupe Francophone du Myélome also developed an expression-based multivariate model that predicts disease outcome using a 15-gene model.[109] The high-risk group showed chromosome instability and overexpression of the genes controlling essential cell cycle processes whereas the low-risk group overexpressed genes involved in hyperdiploidy and protein biosynthesis. Interestingly, the 15-gene model and the 17-gene model had no genes in common, reflecting differences in the clinical trials, the platforms used, and the redundancy of the biological processes that control cell growth, proliferation, and apoptosis.[114]

Given the limited microarray data available, international cooperation is needed to validate a unified molecular genetic model that can predict outcome and high-risk MM early in the disease. New therapies that target the pathways unique to high-risk disease, including NF-κB inhibitors, *FGFR3* inhibitors, and *MEK* inhibitors, are in preclinical trials. The genetic changes identified in MM at all levels of risk and the initial molecular classifications of myeloma are providing the rationale for other molecular targeted clinical trials.[20] Moreover, emerging data from microRNA profiling, whole genome and exome sequencing, and studies associating SNPs with drug metabolism and tolerance are beginning to reveal the need to consider the genomes of both the patient and the PC clone when making clinical decisions.[113,115,116]

SUMMARY AND CONSENSUS RECOMMENDATIONS

Analysis of the cytogenetic alterations that occur in the clonal plasma cells of MM patients, and correlation of those alterations with disease course and treatment response, enables genetic risk stratification. Despite the great progress in therapeutic advances that has been made in last decade, many questions remain as to which patient will benefit from which treatments, and when. Refining risk stratification is the key to approaching such problems. Investigators proposing consensus guidelines for the workup of patients with suspected MM have included guiding principles for risk stratification.

Investigators have also proposed guidelines for standardized criteria for reporting clinical trials and recommendations for allogeneic stem cell transplantation.[6,16–18] All of these guidelines will pave the way for comparing and consolidating studies on an international level to define a unifying molecular classification system. Prognostic factors such as disease stage and cytogenetics (metaphase and I-FISH) findings are recommended for the initial workup of newly diagnosed patients. Although any cytogenetic abnormality suggests elevated risk, known poor-risk abnormalities include hypodiploidy, monosomy 13, or deletion 13q and del(17p) when detected by conventional cytogenetics and the detection of t(4;14), t(14;16) and del(17p) by FISH (see **Table 2** and **Fig. 3**). Because the genetic abnormalities predictive of poor outcome at diagnosis may be similarly predictive at relapse, patients with standard or low-risk disease should be reevaluated periodically for del(17p) and other cytogenetic features indicative of clonal evolution. FISH testing for chromosome 1 aberrations and microarray-based studies are currently limited to clinical trials. Moreover, emerging data from GEP and DNA-based microarray studies are unraveling the complex molecular network of plasma cell tumorigenesis. Together, these new genetic diagnostic tools in combination with novel therapeutic agents will permit the development of therapies that target the characteristics of individual tumor types and define the patient population likely to respond.

ACKNOWLEDGMENTS

I thank Sandra Wolman, MD, for her careful review and editing contributions and Miriam Bloom, PhD, for professional editing.

REFERENCES

1. Jemal A, Siegel R, Ward E, et al. Cancer statistics, 2009. CA Cancer J Clin 2009;59:225–49.
2. Bray F, Sankila R, Ferlay J, et al. Estimates of cancer incidence and mortality in Europe in 1995. Eur J Cancer 2002;38:99–166.
3. Alexander DD, Mink PJ, Adami HO, et al. Multiple myeloma: a review of the epidemiologic literature. Int J Cancer 2007;120(Suppl 12):40–61.
4. Landgren O, Kyle RA, Pfeiffer RM, et al. Monoclonal gammopathy of undetermined significance (MGUS) consistently precedes multiple myeloma: a prospective study. Blood 2009;113:5412–7.
5. Weiss BM, Abadie J, Verma P, et al. A monoclonal gammopathy precedes multiple myeloma in most patients. Blood 2009;113:5418–22.
6. Dimopoulos M, Kyle R, Fermand JP, et al. Consensus recommendations for standard investigative workup: report of the International Myeloma Workshop Consensus Panel 3. Blood 2011;117:4701–5.
7. Bergsagel PL, Kuehl WM, Zhan F, et al. Cyclin D dysregulation: an early and unifying pathogenic event in multiple myeloma. Blood 2005;106:296–303.

8. Landgren O, Kyle RA, Rajkumar SV. From myeloma precursor disease to multiple myeloma: new diagnostic concepts and opportunities for early intervention. Clin Cancer Res 2011;17:1243–52.

9. Gonzalez D, van der Burg M, Garcia-Sanz R, et al. Immunoglobulin gene rearrangements and the pathogenesis of multiple myeloma. Blood 2007;110:3112–21.

10. Kyle RA, Rajkumar SV. Multiple myeloma. Blood 2008;111:2962–72.

11. Bergsagel PL, Kuehl WM. Chromosome translocations in multiple myeloma. Oncogene 2001;20:5611–22.

12. Fonseca R, Bailey RJ, Ahmann GJ, et al. Genomic abnormalities in monoclonal gammopathy of undetermined significance. Blood 2002;100:1417–24.

13. Sirohi B, Powles R. Epidemiology and outcomes research for MGUS, myeloma and amyloidosis. Eur J Cancer 2006;42:1671–83.

14. Prince HM, Schenkel B, Mileshkin L. Assessing response rates in clinical trials of treatment for relapsed or refractory multiple myeloma: a study of bortezomib and thalidomide. Leukemia 2007;21:818–20.

15. Kumar SK, Rajkumar SV, Dispenzieri A, et al. Improved survival in multiple myeloma and the impact of novel therapies. Blood 2008;111:2516–20.

16. Lokhorst H, Einsele H, Vesole D, et al. International Myeloma Working Group consensus statement regarding the current status of allogeneic stem-cell transplantation for multiple myeloma. J Clin Oncol 2010;28:4521–30.

17. Rajkumar SV, Harousseau JL, Durie B, et al. Consensus recommendations for the uniform reporting of clinical trials: report of the International Myeloma Workshop Consensus Panel 1. Blood 2011;117:4691–5.

18. Munshi NC, Anderson KC, Bergsagel PL, et al. Consensus recommendations for risk stratification in multiple myeloma: report of the International Myeloma Workshop Consensus Panel 2. Blood 2011;117:4696–4700.

19. Avet-Loiseau H, Li C, Magrangeas F, et al. Prognostic significance of copy-number alterations in multiple myeloma. J Clin Oncol 2009;27:4585–90.

20. Annunziata CM, Hernandez L, Davis RE, et al. A mechanistic rationale for MEK inhibitor therapy in myeloma based on blockade of MAF oncogene expression. Blood 2011;117:2396–2404.

21. Dewald GW, Kyle RA, Hicks GA, et al. The clinical significance of cytogenetic studies in 100 patients with multiple myeloma, plasma cell leukemia, or amyloidosis. Blood 1985;66:380–90.

22. Sawyer JR, Waldron JA, Jagannath S, et al. Cytogenetic findings in 200 patients with multiple myeloma. Cancer Genet Cytogenet 1995;82:41–9.

23. Lai JL, Zandecki M, Mary JY, et al. Improved cytogenetics in multiple myeloma: a study of 151 patients including 117 patients at diagnosis. Blood 1995;85:2490–7.

24. Smadja NV, Fruchart C, Isnard F, et al. Chromosomal analysis in multiple myeloma: cytogenetic evidence of two different diseases. Leukemia 1998;12:960–9.

25. Rajkumar SV, Fonseca R, Dewald GW, et al. Cytogenetic abnormalities correlate with the plasma cell labeling index and extent of bone marrow involvement in myeloma. Cancer Genet Cytogenet 1999;113:73–7.

26. Calasanz MJ, Cigudosa JC, Odero MD, et al. Cytogenetic analysis of 280 patients with multiple myeloma and related disorders: primary breakpoints and clinical correlations. Genes Chromosomes Cancer 1997;18:84–93.

27. Seong C, Delasalle K, Hayes K, et al. Prognostic value of cytogenetics in multiple myeloma. Br J Haematol 1998;101:189–94.

28. Dewald GW, Therneau T, Larson D, et al. Relationship of patient survival and chromosome anomalies detected in metaphase and/or interphase cells at diagnosis of myeloma. Blood 2005;106:3553–8.

29. Fonseca R, Debes-Marun CS, Picken EB, et al. The recurrent IGH translocations are highly associated with nonhyperdiploid variant multiple myeloma. Blood 2003;102: 2562–7.
30. Zhan F, Huang Y, Colla S, et al. The molecular classification of multiple myeloma. Blood 2006;108:2020–8.
31. Carrasco DR, Tonon G, Huang Y, et al. High-resolution genomic profiles define distinct clinico-pathogenetic subgroups of multiple myeloma patients. Cancer Cell 2006;9:313–25.
32. Xiong W, Wu X, Starnes S, et al. An analysis of the clinical and biologic significance of TP53 loss and the identification of potential novel transcriptional targets of TP53 in multiple myeloma. Blood 2008;112:4235–46.
33. Walker BA, Leone PE, Chiecchio L, et al. A compendium of myeloma-associated chromosomal copy number abnormalities and their prognostic value. Blood 2010; 116:e56–e65.
34. Shaughnessy JD Jr, Zhan F, Burington BE, et al. A validated gene expression model of high-risk multiple myeloma is defined by deregulated expression of genes mapping to chromosome 1. Blood 2007;109:2276–84.
35. Broyl A, Hose D, Lokhorst H, et al. Gene expression profiling for molecular classification of multiple myeloma in newly diagnosed patients. Blood 2010;116:2543–53.
36. Mercer BR, Rayeroux KC. Detection of chromosome abnormalities using cytoplasmic immunoglobulin staining and FISH in myeloma. Methods Mol Biol 2011;730: 159–71.
37. Slovak ML, Bedell V, Pagel K, et al. Targeting plasma cells improves detection of cytogenetic aberrations in multiple myeloma: phenotype/genotype fluorescence in situ hybridization. Cancer Genet Cytogenet 2005;158:99–109.
38. Gonzalez D, Gonzalez M, Alonso ME, et al. Incomplete DJH rearrangements as a novel tumor target for minimal residual disease quantitation in multiple myeloma using real-time PCR. Leukemia 2003;17:1051–7.
39. Sarasquete ME, Garcia-Sanz R, Gonzalez D, et al. Minimal residual disease monitoring in multiple myeloma: a comparison between allelic-specific oligonucleotide real-time quantitative polymerase chain reaction and flow cytometry. Haematologica 2005;90:1365–72.
40. Wuilleme S, Robillard N, Lode L, et al. Ploidy, as detected by fluorescence in situ hybridization, defines different subgroups in multiple myeloma. Leukemia 2005;19: 275–8.
41. Cremer FW, Bila J, Buck I, et al. Delineation of distinct subgroups of multiple myeloma and a model for clonal evolution based on interphase cytogenetics. Genes Chromosomes Cancer 2005;44:194–203.
42. Fonseca R, Bergsagel PL, Drach J, et al. International Myeloma Working Group molecular classification of multiple myeloma: spotlight review. Leukemia 2009;23: 2210–21.
43. Smadja NV, Bastard C, Brigaudeau C, et al. Hypodiploidy is a major prognostic factor in multiple myeloma. Blood 2001;98:2229–38.
44. Smadja NV, Leroux D, Soulier J, et al. Further cytogenetic characterization of multiple myeloma confirms that 14q32 translocations are a very rare event in hyperdiploid cases. Genes Chromosomes Cancer 2003;38:234–9.
45. Kuehl WM, Bergsagel PL. Multiple myeloma: evolving genetic events and host interactions. Nat Rev Cancer 2002;2:175–87.
46. Gabrea A, Martelli ML, Qi Y, et al. Secondary genomic rearrangements involving immunoglobulin or MYC loci show similar prevalences in hyperdiploid and nonhyperdiploid myeloma tumors. Genes Chromosomes Cancer 2008;47:573–90.

47. Tonon G. Molecular pathogenesis of multiple myeloma. Hematol Oncol Clin North Am 2007;21:985–1006, vii.

48. Fonseca R, Barlogie B, Bataille R, et al. Genetics and cytogenetics of multiple myeloma: a workshop report. Cancer Res 2004;64:1546–58.

49. Kuehl WM, Bergsagel PL. Early genetic events provide the basis for a clinical classification of multiple myeloma. Hematology Am Soc Hematol Educ Program 2005;346–52.

50. Keats JJ, Reiman T, Maxwell CA, et al. In multiple myeloma, t(4;14)(p16;q32) is an adverse prognostic factor irrespective of FGFR3 expression. Blood 2003;101: 1520–9.

51. Santra M, Zhan F, Tian E, et al. A subset of multiple myeloma harboring the t(4;14)(p16;q32) translocation lacks FGFR3 expression but maintains an IGH/ MMSET fusion transcript. Blood 2003;101:2374–6.

52. Avet-Loiseau H, Facon T, Grosbois B, et al. Oncogenesis of multiple myeloma: 14q32 and 13q chromosomal abnormalities are not randomly distributed, but correlate with natural history, immunological features, and clinical presentation. Blood 2002;99:2185–91.

53. Karlin L, Soulier J, Chandesris O, et al. Clinical and biological features of t(4;14) multiple myeloma: a prospective study. Leuk Lymphoma 2011;52:238–46.

54. Gertz MA, Lacy MQ, Dispenzieri A, et al. Clinical implications of t(11;14)(q13;q32), t(4;14)(p16.3;q32), and -17p13 in myeloma patients treated with high-dose therapy. Blood 2005;106:2837–40.

55. Gutierrez NC, Castellanos MV, Martin ML, et al. Prognostic and biological implications of genetic abnormalities in multiple myeloma undergoing autologous stem cell transplantation: t(4;14) is the most relevant adverse prognostic factor, whereas RB deletion as a unique abnormality is not associated with adverse prognosis. Leukemia 2007;21:143–50.

56. Avet-Loiseau H, Leleu X, Roussel M, et al. Bortezomib plus dexamethasone induction improves outcome of patients with t(4;14) myeloma but not outcome of patients with del(17p). J Clin Oncol 2010;28:4630–4.

57. Hoyer JD, Hanson CA, Fonseca R, et al. The (11;14)(q13;q32) translocation in multiple myeloma. A morphologic and immunohistochemical study. Am J Clin Pathol 2000;113:831–7.

58. Garand R, Avet-Loiseau H, Accard F, et al. t(11;14) and t(4;14) translocations correlated with mature lymphoplasmacytoid and immature morphology, respectively, in multiple myeloma. Leukemia 2003;17:2032–5.

59. Fonseca R, Blood EA, Oken MM, et al. Myeloma and the t(11;14)(q13;q32); evidence for a biologically defined unique subset of patients. Blood 2002;99:3735–41.

60. Rasmussen T, Kuehl M, Lodahl M, et al. Possible roles for activating RAS mutations in the MGUS to MM transition and in the intramedullary to extramedullary transition in some plasma cell tumors. Blood 2005;105:317–23.

61. Chng WJ, Gonzalez-Paz N, Price-Troska T, et al. Clinical and biological significance of RAS mutations in multiple myeloma. Leukemia 2008;22:2280–4.

62. Shaughnessy J Jr, Gabrea A, Qi Y, et al. Cyclin D3 at 6p21 is dysregulated by recurrent chromosomal translocations to immunoglobulin loci in multiple myeloma. Blood 2001;98:217–23.

63. Kumar SK, Mikhael JR, Buadi FK, et al. Management of newly diagnosed symptomatic multiple myeloma: updated Mayo Stratification of Myeloma and Risk-Adapted Therapy (mSMART) consensus guidelines. Mayo Clin Proc 2009;84:1095–1110.

64. Fonseca R, Blood E, Rue M, et al. Clinical and biologic implications of recurrent genomic aberrations in myeloma. Blood 2003;101:4569–75.

65. Ross FM, Chiecchio L, Dagrada G, et al. The t(14;20) is a poor prognostic factor in myeloma but is associated with long-term stable disease in monoclonal gammopathies of undetermined significance. Haematologica 2010;95:1221–5.

66. Avet-Loiseau H, Malard F, Campion L, et al. Translocation t(14;16) and multiple myeloma: is it really an independent prognostic factor? Blood 2011;117:2009–2011.

67. Hurt EM, Wiestner A, Rosenwald A, et al. Overexpression of c-maf is a frequent oncogenic event in multiple myeloma that promotes proliferation and pathological interactions with bone marrow stroma. Cancer Cell 2004;5:191–9.

68. Nair B, van RF, Shaughnessy JD Jr, et al. Superior results of Total Therapy 3 (2003–33) in gene expression profiling-defined low-risk multiple myeloma confirmed in subsequent trial 2006–66 with VRD maintenance. Blood 2010;115:4168–73.

69. Krummel KA, Roberts LR, Kawakami M, et al. The characterization of the common fragile site FRA16D and its involvement in multiple myeloma translocations. Genomics 2000;69:37–46.

70. Jenner MW, Leone PE, Walker BA, et al. Gene mapping and expression analysis of 16q loss of heterozygosity identifies WWOX and CYLD as being important in determining clinical outcome in multiple myeloma. Blood 2007;110:3291–3300.

71. Le Baccon P, Leroux D, Dascalescu C, et al. Novel evidence of a role for chromosome 1 pericentric heterochromatin in the pathogenesis of B-cell lymphoma and multiple myeloma. Genes Chromosomes Cancer 2001;32:250–64.

72. Sawyer JR, Tricot G, Mattox S, et al. Jumping translocations of chromosome 1q in multiple myeloma: evidence for a mechanism involving decondensation of pericentromeric heterochromatin. Blood 1998;91:1732–41.

73. Sawyer JR, Tricot G, Lukacs JL, et al. Genomic instability in multiple myeloma: evidence for jumping segmental duplications of chromosome arm 1q. Genes Chromosomes Cancer 2005;42:95–106.

74. Hanamura I, Stewart JP, Huang Y, et al. Frequent gain of chromosome band 1q21 in plasma-cell dyscrasias detected by fluorescence in situ hybridization: incidence increases from MGUS to relapsed myeloma and is related to prognosis and disease progression following tandem stem-cell transplantation. Blood 2006;108:1724–32.

75. Qazilbash MH, Saliba RM, Ahmed B, et al. Deletion of the short arm of chromosome 1 (del 1p) is a strong predictor of poor outcome in myeloma patients undergoing an autotransplant. Biol Blood Marrow Transplant 2007;13:1066–72.

76. Wu KL, Beverloo B, Velthuizen SJ, et al. Sequential analysis of chromosome aberrations in multiple myeloma during disease progression. Clin Lymphoma Myeloma 2007;7:280–5.

77. Leone PE, Walker BA, Jenner MW, et al. Deletions of CDKN2C in multiple myeloma: biological and clinical implications. Clin Cancer Res 2008;14:6033–41.

78. Chang H, Qi X, Jiang A, et al. 1p21 deletions are strongly associated with 1q21 gains and are an independent adverse prognostic factor for the outcome of high-dose chemotherapy in patients with multiple myeloma. Bone Marrow Transplant 2010;45:117–21.

79. Chang H, Jiang A, Qi C, et al. Impact of genomic aberrations including chromosome 1 abnormalities on the outcome of patients with relapsed or refractory multiple myeloma treated with lenalidomide and dexamethasone. Leuk Lymphoma 2010;51:2084–91.

80. Chng WJ, Gertz MA, Chung TH, et al. Correlation between array-comparative genomic hybridization-defined genomic gains and losses and survival: identification of 1p31–32 deletion as a prognostic factor in myeloma. Leukemia 2010;24:833–42.

81. Inoue J, Otsuki T, Hirasawa A, et al. Overexpression of PDZK1 within the 1q12–q22 amplicon is likely to be associated with drug-resistance phenotype in multiple myeloma. Am J Pathol 2004;165:71–81.

82. Shaughnessy J. Amplification and overexpression of CKS1B at chromosome band 1q21 is associated with reduced levels of p27Kip1 and an aggressive clinical course in multiple myeloma. Hematology 2005;10(Suppl 1):117–26.

83. Zhan F, Colla S, Wu X, et al. CKS1B, overexpressed in aggressive disease, regulates multiple myeloma growth and survival through. Blood 2007;109:4995–5001.

84. Rosinol L, Carrio A, Blade J, et al. Comparative genomic hybridisation identifies two variants of smoldering multiple myeloma. Br J Haematol 2005;130:729–32.

85. Fonseca R, Van Wier SA, Chng WJ, et al. Prognostic value of chromosome 1q21 gain by fluorescent in situ hybridization and increase CKS1B expression in myeloma. Leukemia 2006;20:2034–40.

86. Nemec P, Zemanova Z, Greslikova H, et al. Gain of 1q21 is an unfavorable genetic prognostic factor for multiple myeloma patients treated with high-dose chemotherapy. Biol Blood Marrow Transplant 2010;16:548–54.

87. Avet-Loiseau H, Gerson F, Magrangeas F, et al. Rearrangements of the c-myc oncogene are present in 15% of primary human multiple myeloma tumors. Blood 2001;98:3082–6.

88. Shou Y, Martelli ML, Gabrea A, et al. Diverse karyotypic abnormalities of the c-myc locus associated with c-myc dysregulation and tumor progression in multiple myeloma. Proc Natl Acad Sci USA 2000;97:228–33.

89. Guikema JE, Hovenga S, Vellenga E, et al. CD27 is heterogeneously expressed in multiple myeloma: low CD27 expression in patients with high-risk disease. Br J Haematol 2003;121:36–43.

90. Moreau P, Robillard N, Jego G, et al. Lack of CD27 in myeloma delineates different presentation and outcome. Br J Haematol 2006;132:168–70.

91. Morgan TK, Zhao S, Chang KL, et al. Low CD27 expression in plasma cell dyscrasias correlates with high-risk disease: an immunohistochemical analysis. Am J Clin Pathol 2006;126:545–51.

92. Shaughnessy J, Tian E, Sawyer J, et al. High incidence of chromosome 13 deletion in multiple myeloma detected by multiprobe interphase FISH. Blood 2000;96:1505–11.

93. Zojer N, Konigsberg R, Ackermann J, et al. Deletion of 13q14 remains an independent adverse prognostic variable in multiple myeloma despite its frequent detection by interphase fluorescence in situ hybridization. Blood 2000;95:1925–30.

94. Chiecchio L, Dagrada GP, Ibrahim AH, et al. Timing of acquisition of deletion 13 in plasma cell dyscrasias is dependent on genetic context. Haematologica 2009;94:1708–13.

95. Kapanadze B, Kashuba V, Baranova A, et al. A cosmid and cDNA fine physical map of a human chromosome 13q14 region frequently lost in B-cell chronic lymphocytic leukemia and identification of a new putative tumor suppressor gene, Leu5. FEBS Lett 1998;426:266–70.

96. Drach J, Ackermann J, Fritz E, et al. Presence of a p53 gene deletion in patients with multiple myeloma predicts for short survival after conventional-dose chemotherapy. Blood 1998;92:802–9.

97. Chang H, Qi C, Yi QL, et al. p53 gene deletion detected by fluorescence in situ hybridization is an adverse prognostic factor for patients with multiple myeloma following autologous stem cell transplantation. Blood 2005;105:358–60.

98. Avet-Loiseau H, Li JY, Godon C, et al. P53 deletion is not a frequent event in multiple myeloma. Br J Haematol 1999;106:717–9.

99. Neri A, Baldini L, Trecca D, et al. p53 gene mutations in multiple myeloma are associated with advanced forms of malignancy. Blood 1993;81:128–35.

100. Avet-Loiseau H. Role of genetics in prognostication in myeloma. Best Pract Res Clin Haematol 2007;20:625–35.

101. Avet-Loiseau H. Ultra high-risk myeloma. Hematology Am Soc Hematol Educ Program 2010;2010:489–93.

102. Reece D, Song KW, Fu T, et al. Influence of cytogenetics in patients with relapsed or refractory multiple myeloma treated with lenalidomide plus dexamethasone: adverse effect of deletion 17p13. Blood 2009;114:522–5.

103. Dimopoulos MA, Kastritis E, Christoulas D, et al. Treatment of patients with relapsed/refractory multiple myeloma with lenalidomide and dexamethasone with or without bortezomib: prospective evaluation of the impact of cytogenetic abnormalities and of previous therapies. Leukemia 2010;24:1769–78.

104. Klein U, Jauch A, Hielscher T, et al. Chromosomal aberrations +1q21 and del(17p13) predict survival in patients with recurrent multiple myeloma treated with lenalidomide and dexamethasone. Cancer 2011;117:2136–44.

105. Govindarajan R, Jagannath S, Flick JT, et al. Preceding standard therapy is the likely cause of MDS after autotransplants for multiple myeloma. Br J Haematol 1996;95:349–53.

106. Nilsson T, Nilsson L, Lenhoff S, et al. MDS/AML-associated cytogenetic abnormalities in multiple myeloma and monoclonal gammopathy of undetermined significance: evidence for frequent de novo occurrence and multipotent stem cell involvement of del(20q). Genes Chromosomes Cancer 2004;41:223–31.

107. Jacobson J, Barlogie B, Shaughnessy J, et al. MDS-type abnormalities within myeloma signature karyotype (MM-MDS): only 13% 1–year survival despite tandem transplants. Br J Haematol 2003;122:430–40.

108. Barlogie B, Tricot G, Haessler J, et al. Cytogenetically defined myelodysplasia after melphalan-based autotransplantation for multiple myeloma linked to poor hematopoietic stem-cell mobilization: the Arkansas experience in more than 3,000 patients treated since 1989. Blood 2008;111:94–100.

109. Decaux O, Lode L, Magrangeas F, et al. Prediction of survival in multiple myeloma based on gene expression profiles reveals cell cycle and chromosomal instability signatures in high-risk patients and hyperdiploid signatures in low-risk patients: a study of the Intergroupe Francophone du Myelome. J Clin Oncol 2008;26:4798–805.

110. Annunziata CM, Davis RE, Demchenko Y, et al. Frequent engagement of the classical and alternative NF-kappaB pathways by diverse genetic abnormalities in multiple myeloma. Cancer Cell 2007;12:115–30.

111. Keats JJ, Fonseca R, Chesi M, et al. Promiscuous mutations activate the noncanonical NF-kappaB pathway in multiple myeloma. Cancer Cell 2007;12:131–44.

112. Demchenko YN, Glebov OK, Zingone A, et al. Classical and/or alternative NF-kappaB pathway activation in multiple myeloma. Blood 2010;115:3541–52.

113. Chapman MA, Lawrence MS, Keats JJ, et al. Initial genome sequencing and analysis of multiple myeloma. Nature 2011;471:467–72.

114. Munshi NC, Avet-Loiseau H. Genomics in multiple myeloma. Clin Cancer Res 2011;17:1234–42.

115. Gutierrez NC, Sarasquete ME, Misiewicz-Krzeminska I, et al. Deregulation of microRNA expression in the different genetic subtypes of multiple myeloma and correlation with gene expression profiling. Leukemia 2010;24:629–37.

116. Johnson DC, Corthals SL, Walker BA, et al. Genetic factors underlying the risk of thalidomide-related neuropathy in patients with multiple myeloma. J Clin Oncol 2011;29:797–804.

117. Shaughnessy J, Jacobson J, Sawyer J, et al. Continuous absence of metaphase-defined cytogenetic abnormalities, especially of chromosome 13 and hypodiploidy, ensures long-term survival in multiple myeloma treated with Total Therapy I: interpretation in the context of global gene expression. Blood 2003;101:3849–56.

118. Barlogie B, Anaissie E, van Rhee F, et al. Incorporating bortezomib into upfront treatment for multiple myeloma: early results of total therapy 3. Br J Haematol 2007;138:176–85.

Lymphoma Cytogenetics

Bhavana J. Dave, PhD[a,b,*], Marilu Nelson, MS, CG, MB (ASCP)[CM][b],
Warren G. Sanger, PhD[a,b]

KEYWORDS

- Lymphoma • Cytogenetics
- Fluorescence in situ hybridization • Microarray • Diagnosis
- Disease progression • Prognosis

The historical significance of lymphoma cytogenetics is accentuated by the fact that a distinct chromosomal abnormality, "14q+", was first identified and associated with Burkitt lymphoma.[1] This triggered numerous investigations in search of specific chromosomal abnormalities in various malignancies. However, the maximum success came from chromosome studies in hematologic malignancies because they readily lent themselves to cytogenetic analysis. The characterization of t(8;14)(q24;q32) and its association with Burkitt lymphoma[2] led to focused genetic studies in various subtypes of lymphomas. Since then, cytogenetics has played a crucial role in providing substantial insight into the genetic mechanisms of lymphomagenesis. Consistent chromosomal alterations in lymphomas, specifically, non-Hodgkin lymphomas (NHLs), have greatly impacted the classification of NHLs in general, especially the B-cell lymphomas,[3–5] and has sometimes even helped establish a distinct subtype as in mantle cell lymphoma.[6] Clonal and relatively complex chromosome abnormalities exist in the majority of NHLs.[7] A number of recurring cytogenetic abnormalities have now been associated with various subtypes of lymphomas; these include the t(14;18) in follicular lymphoma, t(8;14) and variants in Burkitt lymphoma, t(3;14) in diffuse large B-cell lymphoma, t(11;14) in mantle cell lymphoma, and t(2;5) and variants in anaplastic large-cell

The study was partly supported by National Institutes of Health (UO1 CA84967), Leukemia and Lymphoma Society of America (6032-99), John A. Weibe Jr. Children's Healthcare Foundation (00-02102), University of Nebraska Medical Center Dean's Research grant, and the internal Cytogenetics Research and Development Fund.

[a] Departments of Pediatrics, Pathology/Microbiology, Munroe Meyer Institute for Genetics and Rehabilitation, University of Nebraska Medical Center, 985440 Nebraska Medical Center, Omaha, NE 68198-5440, USA

[b] Human Genetics Laboratories, Munroe Meyer Institute for Genetics and Rehabilitation, 955440 Nebraska Medical Center, University of Nebraska Medical Center, Omaha, NE 68198-5440, USA

* Corresponding author. Departments of Pediatrics, Pathology/Microbiology, Munroe Meyer Institute for Genetics and Rehabilitation, University of Nebraska Medical Center, 985440 Nebraska Medical Center, Omaha, NE 68198-5440.

E-mail address: bdave@unmc.edu.

Clin Lab Med 31 (2011) 725–761

doi:10.1016/j.cll.2011.08.001

0272-2712/11/$ – see front matter © 2011 Elsevier Inc. All rights reserved.

lymphoma.[8] In many instances, however, the association of a chromosomal alteration with a histologic subtype is not absolute, and NHLs have continued to be reclassified based on collective analysis of characteristic morphologic, immunologic, and genetic features.

With the advent of fluorescence in situ hybridization (FISH) technologies and their implementation in paraffin-embedded tissues to interrogate the existence of specific genetic alterations in defined chromosomal regions, the feasibility of achieving genetic information for specific abnormalities has increased. Retrospective molecular cytogenetic studies and newer and more insightful techniques such as array comparative genomic hybridization (aCGH)[9,10] and gene expression microarrays have helped determine various other gains, deletions, and amplifications and elucidated the pathways of activation and transformation.[11–17] The World Health Organization (WHO) classification has therefore approved of a multiparametric approach of utilizing the clinical, morphologic, immunophenotypic, and genetic features. This has enhanced precise interpretation of clinical and translational investigations, leading to a better molecular understanding of lymphoid malignancies.[18–20] Hence cytogenetic and molecular cytogenetic studies are necessary if not imperative components in lymphoma diagnosis and progression. Here we address and adhere to the various cytogenetic and molecular cytogenetic alterations as they present in the different subtypes of lymphomas and the approaches to detect these abnormalities in lymphoid malignancies, including the mature B-cell and T-cell neoplasms and Hodgkin lymphoma (HL).

METHODS
Cytogenetics

To yield an accurate chromosomal picture, it is crucial that cytogenetic investigations be performed on the tissue representative of tumor and not on the adjacent nonmalignant (stromal) tissue and that appropriate culture methods be utilized for the growth of tumor cells. When sufficient tissue is available, selected tumor material should be divided for morphologic, immunologic, and cytogenetic studies. For best results and to retain viability, the lymphoid tissue should be transported in sterile media at room temperature to the cytogenetics laboratory as quickly as possible. *The tissue should never be fixed or frozen.* Any necrotic tissue should be removed before disaggregation. The tissue is mechanically disaggregated, which can be followed by enzymatic disaggregation if deemed necessary. The minced tissue is divided between the appropriate cultures containing RPMI 1640 (Irvine Scientific, Santa Ana, CA, USA) with 20% fetal bovine serum (FBS), HEPES, glutamine, penicillin, streptomycin, and heparin. Tumor cells are spontaneously dividing; hence the cultures do not require mitogens to achieve metaphase preparations. Depending on the availability of the tissue material for cytogenetic preparations, the unstimulated cultures are set up in the following preference: direct-overnight with 10 μL of a low concentration (10 μg/mL) of Colcemid (Irvine Scientific, Santa Ana, CA, USA) overnight, 24-hour, and 48-hour cultures and incubated at 37°C.

Approximately 40 minutes before the initiation of harvest, the cells are treated with Colcemid, 0.2 μg/mL. After hypotonic treatment (0.4% KCl solution for 20 minutes at 37°C), the cells are prefixed by adding 2 mL of freshly prepared chilled 3:1 methanol–glacial acetic acid fixative and gently inverting the tubes. This is followed by three additional fixation cycles and air-dried slide preparation. The slides are generally "aged" in a hot oven (100°C) for 30 minutes or in a 60°C oven overnight. The slides are then G-banded with a trypsin pretreatment. When available, at least 20 metaphases are analyzed. Karyotypes of Giemsa-banded metaphase chromosomes are typically described according to the most recent version of the International System of Cytogenetic Nomenclature (ISCN 2009).[21] Abnormal clones are defined as either two or more cells with the same structural abnormality or gain of the same chromosome, or the presence of three or more cells with loss of the same chromosome. However, if an abnormal karyotype contains a known NHL-associated translocation in only one cell, it is included in the nomenclature. All normal cells are also included in the nomenclature.[22–24]

FISH

Depending on the availability and requirement for differential diagnosis, FISH procedures are performed either on cell suspensions prepared from cryopreserved cell pellets or on 4- to 5-μm unstained paraffin embedded tumor tissue sections. FISH probes to investigate the majority of the specific NHL-related translocations or gene disruptions are commercially available. Many laboratories generate homebrew FISH probes for detection of common abnormalities to make the testing more cost effective. The protocol for FISH studies has been outlined in another article by Karen D. Tsuchiya elsewhere in this issue. Our laboratory protocol has been described in detail previously.[22–24]

CYTOGENETIC ABNORMALITIES IN LYMPHOMAS

The core distinction in lymphoid malignancies historically has been HL and NHL. The majority of these are B-cell neoplasms, with fewer than 1% of HLs and 15% of NHLs being T/NK cell diseases. These may present as leukemic forms or as tumors of lymphatic organs. This section accounts for abnormalities that are identified by either conventional cytogenetics or FISH studies. Many of these present as primary abnormalities in some lymphoma subtypes, while being secondary or more downstream in clonal evolution in other subtypes. Often more than one of these abnormalities are seen in different lymphoma subtypes. To facilitate differential diagnosis, the possible existence of two or more abnormalities may need to be verified. **Table 1** presents a list of primary abnormalities in most common lymphoma subtypes and **Table 2** outlines the clinically available techniques to determine these abnormalities. **Fig. 1** illustrates the various characteristic abnormalities and **Table 3** summarizes the various recurrent cytogenetic alterations and those with prognostic implications. The descriptions of various subtypes of lymphomas have been presented in sequential order as they appear in the most recent edition of WHO classification of tumors of hematopoietic malignancies and lymphoid tissues[8] and are limited only to lymphomas (plasma cell neoplasm/multiple myeloma is discussed in a separate article by Marilyn L. Slovack elsewhere in this issue).

B-CELL LYMPHOMAS
Chronic Lymphocytic Leukemia/Small Lymphocytic Lymphoma

A rare disease in Eastern countries and the most common leukemia of adults in Western nations, chronic lymphocytic leukemia/small lymphocytic lymphoma (CLL/SLL) accounts for about 7% of NHL. The term SLL is used for the nodal form with the tissue morphology and immunophenotype of CLL. Of all hematologic malignancies, CLL/SLL shows the highest genetic predisposition.[25] Cytogenetic abnormalities have been detected in nearly 80% of CLL/SLL, specifically by FISH techniques.[26–28] The malignant CLL cells have a poor response to conventional mitogens; thus previous studies identified the cytogenetic abnormalities at a different frequency than those

Table 1
"Characteristic" primary chromosome abnormalities in common B- and T-cell lymphoma subtypes

Chromosome Lesion	Gene Rearrangement	Lymphoma Subtype (other subtypes sometimes containing the abnormality)
Trisomy 12, del(13q), monosomy 13, del(14)(q24q32), t(14q32), del(11q22.3), del(17p13)	IGH rearrangement ATM deletion, TP53 deletion	CLL/SLL (mantle cell lymphoma)
t(2;7)((p12;q21) del(7q), gain 3/(3q)	IGK with CDK6	Splenic marginal zone
t(11;18)(q21;q21) t(14;18)(q32;q21) t(3;14)(p14;q32) t(1;14)(p22;q32)	BIRC3 (API2)/MALT1 IGH/MALT1 FOXP1/IGH BCL10/IGH	Extranodal MALT
t(14;19)(q32;q13)	IGH/BCL3	Nodal marginal zone
t(14;18)(q32;q21) and variants t(2;18)(p12;q21), t(18;22)(q21;q11.2)	IGH/BCL2 IGK/BCL2 BCL2/IGL	Follicular (diffuse large cell)
t(11;14)(q13;q32)	CCND1/IGH	Mantle cell (CLL/SLL; splenic lymphoma with villous lymphocytes)
t(3;14)(q27;q32) and multiple 3q27 partners t(3q27)	BCL6/IGH BCL6 rearrangement	Diffuse large cell (follicular)
t(8;14)(q24;q32) variants t(2;8)(p12;q24) and t(8;22)(q24;q11.2)	MYC/IGH IGK/MYC IGL/MYC	Burkitt (diffuse large cell)
t(2;5)(p23;q35) and multiple 2p23 partners t(2p23)	ALK/NPM ALK rearrangement	Anaplastic large cell
14q11 rearrangements	TCR	Other T-cell lymphomas

observed with specific FISH probes.[27,29–31] Interphase studies demonstrated that del(13q) is the most common abnormality detectable by FISH.[31] This is followed by trisomy 12 and deletions of 11q22–q23, 17p13, and 6q21.[27] The use of mitogenic agents such as CD40L and immunostimulatory CpG-oligonucleotide DSP30 and IL2, has improved the percentage of metaphase chromosome abnormalities in CLL cases. CLL/SLL primarily depicts genomic imbalances; more chromosomal abnormalities and rare reciprocal translocations are observed with an overall karyotypic evaluation than focused FISH studies.[28] The expression of tyrosine kinase ZAP-70 is associated with IGHV unmutated CLL genotype.[17] The distribution of genomic abnormalities varies depending on the mutational status of VH.[25] Trisomy 12, del(13q), del(11q), and del(17p) are frequently observed independent of each other. However, combinations of these abnormalities appearing together are not uncommon. The del(11q) and del(17p) are recurrently noted as secondary changes. Although rare, trisomies of 3, 8, and 18 and del(6q) have been observed, recurrently.[32]

Trisomy 12, frequently associated with atypical morphology,[32] is found in nearly one third of CLL with abnormal karyotypes and in about 15% of all CLL as detected by FISH,[29] with the minimum common gain being 12q13. Other additional recurrent aberrations among the trisomy 12 cases include trisomies of 18 and 19,[33] t(14; 18)(q24;q32) IGH-BCL2 fusion,[34] t(14;19)(q32;q13) leading to IGH–BCL3 fusion,[35]

Table 2
Common B- and T-cell lymphoma subtypes and possible cytogenetics/FISH testing

Lymphoma Subtype (other subtypes sometimes containing the abnormality)	Type of Testing[a]	Informative FISH Probes[b]	Combination of FISH Testing to Refine Differential Diagnosis
CLL/SLL (mantle cell)	*Cytogenetics and FISH* Rearrangement detection with breakapart probe, deletion with locus specific, and trisomy with pericentromeric probes	FISH: Usually panel of the following probes: 12 centromere; D13S319 [13q14.3/13q34]; *ATM* [11q22.3]; *IGH* [14q32]; *TP53* [17p13.1]	FISH panel containing the informative probes described
Splenic marginal zone lymphoma	*Cytogenetics and/or FISH* Rearrangement detection with breakapart probe, deletion with locus specific, and trisomy with pericentromeric probes	7 centromere/D7S486 [7q31], 3 centromere, break-apart *IGK* [2p12]	*MALT1* [18q21]/18 centromere *IGH* [14q32] 7 centromere/D7S486 [7q31]/3 centromere
Extranodal MALT	*Cytogenetics and/or FISH* Translocation detection Rearrangement detection with breakapart probe	*API2/MALT1*[t(11;18)] *MALT1*[18q21]	*MALT1* [18q21]/18 centromere *IGH* [14q32] 3 centromere/12 centromere
Follicular (diffuse large cell)	*Cytogenetics and/or FISH* Translocation detection Rearrangement detection with breakapart probes	*IGH/BCL2* [t(14;18)]; *IGH* [14q32]; *IGK* [2p12]; *IGL* [22q11.2]	*IGH/BCL2, BCL2, BCL6* *BCL2* [18q21]; *BCL6* [3q27]

(continued on next page)

Table 2
(continued)

Lymphoma Subtype (other subtypes sometimes containing the abnormality)	Type of Testing[a]	Informative FISH Probes[b]	Combination of FISH Testing to Refine Differential Diagnosis
Mantle cell (B-CLL/SLL; splenic lymphoma with villous lymphocytes)	*Cytogenetics and/or FISH* Translocation detection Rearrangement detection with breakapart probe	*IGH/CCND1* [t(11;14)] *CCND1* [11q13], *IGH* [14q32]	*IGH/CCND1*
Diffuse large cell (follicular)	*Cytogenetics and/or FISH* Rearrangement detection with breakapart probe	*BCL6* [3q27]; *MYC* [8q24.1] *IGH* [14q32]; *IGK* [2p12]; *IGL* [22q11.2]	*BCL6, IGH/BCL2, MYC*
Burkitt (diffuse large cell)	*Cytogenetics and/or FISH* Translocation detection Rearrangement detection with breakapart probe	*IGH/MYC* [t(8;14)] *MYC* [8q24.1]; *IGH* [14q32]; *IGK* [2p12]; *IGL* [22q11.2]	*MYC*, if *MYC* positive follow-up with *IGH/MYC, BCL6, IGH/BCL2*
Anaplastic large cell	*Cytogenetics and/or FISH* Rearrangement detection with breakapart probe	*ALK* [2p23]	
Other T-cell lymphomas	*Cytogenetics and/or FISH* Rearrangement detection with breakapart probe	*TCR* [14q11]	

[a] Cytogenetics is performed on fresh tumor specimen. Metaphase FISH requires fresh tissue for chromosome preparations. Interphase FISH can be performed on both fixed cell pellet from chromosome preparations or on paraffin-embedded tissue sections.

[b] The table mostly describes commercially available probes. Newer probes are continually available from various vendors. FISH probes with two chromosomes/regions in parentheses typically represent dual fusion FISH signal pattern when translocation positive; probes with one chromosome region in parentheses represent breakapart signal pattern when rearrangement positive. These are used mostly for regions involved in translocations with multiple partners.

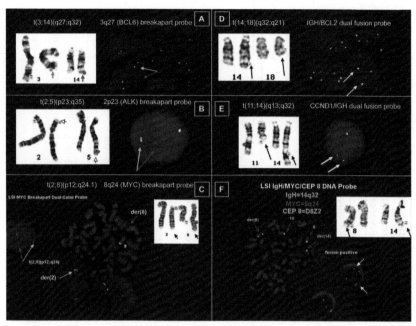

Fig. 1. Common translocations in lymphomas, containing partial karyotypes with FISH signal pattern portrayal and FISH images depicting the detection of various rearrangements and translocations. Figures A, B, and C illustrate FISH examples of breakapart probes for the determination of the rearrangement of specific chromosomal regions and figures D, E, and F illustrate dual fusion probes detecting various translocations. (A) translocation t(3;14)(q27; q32) and rearrangement of 3q27 (BCL6) determined on paraffin embedded tissue; (B) translocation t(2;5)(p23;q35) and rearrangement of 2p23 (ALK) shown in an interphase cell; (C) translocation t(2;8)(p12;q24.1) and rearrangement of 8q24.1 (MYC) as seen in a metaphase spread; (D) chromosome representation of t(14;18)(q32;q21) and its detection in interphase cells in paraffin embedded tissue; (E) partial karyotype of t(11;14)(q13;q32) and its detection in an interphase cell; (F) the t(8;14)(q24.1;q32) and a metaphase FISH image illustrating the translocation.

and del(14)(q24q32) with one breakpoint in *IGH* locus.[36] Variant translocations including the 2p12 and 22q13 (*IGK* and *IGL*, respectively) are also observed. After initial FISH studies,[29] abnormalities of 13/13q were accepted as the most frequent alteration in CLL/SLL. These are observed in 50% of CLL by FISH and in about 20% of abnormal karyotypes. The critical deletion region involves 13q14 and excludes the *RB1* gene.[37,38] Monoallelic as well as biallelic losses of 13q14, and monosomy/ nullisomy of 13, have been observed in CLL/SLL. Deletions of 11q, involving the minimum deletion region 11q22–q23 which included the *ATM* gene, are observed mostly by interphase FISH studies.[27,30,39] Structural abnormalities of 17p including deletions of *TP53* are also seen in CLL/SLL and are associated with an unfavorable prognosis.[28,40] Most cases containing translocation t(11;14)(q13;q32) linking the *IGH–CCND1* genes may now be classified as mantle cell lymphoma (MCL); however, this may also rarely be noted CLL/SLL.

Progression of CLL/SLL to B-PLL is rare; however, an acute transformation to a diffuse large cell lymphoma, known as Ritcher's syndrome, takes place in some cases and a very low percentage develop HL. Complex karyotypes, deletions of *TP53* and

Table 3
Recurrent cytogenetic abnormalities including those with prognostic relevance in different categorized subtypes of B- and T-cell lymphomas[a]

Lymphoma Subtype	Recurrent Chromosome Abnormalities[a]	Chromosome Abnormalities with Prognostic Relevance[b]
B-Cell Lymphoma		
B-cell chronic lymphocytic leukemia/small lymphocytic lymphoma	*Trisomy/gain:* 3, **12**, 18, 2p24–25, 3q26–27, 8q24 *Monosomy/deletions/loss:* 6q, 11q, **13q**, 14q24–32, 17p, *Rearrangements:* 2p12 (*IGK*), 6q21–23, 11q22–23, 12p13–15, 13q14.3, 14q22, 14q32 (*IGH*), 22q11.2 (*IGL*) *Translocations:* t(8;14)(q24;q32) and variants, t(9;14)(p13; q32), t(11;14)(q13;q32), t(14;18)(q32;q21) and variants, t(14;19)(q32;q13.3)	*Poor prognosis:* del(17p), del(11q), del(6q) t(8q24)/+8q24, del (9)(p21) *Favorable prognosis:* isolated 13q14.3 deletions
B-Promyelocytic	Abnormalities observed in CLL/SLL (trisomy 12 rare) Complex karyotypes	ND
Splenic marginal zone	*Trisomy/gain:* 3q *Monosomy/deletions/loss:* **del(7q31–32)** *Translocations:* t(11;14)(q13;q32), t(2;7)(p12;q21)	*Poor prognosis:* del(7q)
Hairy cell leukemia	*Trisomy/gain:* 5q13–31 *Monosomy/deletions/loss:* 14q22–24 *Rearrangements:* 14q, 15q	ND
Splenic B-cell leukemia/ lymphoma, unclassifiable	*Monosomy/deletions/loss:* 17p13 (*TP53*) *Rearrangements:* 8q24, 14q32, 3q27 *Complex rearrangements*	ND
Lymphoplasmacytic	*Trisomy/gain:* 3 *Deletions/loss:* 6q *Translocations:* t(9;14)(p13;q32)	*Poor prognosis:* del(6q)
Extranodal marginal zone lymphoma of mucosa-associated lymphoid tissue (MALT lymphoma)	*Trisomy/gain:* **3**, **18**, 3q (3q27), 9q (9q34), 18q *Rearrangements:* 2q, 3q27 *Translocations:* **t(1;14)(p22;q32)**, t(1;2)(p22;p12), **t(11;18)(q21;q21)**, **t(14;18)(q32;q21)** (18q21–*MALT1*), **t(3;14)(p14.1;q32)**	*Poor prognosis:* del(9p), del(17p), t(1;14)(p22;q32), partial or complete trisomy of 18

(continued on next page)

Table 3
(continued)

Lymphoma Subtype	Recurrent Chromosome Abnormalities[a]	Chromosome Abnormalities with Prognostic Relevance[b]
Nodal marginal zone	*Trisomy/gain:* 3, 18 *Translocations:* **t(14;19)(q32;q21)** Complex karyotypes	ND
Follicular	*Trisomy/gain:* X, 3, 5, 7, 8, 12 (12q), 18 (18q) *Monosomy/deletions/loss:* 1p36, 6q21, 6q23–26, 9p21, 10q22–24, 17p13 *Rearrangements:* 1p, 3q27, 6q23–26, 11q, 12q13–15, 18q21, frequently as +der(18)t(14;18) *Translocations:* **t(14;18)(q32;q21) and variants** involving (18q21) *BCL2*, t(3;14)(q27;q32) and variants involving (3q27) *BCL6*	*Transformation/aggressive clinical course/poor prognosis:* +X, del(1)(p36) +7, del(6q), del(9)(p21) (*CDKN2A*), 8q24 (*MYC* abnormality), del(10)(q22–q24), +11q, +12, and del(17p) (*TP53*), +18, and +der(18)t(14;18) Total number of abnormalities, presence of polyploidy, and markers
Mantle cell	*Trisomy/gain:* 3 (3q), 12 (12q) *Monosomy/deletions/loss:* Y, 1p, 6q, 9 (9p),10q, 11q, 13 (13q), 17p,18 *Rearrangements:* 1p13–p31, 3q27, 6q11–15, 6q23–27, 7p21, 8q24, 9p21, 10p12–13, 11q22–23, 13q11–13, 13q14–34, and 17p13-pter *Translocations:* **t(11;14)(q13;q32)**, t(12;14)(p13;q32), t(2;12)(p12;p13), t(6;14)(p21;q32) and occasionally translocations involving (3q27) *BCL6*	*Transformation/aggressive clinical course/poor prognosis:* Involvement of (8q24) *MYC* locus +3q, −9q, +12, del(13)(q14), del(17p) *TP53*, karyotypic complexity
Diffuse large-cell lymphoma (DLBCL)	*Trisomy/gain:* X, 3, 7, 9, 12, 18, 1q23–31, 1q32–44, 3q, 6p, 7p, 7q31–32, 8q22–24, 11q12–13, 12q14–24, 18q11–21, and 22q12-qter *Monosomy/deletions/loss:* Y, 4, 6, 13, 15, 17, 1p36-pter, 2p23-pter, 4q32-qter, 6q21–25, 8p12-pter, 9p21-pter, 11q23-qter, 12p12–13, 14q23-qter, 17p12–13, 18q21-qter *Other breakpoints in rearrangements:* 1p22, 1q21, 1q25, 3p21, 3q27, 4q31, 6p21, 7q33, 8q21, 8q24, 9p24, 16p13, 18q21, 19q13 *Translocations:* **t(3;14)(q27;q32)**, t(2;3)(p12;q27), t(3;22)(q27;q11.2), t(8;14)(q24; q32), t(14;18) q32;q21 *Breakpoints involved with* **3q27** (*BCL6*): 4p13, 6p22, 7p13, 8q24, 11q23, 13q14, 15q22, 17q11	*Transformation/aggressive clinical course/poor prognosis:* Del(9)(p21), del(17p), dup(1q), *MYC* rearrangement *Reduced risk:* Trisomy 5, 5q, 7q

(continued on next page)

Table 3
(continued)

Lymphoma Subtype	Recurrent Chromosome Abnormalities[a]	Chromosome Abnormalities with Prognostic Relevance[b]
DLBCL subtypes		
T-histiocyte-rich large cell lymphoma (THRLBCL)	*Trisomy/gain:* Xq, 4q13–28, Xp21–11, 18q21 *Monosomy/deletions/loss:* 17p	ND
Primary DLBCL of central nervous system	*Trisomy/gain:* 12q, 22q, 18q21, with *BCL2* and *MALT1* amplification *Monosomy/deletions/loss:* 6q	ND
Primary cutaneous DLBCL, leg type	*Trisomy/gain:* of 18q21.31–21.33, with *BCL2* and *MALT1* amplification *Monosomy/deletions/loss:* 9p21.3 (*CDKN2A* and *CDKN2B*) *Translocations:* involving *CMYC, BCL6,* and *IGH*	ND
EBV-positive DLBCL in elderly	ND	ND
Other lymphomas of large B cells		
DLBCL associated with chronic inflammation	Complex karyotypes with numerous numeric and structural abnormalities	ND
Lymphoid granulomatosis	Nonrandom cytogenetic aberrations yet to be identified	ND
Primary mediastinal (thymic) large B-cell	*Gains:* 9p24, 2p15, Xp11.4-21 and Xq24-26	ND
Intravascular large B-cell	*Monosomy/deletions/loss:* 6q21-24 *Rearrangements of:* 1, 4, 5, 6, 8, 10 *Translocations:* t(11;14)(q13;q32), t(14;18)(q32;q21)	ND

(continued on next page)

Table 3
(continued)

Lymphoma Subtype	Recurrent Chromosome Abnormalities[a]	Chromosome Abnormalities with Prognostic Relevance[b]
ALK-Positive DLBCL	*Translocations:* t(2;17)(p23;q23)	
Plasmablastic lymphoma	ND	ND
HHV8-associated multicentric Castleman disease	ND	ND
Primary effusion lymphoma (PEL)	*Trisomy/gain:* X, 7, 12(12q) *Rearrangements:* 1q, complex karyotypes *Translocations:* t(8;14)(q24;q32) and variant *MYC* translocations	ND
Burkitt	*Trisomy/gain:* 7(7q), 8, 12, 1q21–25 *Monosomy/deletions/loss:* 6q, 7q, 8q, 13q, 17p *Rearrangements:* 1q23–31, 3q27, 8q24, 14q32, 17p13.1 *Translocations:* **t(2;8)(p11;q24.1), t(8;14)(q24.1;q32), t(8;22)(q24.1;q11.2)**	*Transformation/aggressive clinical course/poor prognosis:* del(13q)
B-cell lymphoma, unclassifiable, with features intermediate between DLBCL and Burkitt lymphoma	*Rearrangements:* 3q27, 8q24, 14q32 *Translocations:* **t(2;8)(p11;q24.1), t(8;14)(q24.1;q32), t(8;22)(q24.1;q11.2), t(14;18)(q32;q21), t(3q27)** *BCL6*	*Transformation/aggressive clinical course/poor prognosis:* *MYC* rearrangement in addition to t(14;18)— "double hit"
T-cell lymphoma		
T-cell prolymphocytic leukemia	*Trisomy/gain:* 6p, 8 (8q) (cytogenetics and CGH) *Monosomy/deletions/loss:* 6q, 8p, 10p (cytogenetics and CGH) *Rearrangements:* i(8)(p11), 11q (*ATM*), 17p, 22q *Translocations:* **t(14;14)(q11;q32), (X;14)(q28;q11)**	ND

(continued on next page)

Table 3
(continued)

Lymphoma Subtype	Recurrent Chromosome Abnormalities[a]	Chromosome Abnormalities with Prognostic Relevance[b]
T-cell large granular lymphocytic leukemia	*Deletions/loss:* 6q *Rearrangements:* 7p, 7q, 14q11 (*TCR loci*)	ND
Chronic lymphoproliferative disorders of NK cells	Usually normal karyotype	*Transformation/aggressive clinical course/poor prognosis:* Presence of karyotypic abnormalities
Aggressive NK cell leukemia	*Trisomy/gain:* By CGH (1p32-pter, 6p, 11q, 12q, 17q, 19p, 20q, and Xp) *Monosomy/deletions/loss:* del(6q21q25), 11p (by CGH, X, 6q16–27, 13q14–34, 11q22–25, 17p13)	ND
EBV-positive T-cell lymphoproliferative disorders of childhood	ND	ND
Adult T-cell	*Trisomy/gains:* 1p36, 1q, 2p, 3p, 4q, 6p25, 7p (7p22), 7q, 14q32 *Monosomy/deletions/loss:* 6q (6q15–21), 10p, 13q, 16q, 18p *Rearrangements:* 1p, 1q, 3q, 5p, 5q, 9q, 10p, 10q, 11q, 12q, 18q *Translocation:* t(14;14)(q11;q32) *Rearrangements with* **14q11:** Xq, 1p, 1q, 3p, 3q, 8q, 10p, 11p, 12q, 18p	ND
Extranodal NK-T cell lymphoma, nasal type	*Gains:* 2q *Loss:* 1p36.23–36.33, 2p16.1–16.3, 4q12 , 4q13.3–32.1, 5p14.1–14.3, 5q34–35.3, 6q16.1–q27, 11q22.3–23.3	ND

(continued on next page)

Table 3
(continued)

Lymphoma Subtype	Recurrent Chromosome Abnormalities[a]	Chromosome Abnormalities with Prognostic Relevance[b]
Enteropathy-associated T-cell lymphpma (EATL)	*Gains:* 1q, 5q, 7q, 9q (9q31.3–qter), 16q12.1 *Classic ETL-linked to celiac disease-gains:* 1q, 5q *Monomorphic variant ETL-gain: MYC locus* *Loss:* 8p, 9p, 13q	ND
Hepatosplenic T-cell lymphoma (HSTL)	*Gain:* 7, i(**7q**), 8 *Loss:* X, Y *Rearrangements:* **7q**	ND
Subcutaneous penniculitis-like T-cell lymphomas (SPTL)	*Trisomy/gain:* 2q, 4q, 5q, 13q *Monosomy/loss:* 1pter, 2pter, 10qter, 11qter, 12qter, 16, 19, 20, 22	ND
Mycosis fungoides (MF) and Sezary syndrome (SS)	*Trisomy/gain:* 7, 8q, 17q, **18** *Monosomy/loss:* 1p, 6q, **9**, **10**, (10q) 10q, 13q, 17p, 19 *Rearrangements:* 1p32–36, 1q, 2q, 6q22–27, 8q22, 10q23–26, 12q21, 12q22, 17p11–13, 19p13.3, complex karyotypes Deletion *NAV3 (POMFIII)* and amplification of *JUNB* in SS (FISH and CGH)	*Transformation/aggressive clinical course/poor prognosis:* Gain of 8q and loss of 6q and 13q
Primary cutaneous CD-30 positive T-cell lymphoproliferative disorders	*Trisomy/gain:* 9 *Monosomy/loss:* 6q21 and 18p11.3	ND
Primary cutaneous peripheral T-cell lymphomas, rare subtypes	ND	ND

(continued on next page)

Table 3
(continued)

Lymphoma Subtype	Recurrent Chromosome Abnormalities[a]	Chromosome Abnormalities with Prognostic Relevance[b]
Primary cutaneous γδT-cell lymphomas	ND	ND
Peripheral T-cell lymphoma not otherwise specified	*Trisomy/gain:* 1q, 3p, 5p, 7q22–31, 8q24-qter, 11q13 17q (17q11–25),12p13, 22q *Monosomy/deletions/loss:* 4q, 5q, 6q22–24, 9p (9p21–q33), 10p13-pter, 10q (10q23–24), 11p11, 12q (12q21–22),13q (13q21) *Translocations:* t(14;19)(q11;q13), t(5;9)(q33;q22)	ND
Angioimmunoblastic T-cell lymphomas	*Trisomy/gain:* X, 3 (3q), 5 (5q), 11p11–q14 (11q13), 19, 21, 22q *Monosomy/deletions/loss:* 6q, 13q	*Transformation/aggressive clinical course/poor prognosis:* +X, aberrations of 1p31–32, and complex abnormalities
Anaplastic large cell (ALCL) *ALK*-positive	*Trisomy/gain:* X, 7, 9, 17p, and 17q24-qter *Monosomy/deletions/loss:* Y, 4q13–21, 6q, 17, 11q14, 13q *Translocations:* **t(2;5)(p23;q35)** *Rearrangements with* **2p23** *(ALK):* 1q25, inv(2)(p23q35) 3q21, 17q23, 19p13.1, 22q11.2, 17q25, Xq11–12	*Favorable prognosis:* t(2;5)(p23;q35) and variants involving *ALK*
Anaplastic large cell lymphoma (ALCL) *ALK*-negative	*Trisomy/gain:* 1q, 3p, 6p21, 7 *Monosomy/deletions/loss:* 6q13–21, 13q, 15, 16pter, 16qter, 17p13	ND

(continued on next page)

Table 3
(continued)

Lymphoma Subtype	Recurrent Chromosome Abnormalities[a]	Chromosome Abnormalities with Prognostic Relevance[b]
Hodgkin Lymphoma		
Nodular lymphocyte predominant Hodgkin Lymphoma (NLPHL)	Similar rearrangements as in DLBCL t(3q27)(*BCl6*) rearrangements Polyploid (triploid to tetraploid)—complex karyotypes	*Poor prognosis: del(13q)*
Classical Hodgkin (cHL)	*Gains:* 4p16, 4q23–q24 and 9p23–p24 *Monosomy/deletions/loss:* 1p, 3p, 6q, 7q *Rearrangements:* 1p36, 6q15, 6q21, 7q22, 7q32, 8q24, 11q23, 12q24, 13p11, 14p11, 14q32, 15p11, 19p13 *Translocation:* t(14;18)(q32;q21) and other 14q32 (*IGH*) translocations with 2p16, 3q27, 8q24, 16p13, 17q12, 19q13 Polyploid (triploid to tetraploid)—complex karyotypes	ND

[a] Primary abnormalities are **bold**. Majority of the abnormalities are those detected by conventional cytogenetics or FISH, or both. In diseases with few comprehensive reports as in T- and NK-cell lymphomas, CGH reports may have been taken into account. ND, none detected.

[b] In all lymphoid malignancies except HL, complex karyotypes in general signify an aggressive clinical course. However, if enough clinical information regarding specific subtype and cytogenetic abnormalities is unavailable, the data have not been included in this table.

ATM, and involvement of 8q24 (*MYC* region) and 9p21 (*CDKN2A*) are indicators of transformation,[41] while isolated 13q14.3 deletions are associated with a favorable prognosis.[27]

B-Cell Prolymphocytic Leukemia

A neoplasm of B prolymphocytes with more than 55% of lymphocytes being prolymphocytes, B-cell prolymphocytic leukemia (B-PLL) is an extremely rare disease, comprising approximately 1% of lymphocytic leukemias.[42] Chromosome abnormalities that are common in CLL/SLL are also characteristic of B-PLL.[26,28,40] Complex karyotypes with nearly 50% cases containing the deletion of 17p including the *TP53* gene have been demonstrated in B-PLL. In addition, deletions of 13q14 are also noted by FISH analysis. Trisomy 12 is rare in B-PLL.[43] The initial finding of nearly 20% cases of B-PLL containing t(11;14)(q13;q32)[44] is now refined, and these cases are more likely considered to be leukemic variants of mantle cell lymphoma.[43,45]

Splenic B-Cell Marginal Zone Lymphoma

Constituting about 2% of the lymphoid neoplasms, splenic B-cell marginal zone lymphoma (SMBZL) is seen mostly among patients older than 50 years of age.[46] SMBZL is composed of small lymphocytes that surround and replace the splenic white pulp germinal center, efface the follicle mantle, and merge with a peripheral (marginal) zone of larger cells. Lymphoma cells may be found in the peripheral blood as villous lymphocytes (splenic lymphoma with circulating villous lymphocytes [SLVLs]).[47] Deletion of 7q is the most frequent abnormality in SMBZL and is observed in nearly 40% of the cases; the critical region is 7q31–32. Gain of 3q and numerous other abnormalities have also been described.[48–50] In addition, dysregulation of *CDK6* gene as a result of a t(2;7)(p12;q21) has been demonstrated in some cases.[51,52] The t(11;18), common in extranodal marginal zone lymphoma of mucosa associated lymphoid tissue (MALT), is absent in SMBZL. The presence of a 7q deletion may be associated with an unfavorable outcome.[47,53]

Hairy Cell Leukemia

An indolent and rare disease of small mature B lymphoid cells with oval nuclei and abundant cytoplasm with "hairy" projections, hairy cell leukemia (HCL) constitutes 2% of lymphoid leukemias, occurring at a median age of 50 years and exhibiting a strong male predominance (5:1 male to female ratio).[54] Structural rearrangements of 14q including translocations involving 14q32 and deletions of 14q22−24 have been described.[55] Further, abnormalities of chromosome 5 including gains in 5q13–31 have been observed.[56,57]

Lymphoplasmacytic Lymphoma

Lymphoplasmacytic lymphoma (LPL) involves small B lymphocytes, plasmacytoid lymphocytes, and plasma cells, usually involving bone marrow and sometimes lymph nodes and spleen. Walderstom macroglobulinemia (WM) is found in a large subset and is usually defined as LPL with BM involvement. These LPLs are characterized by excessive proliferation of an immunoglobulin M (IGM)-producing clone of malignant plasmacytoid cells.[5] The distinction between marginal zone lymphoma (MZL) and LPL is sometimes difficult. These cases may be described as small lymphocytic lymphoma with plasmacytic differentiation.[58] No specific cytogenetic abnormality is currently defined as a hallmark of LPL. Previously these lymphomas were associated with a characteristic translocation t(9;14)((p13;q32) involving the *PAX5/IGH* genes[59]; however, the translocation is rarely observed in LPL and is also observed in other B-cell neoplasms.[60,61] Although deletion of 6q is nonspecific for LPL, it is most frequently noted in LPL/WM (6q21 deletions by FISH).[62] Cases with a deletion of 6q have been associated with an adverse prognosis.

Extranodal Marginal Zone Lymphoma of Mucosa-Associated Lymphoid Tissue (MALT lymphoma)

Composed of morphologically heterogeneous small B cells including marginal zone (centrocyte-like) cells, small lymphocytes, scattered immunoblasts, and centroblast-like cells, MALT lymphoma is an extranodal lymphoma that comprises 7% to 8% of all B-cell lymphomas.[63] The differential diagnosis of MALT lymphoma includes the reactive inflammatory processes including *Helicobactor pylori* gastritis that typically precede the lymphoma and other small B-cell lymphomas (follicular lymphoma, mantle cell lymphoma, small lymphocytic lymphoma). The t(11;18)(q21;q21) is the most frequent translocation that occurs in MALT lymphoma. The *API2 (BRIC3)* gene on 11q21 and the *MALT1* gene on chromosome 18q21 are disrupted and recombined to form a *API2–MALT1* fusion gene on the derivative chromosome 11.[64–66] Most often this appears as a sole abnormality.[67–69] Approximately 15% of MALT lymphomas reveal the t(11;18) when molecular or FISH techniques are utilized; the majority of these are the gastric and pulmonal MALT cases.[70,71] The t(11;18) appears to be specific for MALT lymphomas and has not been observed in nodal and splenic marginal zone B-cell lymphomas.[64,65,72] Three other recurrent and mutually exclusive translocations are observed in MALT lymphoma. The t(14;18)(q32;q21), which deregulates the *MALT1* gene through *IGH* juxtaposition,[73,74] is observed in nearly 11% of MALT lymphomas, more frequently in ocular adnexel and liver lymphomas.[70,71] This translocation can be distinguished from the cytogenetically identical t(14;18)(q32;q21) involving the *IGH* and *BCL2* by using FISH techniques. The t(3;14)(p14.1;q32) resulting in the transcriptional deregulation of *FOXP1* on 3p14.1[72] was identified in 10% of MALT lymphomas of thyroid, ocular adnexae/orbit, and skin. The t(1;14)(p22; q32), which juxtaposes the *BCL10* gene with the *IGH* locus,[75,76] is seen in 2% of MALT lymphomas.[71] A variant t(1;2)(p22;p12) involving the *IGK* locus has also been described.[77]

Trisomies of 3 and 18 are seen in nearly 30% of all MALT lymphomas, including those that are translocation negative. Trisomies are more commonly seen in intestinal, salivary gland, and orbital adnexal lymphomas.[70] Partial gains of 3q (3q27), 9q (9q34), and 18q are common in MALT.[78,79] Deletions of 6q have also been observed in aCGH studies.[80] *MYC* amplifications, del(9p), and del(17p) are seen in progressive disease.[69–71] The t(1;14) and partial or complete trisomy 18 predict adverse clinical behavior.[81] FISH studies on paraffin-embedded tissues help in the differential diagnosis of marginal zone and MALT lymphomas.

Nodal Marginal Zone Lymphoma (Including Pediatric Marginal Zone Lymphoma)

Nodal marginal zone lymphomas (NMZLs) are rare lymphomas and comprise only about 1.8% of all lymphomas. Morphologically, NMZL resembles lymph nodes involved by marginal zone lymphoma of splenic or extranodal types, but does not have the involvement of either of the diseases.[46] Few cytogenetic studies have been reported; however, the majority of them present with complex karyotypes with various structural changes. The t(14;19)(q32;q21) causing the *IGH–BCL3* fusion has been reported as a recurrent change.[35] Other consistent changes include structural abnormalities involving chromosome 3 and partial or complete trisomy of chromosome 18.[49,64,82] Cytogenetic changes do not include the translocations typically observed in extranodal marginal zone lymphoma of MALT type.[64]

Follicular Lymphomas (Including Pediatric Follicular Lymphoma and Primary Cutaneous Follicle Center Lymphoma)

Follicular lymphoma (FL), a neoplasm composed of follicle center (germinal center) B-cells, accounts for 20% of all lymphomas, with the highest incidence in the United States and western Europe.[83] Most cases of FL have a predominantly follicular pattern with closely packed follicles that efface the nodal architecture. Any area of diffuse large B-cell lymphoma (DLBCL) in a FL is typically reported as the primary diagnosis with an estimate of the proportion of DLBCL and FL present.[83] FL is genetically characterized by t(14;18)(q32;q21) and BCL2 gene rearrangements.

The t(14;18)(q32;q21) is the most common cytogenetic abnormality in lymphomas, with considerable geographic differences.[84] This rearrangement is almost always associated with a B-cell phenotype. Although a characteristic translocation found in 80% to 90% of FLs, it is also observed in approximately 30% of DLBCLs,[3] and sometimes in SLL (CLL). Rarely one of the variant translocations involving BCL2 with IGK or IGL t(2;18)(p12;q21) or t(18;22)(q21;q11.2) may be observed in FL.[85] It is noteworthy that t(14;18) is extremely rare in pediatric FL.[86] The t(14;18) juxtaposes the IGH gene on 14q32 with the BCL-2 oncogene on 18q21 during early B-cell development, resulting in overexpression of BCL-2 protein[87] inhibition of programmed cell death and extending cell survival.[88,89] This translocation is cytogenetically identical to the t(14;18) seen in MALT lymphomas but is molecularly different. The breakpoints on 14q are tightly clustered, as are the majority of the breakpoints on 18q. The 18q21 breakpoint region includes the 2.8-kb major (MBR) and the minor (MCR) breakpoint regions, accounting for 66% and 16%, respectively, of the t(14;18) rearrangements. A third intermediate cluster region as well as several small breakpoint clusters have also been reported.[90] The less common variant translocations t(2;18) and t(18;22) involve the IGK and IGL loci, respectively. Unlike the t(14;18), where the breakpoint of the BCL2 locus is at the 3′ end, in the variant translocations, the breakpoint is located at the 5′ end of BCL2. It is not clear whether the cases with variant translocation follow the same clinical course as those with the t(14;18). The (14;18) is often accompanied by a series of recurrent secondary abnormalities in FL. Complex karyotypes containing additional abnormalities frequently include +X, add(1)(p36), +1q21−44, del(6q), +7, del(10)(q22−24), +12q, del(17p) +18, and polyploidy in more than 10% of the cases, the most frequent being an additional der(18)t(14;18).[91,92] Evidence suggests multiple common pathways with distinct temporal pattern order and frequent parallel clonal evolution in the t(14;18)-positive follicular lymphoma. The abnormalities governing the temporal sequence include +(18)t(14;18), +7, or del (6q).[91,92]

Several reports have documented the higher incidence of translocations involving 3q27 in the t(14;18)-negative FL, which mostly comprise FL grade 3. The t(3;14)(q27; q32) and variants t(2;3)(p12;q27) and t(3;22)(q27;q11.2) are less common in FL grades 1 and 2 and most frequent in FL grade 3b with a DLBCL.[93,94] The BCL6 gene (LAZ3) located within 3q27, one of the most promiscuous loci in B-cell lymphoma, encodes a transcriptional regulator involved in germinal center formation[95] and is deregulated by juxtaposition with IGH or variants IGL and IGK or other various partners. When the BCL6 promoter is substituted, its negative autoregulation is interrupted.[96] Molecular studies have recognized the major breakpoint region (MBR) and the alternate breakpoint region (ABR) in the *BCL6* gene region.[97] FLs exhibit predominant involvement of the ABR region[98]; specifically the t(14;18)-negative FL has a higher incidence of ABR rearrangement.[99]

FL is frequently characterized by complex karyotypes including multiple other abnormalities in addition to the t(14;18). The most common and those impacting the prognosis include +X, del(1)(p36) +7, del(6q), del(9p21), del(10)(q22–24), +11q, +12, and del(17p), +18, and +der(18)t(14;18).[22,91,92,100,101] Transformation or "progression" of FL with poor prognosis is triggered by acquisition of secondary/tertiary abnormalities of 17p (*TP53*), 9p21 (*CDNK2A*), or 8q24 (*MYC*).[98,101–103]

Mantle Cell Lymphoma

Accounting for approximately 3% to 10% of NHLs, mantle cell lymphoma is an aggressive NHL that is more predominant among males and is characterized by monomorphous small- to medium-sized cells. The hallmark translocation t(11;14)(q13;q32) led to the recognition of MCL as a distinct lymphoma entity.[6,104–106] The translocation juxtaposes the *CCND1* (*PRAD1, BCL1*) gene with *IGH* resulting in overexpression of cyclin D1. Rare variants involving the *IGK* and *IGL* regions with *CCND1* have been reported.[107,108] Also, other rare translocations involving the *CCND2* locus on 12p13 and *CCND3* locus on 6p21 have been reported. The recurrent translocations include t(12;14)(p13;q32) and variant t(2;12)(p12;p13).[105,109,110] In addition, translocations involving *CCND3* include t(6;14)(p21;q32) and the other translocations with *IG* variants *IGK* and *IGL*. A high number of nonrandom secondary cytogenetic abnormalities have been seen in MCL. Common whole chromosome losses frequently include Y, 13, 9, and 18, and gains include 3 and 12. Recurrent structural abnormalities demonstrate gains of 3q and 12q and deletions of 6q, 1p, 9p, 10q, 13q, 11q, and 17p. Specifically, the breakpoint cluster regions were 1p21–22, 1p31–32, 1q21, 3q27, 6q11–15, 6q23–27, 8q24, 9p21, 10p12–13, 11q22–23, 13q11–13, 13q14–34, and 17p13-pter.[5,10,111,112] Recent aCGH studies also confirm the cytogenetically observed gains and losses.[10,113] In addition, translocations involving *BCL6* (3q27) have also been reported in MCL. Translocations involving the *MYC* locus (8q24) in MCL are associated with an aggressive clinical course. Gains of 3q and losses of 9q, trisomy12, karyotypic complexity, loss of 13q14, and *TP53* mutations are associated with adverse clinical outcome.[112,114,115]

Diffuse Large B-Cell Lymphoma

Diffuse large B-cell lymphomas (DLBCLs) are a morphologically, biologically, and clinically heterogeneous group that constitutes 30% to 40% of all B-cell lymphomas. DLBCLs may be systemic or site specific. Others, for which there are no clear and accepted criteria for subdivision, are categorized as DLBCL not otherwise specified (DLBCL-NOS). Cytogenetic studies focusing on these various site-specific DLBCL are limited. Further, there are variants, subgroups, and subtypes of DLBCL and other entities of large B-cell lymphomas that are currently grouped together under "other large cell lymphomas" and listed as DLBCL.[116] The DLBCL subtypes include (1) T-histiocyte-rich large-cell lymphoma (THRLBCL); (2) primary DLBCL of the central nervous system; (3) primary cutaneous DLBCL, leg type (PCLBCL); and (4) Epstein–Barr virus (EBV)-positive DLBCL in elderly patients. Other lymphomas of large B cells include (1) DLBCL associated with chronic inflammation: pyothorax-associated lymphomas (PAL), (2) lymphoid granulomatosis, (3) primary mediastinal (thymic) large B-cell lymphoma; (4) intravascular large B-cell lymphoma (IVBCL); (5) anaplastic lymphoma kinase (ALK)-positive DLBCL; (6) plasmablastic lymphoma; (7) large B-cell lymphoma arising in HHV8-associated multicentric Castleman disease; and (8) primary effusion lymphoma (PEL). These have not been individually discussed in the text; however, available cytogenetic information on recurrent abnormalities in these groups is provided in **Table 3**.

Diffuse Large B-Cell Lymphoma Not Otherwise Specified

Diffuse large B-cell lymphoma not otherwise specified (DLBCL-NOS) is a heterogeneous group of NHLs that constitutes nearly 30% of all adult NHLs in Western countries.[116] DLBCL may arise de novo or can represent progression or transformation of a less aggressive lymphoma. Lymph nodes demonstrate a diffuse proliferation of large lymphoid cells that have effaced the architecture. Cytomorphologically, DLBCL-NOS is diverse and can be divided into common and rare morphologic variants.[116] The gene expression profiling studies outlined two cell-of-origin subgroups, the activated B-cell type (ABC)-DLBCL associated with an unfavorable prognosis and the germinal-center B-cell type (GCB)-type associated with a favorable prognosis.[15,117]

Many of the generally lymphoma-associated rearrangements are prominent in DLBCL; however, none is absolutely specific. Translocations of 14q32 involving the *IGH* locus most often observed in DLBCL include t(3;14)(q27;q32) involving *BCL6*, the t(14;18)(q21;q32) involving *BCL2*, and t(8;14)(q24;q32) involving *MYC*. One or more of these are found in nearly 50% of DLBCLs.[118] Abnormalities of 3q27 including t(3;14)(q27;q32) and variants involving the *BCL6* locus are seen in nearly 30% of DLBCLs.[119,120] In addition to the t(3;14)(q27;q32), which juxtaposes the *BCL6* gene with *IGH*,[121] variant translocations most often include the involvement of *BCL6* with *IGK* in the t(2;3)(p12;q27) and with *IGL* in the t(3;22)(q27;q11.2). Other variant translocations occurring with 4p13, 6p22, 7p13, 8q24, 11q23, 13q14, 15q22, and 17q11[5] have also been observed. The t(14;18)(q21;q32), the hallmark translocation of FL, is noted in 20% to 30% DLBCL cases.[15,122] These cases are almost exclusively the GCB type.[15,123,124] *MYC* rearrangement involving the 8q24 region is observed in about 10% DLBCLs[12,122] DLBCLs with *MYC* rearrangements generally demonstrate complex karyotypic changes.[122] A concurrent *BCL6* rearrangement or t(14;18) is noted in about 20% of these *MYC* rearrangement DLBCLs.[122,125] and these may best be described as "B-cell lymphomas with features intermediate between DLBCL and Burkitt lymphoma." Recently the term "double-hit B-cell lymphomas" has been applied to lymphomas that in addition to *MYC* disruption have the involvement of *BCL2*, and less frequently *BCL6*, or both (triple-hit). The combination of *MYC* with *BCL2*, and/or *BCL6*, expression and high genomic complexity play a role in poor outcome.[126]

Other frequently recurring abnormalities in DLBCL include trisomies of X, 3, 7, 9, 12, and 18 and losses of Y, 4, 6, 13, 15, and 17. Most frequently duplicated regions include 1q23–31, 1q32–44, 3q, 6p, 7p, 7q31–32, 8q22–24, 11q12–13, 12q14–24, 18q11–21, and 22q12-qter. Most commonly deleted regions include 1p36-pter, 2p23-pter, 4q32-qter, 6q21–25, 7q33, 8p12-pter, 9p21-pter, 11q23-qter, 12p12–13, 14q23-qter, 16p13, 17p12–13, and 18q21-qter. Other reported recurrent breakpoints include 1p22, 1q21, 1q25, 3p21, 3q27, 4q31, 6p21, 7q33, 8q21, 8q24, 9p24, 16p13, 18q21, and 19q13.[5,22–24,85,123,127] More recently, the aCGH data imply that distinct chromosomal imbalances occur in different subgroups of DLBCLs. Clinical correlations in DLBCL should be dealt with cautiously owing to heterogeneity of this subtype and because some of the studies were performed before the current therapeutic trend (Rituxan therapy). Conflicting data have been obtained for the prognostic significance of t(14;18) and

3q27 abnormalities; however, del(17p) and del(9p) indicate a poor prognosis and trisomy 5, 7q, and 15q are indicators of reduced risk.[123] As discussed earlier, the presence of a *MYC* rearrangement is associated with a poor prognosis.

Burkitt Lymphoma

Burkitt lymphoma (BL), the first lymphoid neoplasm in which the underlying chromosomal rearrangement was characterized, is best described by comprehensive investigation including morphology, immunophenotyping and genetic analysis. These B-cell lymphomas often present at extranodal sites or as an acute leukemia and typically contain a translocation involving the *MYC* gene. There are three clinical variants of these lymphomas: endemic BL, sporadic BL, and immunodeficiency-associated BL. The hallmark translocations t(8;14)(q24;q32), and variants t(2;8)(p12; q24) and t(8;22)(q24;q11.2) were subsequently described after chromosomal banding techniques.[1,2] Molecular consequences involve the deregulation of the *MYC* oncogene by juxtapositioning with one of the *IG* loci, the *IGH* (14q32), the *IGK* (2p12), or the *IGL* (22q11.2). Although cytogenetically the breakpoint is 8q24 in all three translocations, molecular studies revealed that the breakpoint is proximal to the *MYC* gene in the t(8;14) and more distal in the variant translocations. Nearly 90% of the cases of BL involve a *MYC* translocation involving 8q24.[128] Depending on different maturation stages, molecular differences have been noted in the EBV-positive (mainly endemic) and EBV-negative (sporadic) BL.[129] The molecular heterogeneity with differential molecular breakpoints both in *MYC* and *IG* loci should be considered during the diagnosis of BL. However, the characteristic translocations of BL are not exclusive to the disease. Karyotypes of approximately 60% of BL cases demonstrate secondary chromosome rearrangements that are mutually exclusive in disease progression[130]; the frequent ones include partial trisomies of 1q, trisomy 7, and trisomy 12. Other genetic alterations include the involvement of p16[INK4], *TP53*, *TP73*, *BAX*, p130RB2, and *BCL6*.[131,132] The 13q region is also involved in disease progression.[133] A consistent gene expression signature differentiating BL from DLBCL has been outlined by gene profiling studies.[12,122]

B-Cell Lymphoma, Unclassifiable, with Features Intermediate Between DLBCL and BL

This B-cell lymphoma has morphologic features of both DLBCL and BL, and most often contains *MYC* translocations. However, in contrast to classic BL, these cases are of significantly older age and present with complex karyotypes.[122,130] Other recurrent *IG* translocations, including the t(14;18)(q32;q21) and the 3q27 (*BCL6*) rearrangements, may occur in the "double-hit" cases.[12,122,126] Moreover, other *MYC* translocations including the t(3;8)(q27;q24) involving the *MYC* and *PAX5* genes, or the t(3;8)(q27;q24) involving *MYC* and *BCL6*,[122,134,135] may occur in these lymphomas. The revelation of a "double hit" in a complex karyotype containing a *MYC*-related translocation and a non-*IG-MYC* translocation with a *BCL2* involvement, especially in elderly patients should be cautiously reviewed because these may represent aggressive, therapy-resistant lymphomas.[122,126]

T-CELL LYMPHOMAS

Specific genetic abnormalities have been observed in only a few T-cell lymphomas. Because the T- and NK-cell lymphomas constitute only 15% of all lymphomas, fewer genetic studies are available in this group. This text includes only those whose relative frequencies in the adult population are at least 5% of all T-cell lymphomas.[136,137] Relevant information on all other T-cell lymphomas is provided in **Table 3**. These include (1) T-cell large granular lymphocytic leukemia (T-LGL); (2) chronic lymphopro-liferative disorders of NK cells (CLPD-NK); (3) aggressive NK cell leukemia; (4) EBV-positive T-cell lymphoproliferative disorders of childhood; (5) hepatosplenic T-cell lymphoma (HSTL); (6) subcutaneous penniculitis-like T-cell lymphomas (SPTLs); (7) primary cutaneous CD30-positive T-cell lymphoproliferative disorders; (8) primary cutaneous peripheral T-cell lymphomas, rare subtypes; and (9) primary cutaneous γδT-cell lymphomas.

T-Cell Prolymphocytic Leukemia

T-cell prolymphocytic leukemia (T-PLL), which may involve peripheral blood, bone marrow, spleen, lymph nodes, liver, and skin, is defined by proliferation of small to medium-sized lymphocytes with a mature postthymic T-cell phenotype. The disease constitutes about 2% of mature lymphocytic leukemias.[138] The most frequent cytogenetic abnormalities involve rearrangements that include 14q11, 14q32 mostly as a t(14;14)(q11;q32)[139,140] juxtaposing the TRA with oncogenes TCL1A and TCL1B at 14q32.1.[141] Another translocation that is not as frequent is the t(X;14)(q28;q11) involving a MTCP1 oncogene on Xq28 with the TCA.[142] These TCR-associated alterations are considered to be the primary event. Abnormalities of chromosome 8 including trisomy of 8, gain of 8q, idic(8p11), and t(8;8)(p11-12;q12) frequently resulting in gain of 8q and loss of 8p are observed in as many as 80% of cases.[141] Rearrangements of chromosome 6 leading to gain of 6p and loss of 6q, abnormalities of 17 disrupting TP53, aberrations of 11q leading to loss of one copy of the ATM gene, recurrent deletions of 10p and 8p, and structural alterations of 22q are other common secondary abnormalities determined by conventional cytogenetics and chromosomal CGH.[139,143,144] Deletions of 12p13 and 11q22.3 (ATM) have been observed by FISH studies.[143,145] Gene expression patterns correlate well with the reported genomic changes in T-PLL.[146] Recent studies have suggested high expression of TCL1 and AKT are poor prognostic indicators.[147]

Adult T-Cell Leukemia/Lymphoma

Adult T-cell leukemia/lymphoma (ATLL), a T-cell neoplasm composed mostly of highly pleomorphic lymphoid cells, is endemic in several regions of the world, particularly in southwestern Japan, the Caribbean basin, and parts of Central Africa, and is closely linked to the prevalence of HTLV-1 in the population.[148] Complex and multiple chromosome aberrations are found in about 90% of ATLL cases. Nonrandom rearrangements involving chromosome 14, either as a rearranged 14 or recombining with other chromosomes, especially involving the 14q11 region, have been consis-tently noted. A del(6q) with breakpoints mostly localized to bands q15 and q21 is seen in ATLL. Frequent gains of 7q and 3p and losses of 6q and 13q were detected by CGH studies.[149,150] The ATLL lymphoma type has gains of 1q, 2p, 4q, 7p, and 7q and losses of 10p, 13q, 16q, and 18p. Amplification of 1p36, 6p25, 7p22, 7q, and 14q32 was observed in CGH studies comparing the acute and the lymphoma types.[150]

Extranodal NK/T-Cell Lymphoma, Nasal Type

Often associated with EBV, this predominantly extranodal lymphoma is characterized by vascular damage and prominent necrosis.[151] A variety of chromosomal alterations have been reported but none so far have been considered specific to the disease. The most frequent abnormality is deletion of 6q observed as del(6)(q21q25) or i(6)(p10).[152–154] Array-based comparative genomic hybridization showed gains of 2q and losses of 1p36.23–36.33, 2p16.1–16.3, 4q12 and 4q13.3–32.1, 5p14.1–14.3,

5q34–35.3, 6q16.1–27, and 11q22.3–23.3.[155] The prognostic significance of these genetic changes is unknown.

Enteropathy-Associated T-Cell Lymphoma

Enteropathy-associated T-cell lymphoma (EATL; synonyms: intestinal T-cell lymphoma, with and without enteropathy), an intestinal tumor, usually presents as a tumor of intraepithelial T lymphocytes demonstrating variable transformation.[156] Few cytogenetic studies have been reported in this lymphoma. Chromosomal CGH studies showed recurrent gains of 9q, 7q, 5q, and 1q and losses of 8p, 13q, and 9p. Complex segmental amplification of 9q31.3-qter or losses of 16q12.1, exclusive of each other, were observed in aCGH. There are two distinct groups of ETL: (1) The classic ETL-linked to celiac disease, which is characterized by gains of 1q and 5q and (2) the monomorphic variant ETL, which characteristically shows gains of the *MYC* locus.[157–159]

Peripheral T-Cell Lymphoma Not Otherwise Specified

Nodal or extranodal mature T-cell lymphomas, which do not correspond to any of the currently defined entities of mature T-cell lymphomas, are included in this heterogeneous group of diseases. Translocations involving TCR regions are not common in peripheral T-cell lymphoma not otherwise specified (PTCL-NOS); however, the t(14;19)(q11;q13) that involves the *PVRL2* to *TCRA* locus has been observed in rare cases of PTCL-NOS including Lennert's lymphoma.[160,161] The t(5;9)(q33;q22) resulting in *ITK–SYK* fusion is another recurrent translocation seen in PTCL-NOS.[162] Complex karyotypes with numerous abnormalities are typically seen in PTCL-NOS. Frequent gains of 1q, 3p, 5p, 7q22–31, 8q24-qter, 11q13, 17q (17q11–25), 12p13, 22q, and losses of 4q, 5q, 6q22–24, 9p (9p21–33), 10p13-pter, 10q (10q23–24), 11p11, 12q (12q21–22), and 13q (13q21) have been reported.[163–167] aCGH investigations in 20 cases revealed gains of 17, specifically 17q11–25, 8 (including the *MYC* locus 8q24), 11q13, and 22q and losses of 13q, 6q (6q16–22), 11p11, and 9 (9p21–q33).[168] The genetic imbalances and the genetic signature of PTCL-NOS differ from those of other T-cell lymphomas.[167–170] No conclusive correlations have been observed between cytogenetic changes and PTCL-NOS subtypes or clinical outcome. Two other variants of PTCL-NOS include the lymphoepithelioid (Lenner lymphoma), follicular, and T-zone variants.

Angioimmunoblastic T-Cell Lymphomas

Previously thought to be an atypical reactive process, angioimmunoblastic lymphadenopathy is characterized by an increased risk of progression to lymphoma. Angioimmunoblastic T-cell lymphomas (AITLs) constitute nearly 15% to 20% of peripheral T-cell lymphomas.[171] A distinguishing cytogenetic feature of AILT is the presence of unrelated clones in the karyotype.[164–166,172] Numeric gains of chromosome 3, 5, and X have been reported as the most frequent cytogenetic changes in AITL[172,173]; however, structural alterations including gain of 5q21, and 3q and loss of 6q have also been described.[163] Gains of 11p11–q14 (11q13), 19, and partial gains of 22q, and losses of 13q have been observed in CGH studies.[168] Most often translocations affecting *TCR* loci are not present.[161,174] The presence of complex cytogenetic abnormalities has independent prognostic implications; specifically, gain of X and aberrations of 1p31–32 were associated with poor therapeutic response and shorter survival.[175]

Anaplastic Large-Cell Lymphoma, ALK-Positive

The ALK-positive anaplastic large-cell lymphoma (ALCL) is a T-cell lymphoma that accounts for approximately 10% to 20% of childhood lymphomas.[176] It is most common in the first three decades of life.[177–179] The characteristic CD30 (Ki-1)-positivity distinguishes ALK-positive ALCL from a rare distinct DLBCL with immuno-blastic/plasmablastic features, which shares some morphologic features of ALK-positive ALCL. A great majority of ALK-positive ALCLs show clonal gene rearrangement of a T-cell receptor (TCR) loci.[180] The chromosomal translocation t(2;5)(p23;q35) resulting in the fusion of the ALK gene with the nucleophosmin (NPM) gene on 5q35 represents the most frequent genetic alteration in ALCL. ALK rearrangement also results from multiple different translocations of 2p23 (ALK) with other chromosomal partners including 1q25 (TPM3), inv(2)(p23q35) (ATIC), 3q21 (TF6), 17q23 (CLTC), Xq11–12 (MSN), 19p13.1 (TPM4), 22q11.2 (MYH9), and 17q25 (ALO17) as reviewed in Refs.[5,181,182] No prognostic differences are found between NPM–ALK-positive cases and those carrying the variant translocations. Frequent secondary changes in ALK-positive ALCL include losses of Y, 4q13–21, 6q, 17, 11q14, and 13q and gains of 7, 9, 17p, 17q24-qter, and X.[85,183,184]

Anaplastic Large-Cell Lymphoma, ALK-Negative

ALK-negative ALCL is not distinctly characterized by specific features that distinguishes it from ALK-positive ALCL or PTCL-NOS and hence is listed as a provisional entity by current WHO classification.[185] Predominantly seen in older (40–65 years) individuals, ALK-negative ALCL has a generally more aggressive clinical course because patients present at a more advanced stage.[186] Clonal T-cell receptor (TCR) rearrangements are found in the majority of the cases. Recurrent cytogenetic abnormalities are not noted; however, some of the losses and gains of the chromosomes are distinct from PTCL-NOS and ALK-positive ALCL.[167,183] Gains of 1q, 3p, 6p21, and 7 and losses of 6q13–21, 13q, 15, 16pter, 16qter, and 17p13 are frequent in ALK-negative ALCL.[163,167,183] The clinical outcome of ALK-negative ALCL is poorer than that of ALK-positive ALCL with conventional therapy.[186,187]

HODGKIN LYMPHOMA

HL is subdivided into two main entities: (1) nodular lymphocyte predominant Hodgkin lymphoma (NLPHL) and (2) classical Hodgkin lymphoma (CHL).[188–190] These two entities have different morphologic and immunologic presentations.

Nodular Lymphocyte Predominant Hodgkin Lymphoma

Representing approximately 5% of all HLs, nodular lymphocyte predominant Hodgkin lymphoma (NLPHL) is a B-cell neoplasm characterized by nodular or nodular and diffuse proliferation of the lymphocytic or histiocytic Reed-Sternberg cells, or both. There is an overlap in the morphologic presentation of NLPHL and T-cell–rich large B-cell lymphoma (TCRBCL). The translocations involving BCL6 with IG, IKAROS, and ABR, have been noted.[191–193] An association of 13q deletions with poor prognosis has been observed in one study.[194]

Classical Hodgkin Lymphoma

Accounting for 95% of all HLs, CHL is characterized by multinucleated Reed-Sternberg (HRS) cells and Hodgkin cells in a variable mixture of other non-neoplastic cells. Depending on the morphology of the HRS cells, the disease is classified into four subtypes: (1) nodular sclerosis (NSCHL), (2) mixed cellularity (MCCHL), (3) lymphocyte-rich (LRCHL), and (4) lymphocyte-depleted (LDCHL). Although the immunophenotypes of the tumor cells are the same, the four subtypes of CHL vary in site specificity, growth pattern, and cellular background.[195] Conventional cytogenetics and FISH show aneuploidy and hyperdiploidy; however, no recurrent aberrations are noted in CHL.[165,196] The t(14;18) may sometimes be seen in CHL arising from follicular lymphoma.[197] The *IGH* breakpoints have been involved in some HRS cells in CHL.[198] The frequent partner regions are 2p16 (*REL*), 3q27 (*BCL6*) and 8q24 (*MYC*), 16p13 (*C2TA*), 17q12, and 19q13 (*BCL3*).[198,199] CGH studies show gains of 4p16, 4q23–24, and 9p23–24.[200] Because the neoplastic cells are very rare and scattered in HL, cytogenetic studies frequently yield normal karyotypes; however, investigations utilizing combined Fluorescence Immunophenotyping and Interphase Cytogenetics as a Tool for the Investigation of Neoplasms (FICTION) have shown that the HRS cells are composed of very complex karyotypes with multiple complete and segmental gains and losses[198,200–204] Some of the frequently involved breakpoints reported include 1p36, 6q15, 6q21, 7q22, 7q32, 8q24, 11q23, 12q24, 13p11, 14p11, 14q32, 15p11, and 19p13.[205]

SUMMARY

In summary, cytogenetics has played a critical and often a defining role not only at the diagnosis of lymphomas, but also during disease progression. Conventional cytogenetics has helped in categorizing various subtypes of lymphomas, specifically the B-cell NHLs, and has historically been part of the multiparametric approach in reaching accurate diagnosis. Cytogenetic information at diagnosis and during disease progression has benefited our understanding of the genetic changes that have prognostic implication in lymphomas. With refinement of NHL classification, cytogenetic abnormalities considered to be recurrent in broad categories of NHL are now being associated with more specific histopathology within an NHL subtype. FISH studies on paraffin-embedded tissues have specifically facilitated the differential diagnosis of NHL, most importantly when diagnostic chromosome studies are unavailable. The clinical applicability of FISH on individual cases depends on whether it is being utilized as an independent adjunct to histopathology to verify the presence of a translocation or it is performed in conjunction with conventional cytogenetics to determine subtle chromosomal alterations that have clinical implications, as in B-CLL/SLL. Regardless, both cytogenetics and FISH have a proven value in NHL diagnosis, progression, and prognosis. More recently, technical advances including genomic arrays and gene expression array have demonstrated the utility of genetic studies in defining genetically distinct groups within lymphoma subtypes that may have a variable clinical course and response to therapies. These approaches have found their niche particularly in therapeutic stratification; however, they are currently being utilized in research investigations and are unavailable for individual clinical testing. With improved therapeutic approaches in the common subtypes of lymphomas, these newer techniques providing whole genome information at a higher resolution will likely be incorporated in the multifaceted testing approach in prospective investigations.

ACKNOWLEDGMENTS

The authors thank Kersten Higgins for her assistance.

REFERENCES

1. Manolov G, Manolova Y. Marker band in one chromosome 14 from Burkitt lymphomas. Nature 1972;237:33–4.
2. Zech L, Haglund U, Nilsson K, et al. Characteristic chromosomal abnormalities in biopsies and lymphoid-cell lines from patients with Burkitt and non-Burkitt lymphomas. Int J Cancer 1976;17:47–56.
3. Sanger WG, Dave BJ, Bishop MR. Cytogenetics. In: Hancock B, Selby K, MacLennan K, et al, editors. Malignant Lymphoma. London: Arnold; 2000. p. 91–103.
4. Jaffe ES, Harris NL, Stein H, et al. Introduction and overview of the classification of the lymphoid neoplasms. In: Swerdlow SH, Campo E, Harris NL, et al, editors. WHO classification of tumours of haematopoietic and lymphoid tissues. 4th edition. Geneva (Switzerland): IARC; 2008. p. 158–66.
5. Siebert R. Mature B- and T-cell Neoplasms and Hodgkin lymphoma. In: Heim S, Mitelman F, editors. Cancer cytogenetics. 3rd edition. Hoboken (NJ): John Wiley & Sons; 2009. p. 297–374.
6. Banks PM, Chan J, Cleary ML, et al. Mantle cell lymphoma. A proposal for unification of morphologic, immunologic, and molecular data. Am J Surg Pathol 1992;16:637–40.
7. Mitelman F, Johansson B, Mertens F, editors. Mitelman Database of Chromosome Aberrations in Cancer. Available at: http://cgap.nci.nih.gov/Chromosomes/Mitelman. Accessed May, 2011.
8. Swerdlow SH, Campo E, Harris NL, et al. WHO classification of tumours of haematopoietic and lymphoid tissues. 4th edition. Geneva (Switzerland): IARC; 2008.
9. Martin-Subero JI, Kreuz M, Bibikova M, et al. New insights into the biology and origin of mature aggressive B-cell lymphomas by combined epigenomic, genomic, and transcriptional profiling. Blood 2009;113:2488–97.
10. Bea S, Campo E. Secondary genomic alterations in non-Hodgkin's lymphomas: tumor-specific profiles with impact on clinical behavior. Haematologica 2008;93: 641–5.
11. Dave SS, Wright G, Tan B, et al. Prediction of survival in follicular lymphoma based on molecular features of tumor-infiltrating immune cells. N Engl J Med 2004;351:2159–69.
12. Dave SS, Fu K, Wright GW, et al. Molecular diagnosis of Burkitt's lymphoma. N Engl J Med 2006;354:2431–42.
13. Davies AJ, Rosenwald A, Wright G, et al. Transformation of follicular lymphoma to diffuse large B-cell lymphoma proceeds by distinct oncogenic mechanisms. Br J Haematol 2007;136:286–93.
14. Monti S, Savage KJ, Kutok JL, et al. Molecular profiling of diffuse large B-cell lymphoma identifies robust subtypes including one characterized by host inflammatory response. Blood 2005;105:1851–61.
15. Rosenwald A, Wright G, Chan WC, et al. The use of molecular profiling to predict survival after chemotherapy for diffuse large-B-cell lymphoma. N Engl J Med 2002; 346:1937–47.
16. Savage KJ, Monti S, Kutok JL, et al. The molecular signature of mediastinal large B-cell lymphoma differs from that of other diffuse large B-cell lymphomas and shares features with classical Hodgkin lymphoma. Blood 2003;102:3871–9.
17. Rosenwald A, Alizadeh AA, Widhopf G, et al. Relation of gene expression phenotype to immunoglobulin mutation genotype in B cell chronic lymphocytic leukemia. J Exp Med 2001;194:1639–47.

18. The Non-Hodgkin's Lymphoma Classification Project. A clinical evaluation of the International Lymphoma Study Group classification of non-Hodgkin's lymphoma. Blood 1997;89:3909–18.

19. Morton LM, Wang SS, Devesa SS, et al. Lymphoma incidence patterns by WHO subtype in the United States, 1992–2001. Blood 2006;107:265–76.

20. Savage KJ, Harris NL, Vose JM, et al. ALK-anaplastic large-cell lymphoma is clinically and immunophenotypically different from both ALK+ ALCL and peripheral T-cell lymphoma, not otherwise specified: report from the International Peripheral T-Cell Lymphoma Project. Blood 2008;111:5496–504.

21. Schaffer LG, Slovack ML, Campbell LJ. ISCN 2009. An International System for Human Cytogenetic Nomenclature. Basel (Switzerland): Karger S.; 2009.

22. Dave BJ, Hess MM, Pickering DL, et al. Rearrangements of chromosome band 1p36 in non-Hodgkin's lymphoma. Clin Cancer Res 1999;5:1401–9.

23. Dave BJ, Nelson M, Pickering DL, et al. Cytogenetic characterization of diffuse large cell lymphoma using multi-color fluorescence in situ hybridization. Cancer Genet Cytogenet 2002;132:125–32.

24. Dave BJ, Weisenburger DD, Higgins CM, et al. Cytogenetics and fluorescence in situ hybridization studies of diffuse large B-cell lymphoma in children and young adults. Cancer Genet Cytogenet 2004;153:115–21.

25. Muller-Harmelink HK, Montserrat E, Catovsky D, et al. Chronic lymphocytic leukaemia/small lymphocytic lymphoma. In: Swerdlow SH, Campo E, Harris NL, et al, editors. WHO classification of tumours of haematopoietic and lymphoid tissues. 4th edition. Geneva (Switzerland): IARC; 2008. p. 180–2.

26. Dicker F, Schnittger S, Haferlach T, et al. Immunostimulatory oligonucleotide-induced metaphase cytogenetics detect chromosomal aberrations in 80% of CLL patients: a study of 132 CLL cases with correlation to FISH, IgVH status, and CD38 expression. Blood 2006;108:3152–60.

27. Dohner H, Stilgenbauer S, Benner A, et al. Genomic aberrations and survival in chronic lymphocytic leukemia. N Engl J Med 2000;343:1910–6.

28. Haferlach C, Dicker F, Schnittger S, et al. Comprehensive genetic characterization of CLL: a study on 506 cases analysed with chromosome banding analysis, interphase FISH, IgVH status and immunophenotyping. Leukemia 2007;21:2442–51.

29. Dohner H, Pohl S, Bulgay-Morschel M, et al. Trisomy 12 in chronic lymphoid leukemias—a metaphase and interphase cytogenetic analysis. Leukemia 1993;7: 516–20.

30. Dohner H, Stilgenbauer S, James MR, et al. 11q deletions identify a new subset of B-cell chronic lymphocytic leukemia characterized by extensive nodal involvement and inferior prognosis. Blood 1997;89:2516–22.

31. Stilgenbauer S, Lichter P, Dohner H. Genetic features of B-cell chronic lymphocytic leukemia. Rev Clin Exp Hematol 2000;4:48–72.

32. Dohner H, Stilgenbauer S, Dohner K, et al. Chromosome aberrations in B-cell chronic lymphocytic leukemia: reassessment based on molecular cytogenetic analysis. J Mol Med 1999;77:266–81.

33. Sellmann L, Gesk S, Walter C, et al. Trisomy 19 is associated with trisomy 12 and mutated IGHV genes in B-chronic lymphocytic leukaemia. Br J Haematol 2007;138: 217–20.

34. Sen F, Lai R, Albitar M. Chronic lymphocytic leukemia with t14;18 and trisomy 12. Arch Pathol Lab Med 2002;126:1543–6.

35. Martin-Subero JI, Ibbotson R, Klapper W, et al. A comprehensive genetic and histopathologic analysis identifies two subgroups of B-cell malignancies carrying a t14;19q32;q13 or variant BCL3-translocation. Leukemia 2007;21:1532–44.

36. Pospisilova H, Baens M, Michaux L, et al. Interstitial del14q involving IGH: a novel recurrent aberration in B-NHL. Leukemia 2007;21:2079–83.

37. Stilgenbauer S, Leupolt E, Ohl S, et al. Heterogeneity of deletions involving RB-1 and the D13S25 locus in B-cell chronic lymphocytic leukemia revealed by fluorescence in situ hybridization. Cancer Res 1995;55:3475–7.

38. Ouillette P, Erba H, Kujawski L, et al. Integrated genomic profiling of chronic lymphocytic leukemia identifies subtypes of deletion 13q14. Cancer Res 2008;68: 1012–21.

39. Austen B, Skowronska A, Baker C, et al. Mutation status of the residual ATM allele is an important determinant of the cellular response to chemotherapy and survival in patients with chronic lymphocytic leukemia containing an 11q deletion. J Clin Oncol 2007;25:5448–57.

40. Mayr C, Speicher MR, Kofler DM, et al. Chromosomal translocations are associated with poor prognosis in chronic lymphocytic leukemia. Blood 2006;107:742–51.

41. Bea S, Lopez-Guillermo A, Ribas M, et al. Genetic imbalances in progressed B-cell chronic lymphocytic leukemia and transformed large-cell lymphoma Richter's syndrome. Am J Pathol 2002;161:957–68.

42. Campo E, Catovsky D, Montserrat E, et al. B-cell prolymphocytic leukaemia. In: Swerdlow SH, Campo E, Harris NL, et al, editors. WHO classification of tumours of haematopoietic and lymphoid tissues. 4th edition. Geneva (Switzerland): IARC; 2008. p. 183–4.

43. Schlette E, Bueso-Ramos C, Giles F, et al. Mature B-cell leukemias with more than 55% prolymphocytes. A heterogeneous group that includes an unusual variant of mantle cell lymphoma. Am J Clin Pathol 2001;115:571–81.

44. Brito-Babapulle V, Pittman S, Melo JV, et al. Cytogenetic studies on prolymphocytic leukemia. 1. B-cell prolymphocytic leukemia. Hematol Pathol 1987;1:27–33.

45. Ruchlemer R, Parry-Jones N, Brito-Babapulle V, et al. B-prolymphocytic leukaemia with t11;14 revisited: a splenomegalic form of mantle cell lymphoma evolving with leukaemia. Br J Haematol 2004;125:330–6.

46. Berger F, Felman P, Thieblemont C, et al. Non-MALT marginal zone B-cell lymphomas: a description of clinical presentation and outcome in 124 patients. Blood 2000;95:1950–6.

47. Issacson PG, Piris MA, Berger F, et al. Splenic B-cell marginal zone lymphoma. In: Swerdlow SH, Campo E, Harris NL, et al, editors. WHO classification of tumours of haematopoietic and lymphoid tissues. 4th edition. Geneva (Switzerland): IARC; 2008. p. 185–7.

48. Sole F, Salido M, Espinet B, et al. Splenic marginal zone B-cell lymphomas: two cytogenetic subtypes, one with gain of 3q and the other with loss of 7q. Haematologica 2001;86:71–7.

49. Callet-Bauchu E, Baseggio L, Felman P, et al. Cytogenetic analysis delineates a spectrum of chromosomal changes that can distinguish non-MALT marginal zone B-cell lymphomas among mature B-cell entities: a description of 103 cases. Leukemia 2005;19:1818–23.

50. Gazzo S, Baseggio L, Coignet L, et al. Cytogenetic and molecular delineation of a region of chromosome 3q commonly gained in marginal zone B-cell lymphoma. Haematologica 2003;88:31–8.

51. Corcoran MM, Mould SJ, Orchard JA, et al. Dysregulation of cyclin dependent kinase 6 expression in splenic marginal zone lymphoma through chromosome 7q translocations. Oncogene 1999;18:6271–7.

52. Brito-Babapulle V, Gruszka-Westwood AM, Platt G, et al. Translocation t(2;7)(p12; q21–22) with dysregulation of the CDK6 gene mapping to 7q21–22 in a non-Hodgkin's lymphoma with leukemia. Haematologica 2002;87:357–62.

53. Algara P, Mateo MS, Sanchez-Beato M, et al. Analysis of the IgVH somatic mutations in splenic marginal zone lymphoma defines a group of unmutated cases with frequent 7q deletion and adverse clinical course. Blood 2002;99:1299–304.

54. Foucar K, Falini B, Catovsky D, et al. Hairy cell leukaemia. In: Swerdlow SH, Campo E, Harris NL et al, editors. WHO classification of tumours of haematopoietic and lymphoid tissues. 4th edition. Geneva (Switzerland): IARC; 2008. p. 188–90.

55. Sambani C, Trafalis DT, Mitsoulis-Mentzikoff C, et al. Clonal chromosome rearrangements in hairy cell leukemia: personal experience and review of literature. Cancer Genet Cytogenet 2001;129:138–44.

56. Nessling M, Solinas-Toldo S, Lichter P, et al. Genomic imbalances are rare in hairy cell leukemia. Genes Chromosomes Cancer 1999;26:182–3.

57. Ostergaard M, Lindbjerg AC, Pedersen B, et al. Recurrent imbalances involving chromosome 5 and 7q22–q35 in hairy cell leukemia: a comparative genomic hybridization study. Genes Chromosomes Cancer 2001;30:218–9.

58. Swerdlow SH, Berger F, Pileri SA. Lymphoplasmacytic lymphoma. In: Jaffe ES, Pileri SA, Stein H, editors. WHO classification of tumours of haematopoietic and lymphoid tissues. 4th edition. Geneva (Switzerland): IARC; 2008. p. 194–5.

59. Iida S, Rao PH, Nallasivam P, et al. The t(9;14)(p13;q32) chromosomal translocation associated with lymphoplasmacytoid lymphoma involves the *PAX-5* gene. Blood 1996;88:4110–7.

60. Cook JR, Aguilera NI, Reshmi-Skarja S, et al. Lack of *PAX5* rearrangements in lymphoplasmacytic lymphomas: reassessing the reported association with t9;14. Hum Pathol 2004;35:447–54.

61. Baro C, Salido M, Domingo A, et al. Translocation t(9;14)(p13;q32) in cases of splenic marginal zone lymphoma. Haematologica 2006;91:1289–91.

62. Schop RF, Kuehl WM, Van Wier SA, et al. Waldenstrom macroglobulinemia neoplastic cells lack immunoglobulin heavy chain locus translocations but have frequent 6q deletions. Blood 2002;100:2996–3001.

63. Issacson PG, Chott A, Nakamura S, et al. Extranodal marginal zone lymphoma of mucosa-associated lymphoid tissue MALT lymphoma. In: Swerdlow SH, Campo E, Harris NL et al, editors. WHO classification of tumours of haematopoietic and lymphoid tissues. 4th edition. Geneva (Switzerland): IARC; 2008. p. 214–7.

64. Dierlamm J, Baens M, Stefanova-Ouzounova M, et al. Detection of t(11;18)(q21;q21) by interphase fluorescence in situ hybridization using API2 and MLT specific probes. Blood 2000;96:2215–8.

65. Akagi T, Motegi M, Tamura A, et al. A novel gene, *MALT1* at 18q21, is involved in t(11;18)(q21;q21) found in low-grade B-cell lymphoma of mucosa-associated lymphoid tissue. Oncogene 1999;18:5785–94.

66. Vega F, Medeiros LJ. Chromosomal translocations involved in non-Hodgkin lymphomas. Arch Pathol Lab Med 2003;127:1148–60.

67. Horsman D, Gascoyne R, Klasa R, et al. t(11;18)(q21;q21.1): a recurring translocation in lymphomas of mucosa-associated lymphoid tissue MALT? Genes Chromosomes Cancer 1992;4:183–7.

68. Ott G, Katzenberger T, Greiner A, et al. The t(11;18)(q21;q21) chromosome translocation is a frequent and specific aberration in low-grade but not high-grade malignant non-Hodgkin's lymphomas of the mucosa-associated lymphoid tissue MALT- type. Cancer Res 1997;57:3944–8.

69. Barth TF, Bentz M, Leithauser F, et al. Molecular-cytogenetic comparison of mucosa-associated marginal zone B-cell lymphoma and large B-cell lymphoma arising in the gastro-intestinal tract. Genes Chromosomes Cancer 2001;31:316–25.

70. Streubel B, Simonitsch-Klupp I, Mullauer L, et al. Variable frequencies of MALT lymphoma-associated genetic aberrations in MALT lymphomas of different sites. Leukemia 2004;18:1722–6.

71. Ye H, Gong L, Liu H, et al. MALT lymphoma with t(14;18)(q32;q21)/IGH-MALT1 is characterized by strong cytoplasmic MALT1 and BCL10 expression. J Pathol 2005;205:293–301.

72. Streubel B, Vinatzer U, Lamprecht A, et al. T(3;14)(p14.1;q32) involving IGH and FOXP1 is a novel recurrent chromosomal aberration in MALT lymphoma. Leukemia 2005;19:652–8.

73. Streubel B, Lamprecht A, Dierlamm J, et al. T(14;18)(q32;q21) involving IGH and MALT1 is a frequent chromosomal aberration in MALT lymphoma. Blood 2003;101:2335–9.

74. Sanchez-Izquierdo D, Buchonnet G, Siebert R, et al. MALT1 is deregulated by both chromosomal translocation and amplification in B-cell non-Hodgkin lymphoma. Blood 2003;101:4539–46.

75. Willis TG, Jadayel DM, Du MQ, et al. Bcl10 is involved in t(1;14)(p22;q32) of MALT B cell lymphoma and mutated in multiple tumor types. Cell 1999;96:35–45.

76. Zhang Q, Siebert R, Yan M, et al. Inactivating mutations and overexpression of BCL10, a caspase recruitment domain-containing gene, in MALT lymphoma with t(1;14)(p22;q32). Nat Genet 1999;22:63–8.

77. Chuang SS, Liu H, Martin-Subero JI, et al. Pulmonary mucosa-associated lymphoid tissue lymphoma with strong nuclear B-cell CLL/lymphoma BCL10 expression and novel translocation t(1;2)(p22;p12)/immunoglobulin kappa chain-BCL10. J Clin Pathol 2007;60:727–8.

78. Zhou Y, Ye H, Martin-Subero JI, et al. Distinct comparative genomic hybridisation profiles in gastric mucosa-associated lymphoid tissue lymphomas with and without t(11;18)(q21;q21). Br J Haematol 2006;133:35–42.

79. Zhou Y, Ye H, Martin-Subero JI, et al. The pattern of genomic gains in salivary gland MALT lymphomas. Haematologica 2007;92:921–7.

80. Honma K, Tsuzuki S, Nakagawa M, et al. TNFAIP3 is the target gene of chromosome band 6q23.3–q24.1 loss in ocular adnexal marginal zone B cell lymphoma. Genes Chromosomes Cancer 2008;47:1–7.

81. Nakamura S, Ye H, Bacon CM, et al. Clinical impact of genetic aberrations in gastric MALT lymphoma: a comprehensive analysis using interphase fluorescence in situ hybridisation. Gut 2007;56:1358–63.

82. Rizzo KA, Streubel B, Pittaluga S, et al. Marginal zone lymphomas in children and the young adult population; characterization of genetic aberrations by FISH and RT-PCR. Mod Pathol 2010;23:866–73.

83. Harris NL, Swerdlow SH, Jaffe ES, et al. Follicular lymphoma. In: Swerdlow SH, Campo E, Harris NL, et al, editors. WHO classification of tumours of haematopoietic and lymphoid tissues. 4th edition. Geneva (Switzerland): IARC; 2008. p. 220–6.

84. Biagi JJ, Seymour JF. Insights into the molecular pathogenesis of follicular lymphoma arising from analysis of geographic variation. Blood 2002;99:4265–75.

85. Johansson B, Mertens F, Mitelman F. Cytogenetic evolution patterns in non-Hodgkin's lymphoma. Blood 1995;86:3905–14.

86. Swerdlow SH. Pediatric follicular lymphomas, marginal zone lymphomas, and marginal zone hyperplasia. Am J Clin Pathol 2004;122(Suppl):S98–109:S98–109.

87. Tsujimoto Y, Finger LR, Yunis J, et al. Cloning of the chromosome breakpoint of neoplastic B cells with the t(14;18) chromosome translocation. Science 1984;226: 1097–9.

88. Zinkel S, Gross A, Yang E. *BCL2* family in DNA damage and cell cycle control. Cell Death Differ 2006;13:1351–9.

89. Letai AG. Diagnosing and exploiting cancer's addiction to blocks in apoptosis. Nat Rev Cancer 2008;8:121–32.

90. Albinger-Hegyi A, Hochreutener B, Abdou MT, et al. High frequency of t(14;18)–translocation breakpoints outside of major breakpoint and minor cluster regions in follicular lymphomas: improved polymerase chain reaction protocols for their detection. Am J Pathol 2002;160:823–32.

91. d'Amore F, Chan E, Iqbal J, et al. Clonal evolution in t(14;18)-positive follicular lymphoma, evidence for multiple common pathways, and frequent parallel clonal evolution. Clin Cancer Res 2008;14:7180–7.

92. Hoglund M, Sehn L, Connors JM, et al. Identification of cytogenetic subgroups and karyotypic pathways of clonal evolution in follicular lymphomas. Genes Chromosomes Cancer 2004;39:195–204.

93. Horsman DE, Okamoto I, Ludkovski O, et al. Follicular lymphoma lacking the t(14;18)(q32;q21): identification of two disease subtypes. Br J Haematol 2003;120: 424–33.

94. Katzenberger T, Ott G, Klein T, et al. Cytogenetic alterations affecting BCL6 are predominantly found in follicular lymphomas grade 3B with a diffuse large B-cell component. Am J Pathol 2004;165:481–90.

95. Jardin F, Ruminy P, Bastard C, et al. The *BCL6* proto-oncogene: a leading role during germinal center development and lymphomagenesis. Pathol Biol [Paris] 2007;55:73–83.

96. Pasqualucci L, Bereschenko O, Niu H, et al. Molecular pathogenesis of non-Hodgkin's lymphoma: the role of Bcl-6. Leuk Lymphoma 2003;44(Suppl 3):S5–12: S5–12.

97. Butler MP, Iida S, Capello D, et al. Alternative translocation breakpoint cluster region 5' to BCL-6 in B-cell non-Hodgkin's lymphoma. Cancer Res 2002;62:4089–94.

98. Bosga-Bouwer AG, Haralambieva E, Booman M, et al. BCL6 alternative translocation breakpoint cluster region associated with follicular lymphoma grade 3B. Genes Chromosomes Cancer 2005;44:301–4.

99. Gu K, Fu K, Jain S, et al. t(14;18)-negative follicular lymphomas are associated with a high frequency of BCL6 rearrangement at the alternative breakpoint region. Mod Pathol 2009;22:1251–7.

100. Tilly H, Rossi A, Stamatoullas A, et al. Prognostic value of chromosomal abnormalities in follicular lymphoma. Blood 1994;84:1043–9.

101. Schwaenen C, Viardot A, Berger H, et al. Microarray-based genomic profiling reveals novel genomic aberrations in follicular lymphoma which associate with patient survival and gene expression status. Genes Chromosomes Cancer 2009;48:39–54.

102. Bosga-Bouwer AG, van den Berg A, Haralambieva E, et al. Molecular, cytogenetic, and immunophenotypic characterization of follicular lymphoma grade 3B; a separate entity or part of the spectrum of diffuse large B-cell lymphoma or follicular lymphoma? Hum Pathol 2006;37:528–33.

103. Christie L, Kernohan N, Levison D, et al. C-MYC translocation in t(14;18) positive follicular lymphoma at presentation: an adverse prognostic indicator? Leuk Lymphoma 2008;49:470–6.

104. Li JY, Gaillard F, Moreau A, et al. Detection of translocation t(11;14)(q13;q32) in mantle cell lymphoma by fluorescence in situ hybridization. Am J Pathol 1999; 154:1449–52.

105. Rosenberg CL, Wong E, Petty EM, et al. PRAD1, a candidate BCL1 oncogene: mapping and expression in centrocytic lymphoma. Proc Natl Acad Sci USA 1991; 88:9638–42.

106. Weisenburger DD, Vose JM, Greiner TC, et al. Mantle cell lymphoma. A clinicopathologic study of 68 cases from the Nebraska Lymphoma Study Group. Am J Hematol 2000;64:190–6.

107. Komatsu H, Yoshida K, Seto M, et al. Overexpression of PRAD1 in a mantle zone lymphoma patient with a t(11;22)(q13;q11) translocation. Br J Haematol 1993;85: 427–9.

108. Wlodarska I, Meeus P, Stul M, et al. Variant t(2;11)(p11;q13) associated with the IgK-CCND1 rearrangement is a recurrent translocation in leukemic small-cell B-non-Hodgkin lymphoma. Leukemia 2004;18:1705–10.

109. Gesk S, Klapper W, Martin-Subero JI, et al. A chromosomal translocation in cyclin D1-negative/cyclin D2–positive mantle cell lymphoma fuses the CCND2 gene to the IGK locus. Blood 2006;108:1109–10.

110. Herens C, Lambert F, Quintanilla-Martinez L, et al. Cyclin D1-negative mantle cell lymphoma with cryptic t(12;14)(p13;q32) and cyclin D2 overexpression. Blood 2008;111:1745–46.

111. Michaux L, Wlodarska I, Theate I, et al. Coexistence of BCL1/CCND1 and CMYC aberrations in blastoid mantle cell lymphoma: a rare finding associated with very poor outcome. Ann Hematol 2004;83:578–83.

112. Rubio-Moscardo F, Climent J, Siebert R, et al. Mantle-cell lymphoma genotypes identified with CGH to BAC microarrays define a leukemic subgroup of disease and predict patient outcome. Blood 2005;105:4445–54.

113. Vater I, Wagner F, Kreuz M, et al. GeneChip analyses point to novel pathogenetic mechanisms in mantle cell lymphoma. Br J Haematol 2009;144:317–31.

114. Salaverria I, Zettl A, Bea S, et al. Specific secondary genetic alterations in mantle cell lymphoma provide prognostic information independent of the gene expression-based proliferation signature. J Clin Oncol 2007;25:1216–22.

115. Sander S, Bullinger L, Leupolt E, et al. Genomic aberrations in mantle cell lymphoma detected by interphase fluorescence in situ hybridization. Incidence and clinicopathological correlations. Haematologica 2008;93:680–7.

116. Stein H, Warnke RA, Chan WC, et al. Diffuse large B-cell lymphoma, not otherwise specified. In: Swerdlow SH, Campo E, Harris NL et al, editors. WHO classification of tumours of haematopoietic and lymphoid tissues. 4th edition. Geneva (Switzerland): IARC; 2008. p. 233–7.

117. Alizadeh AA, Eisen MB, Davis RE, et al. Distinct types of diffuse large B-cell lymphoma identified by gene expression profiling. Nature 2000;403:503–11.

118. Lenz G, Nagel I, Siebert R, et al. Aberrant immunoglobulin class switch recombination and switch translocations in activated B cell-like diffuse large B cell lymphoma. J Exp Med 2007;19;204:633–43.

119. Bastard C, Deweindt C, Kerckaert JP, et al. LAZ3 rearrangements in non-Hodgkin's lymphoma: correlation with histology, immunophenotype, karyotype, and clinical outcome in 217 patients. Blood 1994;83:2423–7.

120. Offit K, Lo CF, Louie DC, et al. Rearrangement of the bcl-6 gene as a prognostic marker in diffuse large-cell lymphoma. N Engl J Med 1994;331:74–80.

121. Ye BH, Rao PH, Chaganti RS, et al. Cloning of bcl-6, the locus involved in chromosome translocations affecting band 3q27 in B-cell lymphoma. Cancer Res 1993;53:2732–5.

122. Hummel M, Bentink S, Berger H, et al. A biologic definition of Burkitt's lymphoma from transcriptional and genomic profiling. N Engl J Med 2006;354:2419–30.

123. Schlegelberger B, Zwingers T, Harder L, et al. Clinicopathogenetic significance of chromosomal abnormalities in patients with blastic peripheral B-cell lymphoma. Kiel-Wien-Lymphoma Study Group. Blood 1999;94:3114–20.

124. Iqbal J, Sanger WG, Horsman DE, et al. BCL2 translocation defines a unique tumor subset within the germinal center B-cell-like diffuse large B-cell lymphoma. Am J Pathol 2004;165:159–66.

125. Ueda C, Nishikori M, Kitawaki T, et al. Coexistent rearrangements of c-MYC, BCL2, and BCL6 genes in a diffuse large B-cell lymphoma. Int J Hematol 2004;79:52–4.

126. Aukema SM, Siebert R, Schuuring E, et al. Double-hit B-cell lymphomas. Blood 2011;117:2319–31.

127. Cigudosa JC, Parsa NZ, Louie DC, et al. Cytogenetic analysis of 363 consecutively ascertained diffuse large B-cell lymphomas. Genes Chromosomes Cancer 1999;25:123–33.

128. Leoncini L, Raphael M, Stein H, et al. Burkitt lymphoma. In: Swerdlow SH, Campo E, Harris NL, et al, editors. WHO classification of tumours of haematopoietic and lymphoid tissues. Geneva (Switzerland): IARC; 2008. p. 262–4.

129. Bellan C, Stefano L, Giulia de F, et al. Burkitt lymphoma versus diffuse large B-cell lymphoma: a practical approach. Hematol Oncol 2010;28:53–6.

130. Boerma EG, Siebert R, Kluin PM, et al. Translocations involving 8q24 in Burkitt lymphoma and other malignant lymphomas: a historical review of cytogenetics in the light of today's knowledge. Leukemia 2009;23:225–34.

131. Sanchez-Beato M, Saez AI, Navas IC, et al. Overall survival in aggressive B-cell lymphomas is dependent on the accumulation of alterations in p53, p16, and p27. Am J Pathol 2001;159:205–13.

132. Lindstrom MS, Wiman KG. Role of genetic and epigenetic changes in Burkitt lymphoma. Semin Cancer Biol 2002;12:381–7.

133. Nelson M, Perkins SL, Dave BJ, et al. An increased frequency of 13q deletions detected by fluorescence in situ hybridization and its impact on survival in children and adolescents with Burkitt lymphoma: results from the Children's Oncology Group study CCG-5961. Br J Haematol 2010;148:600–10.

134. Bertrand P, Bastard C, Maingonnat C, et al. Mapping of MYC breakpoints in 8q24 rearrangements involving non-immunoglobulin partners in B-cell lymphomas. Leukemia 2007;21:515–23.

135. Sonoki T, Tatetsu H, Nagasaki A, et al. Molecular cloning of translocation breakpoint from der(8)t(3;8)(q27;q24) defines juxtaposition of downstream of C-MYC and upstream of BCL6. Int J Hematol 2007;86:196–8.

136. Jaffe ES, Gaulard P, Ralfkiaer E, et al. Subcutaneous panniculitis-like T-cell lymphoma. In: Swerdlow SH, Campo E, Harris NL, et al, editors. WHO classification of tumours of haematopoietic and lymphoid tissues. 4th edition. Geneva (Switzerland): IARC; 2008. p. 294–5.

137. Vose J, Armitage J, Weisenburger D. International peripheral T-cell and natural killer/T-cell lymphoma study: pathology findings and clinical outcomes. J Clin Oncol 2008;26:4124–30.

138. Catovsky D, Muller-Harmelink HK, Ralfkiaer E. T-cell prolymphocytic leukemia. In: Swerdlow SH, Campo E, Harris NL, et al, editors. WHO classification of tumours of haematopoietic and lymphoid tissues. 4th edition. Geneva (Switzerland): IARC; 2008. p. 270–1.

139. Brito-Babapulle V, Catovsky D. Inversions and tandem translocations involving chromosome 14q11 and 14q32 in T-prolymphocytic leukemia and T-cell leukemias in patients with ataxia telangiectasia. Cancer Genet Cytogenet 1991;55:1–9.

140. Maljaei SH, Brito-Babapulle V, Hiorns LR, et al. Abnormalities of chromosomes 8, 11, 14, and X in T-prolymphocytic leukemia studied by fluorescence in situ hybridization. Cancer Genet Cytogenet 1998;103:110–6.

141. Pekarsky Y, Hallas C, Isobe M, et al. Abnormalities at 14q32.1 in T cell malignancies involve two oncogenes. Proc Natl Acad Sci USA 1999;96:2949–51.

142. Stern MH, Soulier J, Rosenzwajg M, et al. MTCP-1: a novel gene on the human chromosome Xq28 translocated to the T cell receptor alpha/delta locus in mature T cell proliferations. Oncogene 1993;8:2475–83.

143. Stilgenbauer S, Schaffner C, Litterst A, et al. Biallelic mutations in the ATM gene in T-prolymphocytic leukemia. Nat Med 1997;3:1155–9.

144. Costa D, Queralt R, Aymerich M, et al. High levels of chromosomal imbalances in typical and small-cell variants of T-cell prolymphocytic leukemia. Cancer Genet Cytogenet 2003;147:36–43.

145. Hetet G, Dastot H, Baens M, et al. Recurrent molecular deletion of the 12p13 region, centromeric to ETV6/TEL, in T-cell prolymphocytic leukemia. Hematol J 2000;1:42–7.

146. Durig J, Bug S, Klein-Hitpass L, et al. Combined single nucleotide polymorphism-based genomic mapping and global gene expression profiling identifies novel chromosomal imbalances, mechanisms and candidate genes important in the pathogenesis of T-cell prolymphocytic leukemia with inv(14)(q11q32). Leukemia 2007;21:2153–63.

147. Herling M, Patel KA, Teitell MA, et al. High TCL1 expression and intact T-cell receptor signaling define a hyperproliferative subset of T-cell prolymphocytic leukemia. Blood 2008;111:328–37.

148. Oshima K, Jaffe ES, Kikuchi M. Adult T-cell leukaemia/lymphoma. In: Swerdlow SH, Campo E, Harris NL, et al, editors. WHO classification of tumours of haematopoietic and lymphoid tissues. 4th edition. Geneva (Switzerland): IARC; 2008. p. 281–4.

149. Tsukasaki K, Krebs J, Nagai K, et al. Comparative genomic hybridization analysis in adult T-cell leukemia/lymphoma: correlation with clinical course. Blood 2001;97:3875–81.

150. Oshiro A, Tagawa H, Ohshima K, et al. Identification of subtype-specific genomic alterations in aggressive adult T-cell leukemia/lymphoma. Blood 2006;107:4500–7.

151. Chan JKC, Quintanilla-Martinez L, Ferry JA, et al. Extranodal NK/T-cell lymphoma, nasal type. In: Swerdlow SH, Campo E, Harris NL et al, editors. WHO classification of tumours of haematopoietic and lymphoid tissues. 4th edition. Geneva (Switzerland): IARC; 2008. p. 285–8.

152. Siu LL, Wong KF, Chan JK, et al. Comparative genomic hybridization analysis of natural killer cell lymphoma/leukemia. Recognition of consistent patterns of genetic alterations. Am J Pathol 1999;155:1419–25.

153. Tien HF, Su IJ, Tang JL, et al. Clonal chromosomal abnormalities as direct evidence for clonality in nasal T/natural killer cell lymphomas. Br J Haematol 1997;97:621–5.

154. Wong KF, Zhang YM, Chan JK. Cytogenetic abnormalities in natural killer cell lymphoma/leukaemia—is there a consistent pattern? Leuk Lymphoma 1999;34:241–50.

155. Nakashima Y, Tagawa H, Suzuki R, et al. Genome-wide array-based comparative genomic hybridization of natural killer cell lymphoma/leukemia: different genomic alteration patterns of aggressive NK-cell leukemia and extranodal Nk/T-cell lymphoma, nasal type. Genes Chromosomes Cancer 2005;44:247–55.

156. Issacson PG, Chott A, Ott G, Stein H. Enteropathy-associated T-cell lymphoma. In: Swerdlow SH, Campo E, Harris NL, et al, editors. WHO classification of tumours of haematopoietic and lymphoid tissues. 4th edition. Geneva (Switzerland): IARC; 2008. p. 289–91.

157. Zettl A, Ott G, Makulik A, et al. Chromosomal gains at 9q characterize enteropathy-type T-cell lymphoma. Am J Pathol 2002;161:1635–45.

158. Baumgartner AK, Zettl A, Chott A, et al. High frequency of genetic aberrations in enteropathy-type T-cell lymphoma. Lab Invest 2003;83:1509–16.

159. Deleeuw RJ, Zettl A, Klinker E, et al. Whole-genome analysis and HLA genotyping of enteropathy-type T-cell lymphoma reveals 2 distinct lymphoma subtypes. Gastroenterology 2007;132:1902–11.

160. Almire C, Bertrand P, Ruminy P, et al. PVRL2 is translocated to the TRA locus in t(14;19)(q11;q13)-positive peripheral T-cell lymphomas. Genes Chromosomes Cancer 2007;46:1011–8.

161. Leich E, Haralambieva E, Zettl A, et al. Tissue microarray-based screening for chromosomal breakpoints affecting the T-cell receptor gene loci in mature T-cell lymphomas. J Pathol 2007;213:99–105.

162. Streubel B, Vinatzer U, Willheim M, et al. Novel t(5;9)(q33;q22) fuses ITK to SYK in unspecified peripheral T-cell lymphoma. Leukemia 2006;20:313–8.

163. Nelson M, Horsman DE, Weisenburger DD, et al. Cytogenetic abnormalities and clinical correlations in peripheral T-cell lymphoma. Br J Haematol 2008;141:461–9.

164. Schlegelberger B, Himmler A, Bartles H, et al. Recurrent chromosome abnormalities in peripheral T-cell lymphomas. Cancer Genet Cytogenet 1994;78:15–22.

165. Schlegelberger B, Himmler A, Godde E, et al. Cytogenetic findings in peripheral T-cell lymphomas as a basis for distinguishing low-grade and high-grade lymphomas. Blood 1994;83:505–11.

166. Lepretre S, Buchonnet G, Stamatoullas A, et al. Chromosome abnormalities in peripheral T-cell lymphoma. Cancer Genet Cytogenet 2000;117:71–9.

167. Zettl A, Rudiger T, Konrad MA, et al. Genomic profiling of peripheral T-cell lymphoma, unspecified, and anaplastic large T-cell lymphoma delineates novel recurrent chromosomal alterations. Am J Pathol 2004;164:1837–48.

168. Thorns C, Bastian B, Pinkel D, et al. Chromosomal aberrations in angioimmunoblastic T-cell lymphoma and peripheral T-cell lymphoma unspecified: a matrix-based CGH approach. Genes Chromosomes Cancer 2007;46:37–44.

169. de LL, Rickman DS, Thielen C, et al. The gene expression profile of nodal peripheral T-cell lymphoma demonstrates a molecular link between angioimmunoblastic T-cell lymphoma AITL and follicular helper T TFH cells. Blood 2007;109:4952–63.

170. Piccaluga PP, Agostinelli C, Califano A, et al. Gene expression analysis of peripheral T cell lymphoma, unspecified, reveals distinct profiles and new potential therapeutic targets. J Clin Invest 2007;117:823–34.

171. Dogan A, Gaulard P, Jaffe ES, et al. Angioimmunoblastic T-cell Lymphoma. In: Swerdlow SH, Campo E, Harris NL, et al, editors. WHO classification of tumours of haematopoietic and lymphoid tissues. 4th edition. Geneva (Switzerland): IARC; 2008. p. 309–11.

172. Schlegelberger B, Zhang Y, Weber-Matthiesen K, et al. Detection of aberrant clones in nearly all cases of angioimmunoblastic lymphadenopathy with dysproteinemia-type T-cell lymphoma by combined interphase and metaphase cytogenetics. Blood 1994;84:2640–8.

173. Dogan A, Attygalle AD, Kyriakou C. Angioimmunoblastic T-cell lymphoma. Br J Haematol 2003;121:681–91.

174. Gesk S, Martin-Subero JI, Harder L, et al. Molecular cytogenetic detection of chromosomal breakpoints in T-cell receptor gene loci. Leukemia 2003;17:738–45.

175. Schlegelberger B, Zwingers T, Hohenadel K, et al. Significance of cytogenetic findings for the clinical outcome in patients with T-cell lymphoma of angioimmunoblastic lymphadenopathy type. J Clin Oncol 1996;14:593–9.

176. Stein H, Foss HD, Durkop H, et al. CD30+ anaplastic large cell lymphoma: a review of its histopathologic, genetic, and clinical features. Blood 2000;96:3681–95.

177. Benharroch D, Meguerian-Bedoyan Z, Lamant L, et al. ALK-positive lymphoma: a single disease with a broad spectrum of morphology. Blood 1998;91:2076–84.

178. Falini B, Pulford K, Pucciarini A, et al. Lymphomas expressing ALK fusion proteins other than NPM-ALK. Blood 1999;94:3509–15.

179. Kinney MC, Higgins RA, Medina EA. Anaplastic large cell lymphoma: twenty-five years of discovery. Arch Pathol Lab Med 2011;135:19–43.

180. Foss HD, Anagnostopoulos I, Araujo I, et al. Anaplastic large-cell lymphomas of T-cell and null-cell phenotype express cytotoxic molecules. Blood 1996;88: 4005–11.

181. Delsol G, Falini B, Muller-Harmelink HK, et al. Anaplastic large cell lymphoma ALCL, ALK-positive. In: Swerdlow SH, Campo E, Harris NL, et al, editors. WHO classification of tumours of haematopoietic and lymphoid tissues. 4th edition. Geneva (Switzerland): IARC; 2008. p. 312–6.

182. Duyster J, Bai RY, Morris SW. Translocations involving anaplastic lymphoma kinase ALK. Oncogene 2001;20:5623–37.

183. Salaverria I, Bea S, Lopez-Guillermo A, et al. Genomic profiling reveals different genetic aberrations in systemic ALK-positive and ALK-negative anaplastic large cell lymphomas. Br J Haematol 2008;140:516–26.

184. Weisenburger DD, Gordon BG, Vose JM, et al. Occurrence of the t(2;5)(p23;q35) in non-Hodgkin's lymphoma. Blood 1996;87:3860–8.

185. Mason DY, Harris NL, Delsol G, et al. Anaplastic large cell lymphoma, ALK-negative. In: Swerdlow SH, Campo E, Harris NL et al, editors. WHO classification of tumours of haematopoietic and lymphoid tissues. 4th edition. Geneva (Switzerland): IARC; 2008. p. 317–9.

186. ten Berge RL, de Bruin PC, Oudejans JJ, et al. ALK-negative anaplastic large-cell lymphoma demonstrates similar poor prognosis to peripheral T-cell lymphoma, unspecified. Histopathology 2003;43:462–9.

187. Gascoyne RD, Aoun P, Wu D, et al. Prognostic significance of anaplastic lymphoma kinase ALK protein expression in adults with anaplastic large cell lymphoma. Blood 1999;93:3913–21.

188. Anagnostopoulos I, Hansmann ML, Franssila K, et al. European Task Force on Lymphoma project on lymphocyte predominance Hodgkin disease: histologic and immunohistologic analysis of submitted cases reveals 2 types of Hodgkin disease with a nodular growth pattern and abundant lymphocytes. Blood 2000;96:1889–99.

189. Diehl V, Sextro M, Franklin J, et al. Clinical presentation, course, and prognostic factors in lymphocyte-predominant Hodgkin's disease and lymphocyte-rich classical Hodgkin's disease: report from the European Task Force on Lymphoma Project on Lymphocyte-Predominant Hodgkin's Disease. J Clin Oncol 1999;17:776–83.

190. Nogova L, Reineke T, Brillant C, et al. Lymphocyte-predominant and classical Hodgkin's lymphoma: a comprehensive analysis from the German Hodgkin Study Group. J Clin Oncol 2008;26:434–9.

191. Atayar C, Kok K, Kluiver J, et al. BCL6 alternative breakpoint region break and homozygous deletion of 17q24 in the nodular lymphocyte predominance type of Hodgkin's lymphoma-derived cell line DEV. Hum Pathol 2006;37:675–83.

192. Renne C, Martin-Subero JI, Hansmann ML, et al. Molecular cytogenetic analyses of immunoglobulin loci in nodular lymphocyte predominant Hodgkin's lymphoma reveal a recurrent *IGH-BCL6* juxtaposition. J Mol Diagn 2005;7:352–6.
193. Wlodarska I, Nooyen P, Maes B, et al. Frequent occurrence of *BCL6* rearrangements in nodular lymphocyte predominance Hodgkin lymphoma but not in classical Hodgkin lymphoma. Blood 2003;101:706–10.
194. Chui DT, Hammond D, Baird M, et al. Classical Hodgkin lymphoma is associated with frequent gains of 17q. Genes Chromosomes Cancer 2003;38:126–36.
195. Stein H, Delsol G, Pileri SA, et al. Classical Hodgkin lymphoma. In: Swerdlow SH, Campo E, Harris NL et al, editors. WHO classification of tumours of haematopoietic and lymphoid tissues. Geneva (Switzerland): IARC; 2008. p. 326–9.
196. Sarris A, Jhanwar SC, Cabanillas F. Cytogenetics of Hodgkin's disease. In: Mauch P, Armitage JO, Diehl V, editors. Hodgkin's disease. Philadelphia: Lippincott Williams & Willkins; 1999. p. 195.
197. Nakamura N, Ohshima K, Abe M, et al. Demonstration of chimeric DNA of *bcl-2* and immunoglobulin heavy chain in follicular lymphoma and subsequent Hodgkin lymphoma from the same patient. J Clin Exp Hematop 2007;47:9–13.
198. Martin-Subero JI, Klapper W, Sotnikova A, et al. Chromosomal breakpoints affecting immunoglobulin loci are recurrent in Hodgkin and Reed-Sternberg cells of classical Hodgkin lymphoma. Cancer Res 2006;66:10332–8.
199. Szymanowska N, Klapper W, Gesk S, et al. *BCL2* and *BCL3* are recurrent translocation partners of the *IGH* locus. Cancer Genet Cytogenet 2008;186:110–4.
200. Joos S, Kupper M, Ohl S, et al. Genomic imbalances including amplification of the tyrosine kinase gene *JAK2* in CD30+ Hodgkin cells. Cancer Res 2000;60:549–52.
201. Schlegelberger B, Weber-Matthiesen K, Himmler A, et al. Cytogenetic findings and results of combined immunophenotyping and karyotyping in Hodgkin's disease. Leukemia 1994;8:72–80.
202. Weber-Matthiesen K, Deerberg J, Poetsch M, et al. Numerical chromosome aberrations are present within the CD30+ Hodgkin and Reed-Sternberg cells in 100% of analyzed cases of Hodgkin's disease. Blood 1995;86:1464–8.
203. Atkin NB. Cytogenetics of Hodgkin's disease. Cytogenet Cell Genet 1998;80:23–7.
204. Schouten HC, Sanger WG, Armitage JO. Chromosomal abnormalities in malignant lymphoma and Hodgkin's disease: a review. Leuk Lymphoma 1991;5:93–100.
205. Falzetti D, Crescenzi B, Matteuci C, et al. Genomic instability and recurrent breakpoints are main cytogenetic findings in Hodgkin's disease. Haematologica 1999;84:298–305.

Myelodysplastic Syndromes

Olatoyosi Odenike, MD[a,b], John Anastasi, MD[b,c],
Michelle M. Le Beau, PhD[a,b,*]

KEYWORDS

- Myelodysplastic syndromes • Cytogenetics
- Molecular genetics • Diagnosis • Prognosis • Classification

The myelodysplastic syndromes (MDS) include a large spectrum of clonal hematopoietic stem cell disorders that are characterized by peripheral cytopenia(s), morphologic dysplasia, ineffective hematopoiesis, and a variable propensity to transform to acute myeloid leukemia (AML).[1,2] The cytopenia can be limited to a single cell line, resulting in anemia, thrombocytopenia, or neutropenia, and can be chronic and somewhat indolent or profound, involving all 3 lineages with life-threatening consequences. The morphologic dysplasia associated with the ineffective hematopoiesis may be subtle and difficult to recognize, but, in some cases, it can be impressive and evident in both the bone marrow and peripheral blood. The variable increase in blasts relates, in part, to the risk for transformation to AML, although progression is not solely dependent on the blast percentage. MDS is a disease of older adults with a median age at diagnosis of approximately 70 years.[3] Other risk factors for the development of MDS include tobacco use and exposure to solvents, such as benzene and agricultural chemicals. In approximately 10% to 15% of cases, the disease arises as a late complication of cytotoxic therapy (radiotherapy or chemotherapy) for a prior disorder, and is referred to as a therapy-related myeloid neoplasm. MDS is frequently associated with clonal cytogenetic abnormalities of significant prognostic[4,5] and emerging therapeutic importance. An in-depth analysis of some of these is providing significant insights into underlying molecular alterations, which may hold clues to unraveling the pathogenesis of these disorders. This review focuses on the key role of cytogenetic analysis in MDS in the context of the diagnosis, prognosis, and molecular pathobiology of these disorders.

This article was supported by Grant No. CA40046 from the National Cancer Institute.
The authors have nothing to disclose.
[a] Department of Medicine, Section of Hematology/Oncology, University of Chicago, 5841 South Maryland, MC2115, Chicago, IL 60637, USA
[b] The Comprehensive Cancer Center, University of Chicago, 5841 South Maryland, MC1140, Chicago, IL 60637, USA
[c] Department of Pathology, Hematopathology and Clinical Hematology Laboratory, University of Chicago, 5841 South Maryland, MC0008, Chicago, IL 60637, USA
* Corresponding author. Department of Medicine, Section of Hematology/Oncology, University of Chicago, 5841 South Maryland, MC2115, Chicago, IL 60637.
E-mail address: mlebeau@bsd.uchicago.edu

Clin Lab Med 31 (2011) 763–784
doi:10.1016/j.cll.2011.08.005
labmed.theclinics.com
0272-2712/11/$ – see front matter © 2011 Elsevier Inc. All rights reserved.

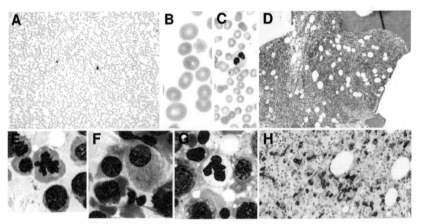

Fig. 1. Morphologic features of a typical case of MDS. (*A–C*) The peripheral smear shows severe pancytopenia (*A*), with a macrocytic anemia (*B*), neutropenia with dysplastic neutrophils and thrombocytopenia with pale platelets (*C*). (*D*) The marrow is typically hypercellular, indicating ineffective hematopoiesis. (*E–H*) The marrow cytology shows dysplasia in the erythroid (*E*), megakaryocytic (*F*), and granulocytic lineage (*G*) as well as increased blasts, which can sometimes be detected by CD34 immunostaining (*H*).

DIAGNOSTIC CONSIDERATIONS
MDS Classification

The earliest recognition of myelodysplastic disorders came with the identification of an anemia that was long standing and refractory, followed by the recognition that these were sometimes preleukemic.[6] The classic myelodysplastic syndrome is exemplified in **Fig. 1**, which illustrates pancytopenia with multilineage dysplasia. Although such a case is classic, it belies the wide pathologic spectrum of MDS, which includes cases that are diagnostically challenging and difficult to distinguish, on one hand, from other benign causes of cytopenia and, on the other hand, from AML and other more aggressive clonal myeloid neoplasms.

The disease spectrum was expanded with the first classification proposed by the French American British (FAB) group in 1982.[7] In this classification scheme, the myelodysplastic disorders were divided into 4 subtypes with increasing blast percentage or as chronic myelomonocytic leukemia (CMML). The 4 entities included refractory anemia (RA), refractory anemia with ring sideroblasts (RARS), refractory anemia with excess of blasts (RAEB), and refractory anemia with excess of blasts in transformation (RAEB-T). These entities differed mainly by the percentage of blasts seen in the bone marrow (**Table 1**). In the FAB scheme, AML was defined by the presence of ≥30% blasts in the blood or marrow.

CMML was included by the FAB in the MDSs, although it was well recognized that CMML differed in that it had a proliferative component with increased circulating and marrow monocytes.[8] At times, the peripheral leukocytosis was particularly elevated in the so-called myeloproliferative type, whereas the process was considered to be a dysplastic type and included in the MDS category when the count was less than 13 K/μL.[9]

The classification of MDS presented by the World Health Organization (WHO) committee in 2001 resulted in significant changes to the classification of both MDS and AML (see **Table 1**).[10] Most notable was the reduction in the blast percentage required for a diagnosis of AML from 30% to 20% leading to the elimination of

Table 1
The evolving classification of MDS

FAB 1982	WHO 2001	WHO 2008 (Current Classification)	Blasts	Other Findings	Cytogenetic Abnormalities
RA	RA	RCUD RA RN RT	<1% PB[a] <5% BM	Uni- or bilineage dysplasia[b] <15% RS	25%
RARS	RARS	RARS	None in PB, <15% BM	At least 15% RS	10%
	RCMD RCMD-RS	RCMD (-RS)	<1% PB[c] < 5% BM	Dysplasia >10% in 2 cell lines, +/− RS, no AR[d]	50%
RAEB	RAEB-1	RAEB-1	<5% PB 5%–9% BM	Cytopenia, <1 K/μL mono; dysplasia in 1 or more lines, no AR[d]	50%–70%
	RAEB-2	RAEB-2	5%–19% PB 10%–19% BM	Cytopenia, <1 K/μL mono, +/− AR; dysplasia in 1 or more lines	50%–70%
		MDS-U	<1% PB <5% BM	Cytopenia, <10% dysplasia; cytogenetic abnormalities present	50%
		MDS with 5q	<1% PB <5% BM	Anemia, nml or incr. platelets, isolated del(5q), hypo-lobated megakaryocytes, no AR	100%
RAEB-T			20%–29% BM		
CMML					

Abbreviations: RCUD, refractory cytopenia with unilineage dysplasia; MDS-U, myelodysplastic syndrome-unclassified; AR, Auer rods; PB, peripheral blood; RS, ring sideroblasts (% indicates percent RS of total nucleated erythroid precursors).

[a] If 1% blasts present, change to MDS-U.
[b] If pancytopenia present, change to MDS-U.
[c] If 2% to 4% PB blasts present, upgrade to RAEB-1.
[d] If AR present, upgrade to RAEB-2.

RAEB-T. The new classification also included a new subtype of MDS that, despite the lack of increased blasts (<5%), had a more aggressive course, probably owing to the presence of more pronounced multilineage dysplasia.[11] This category was called refractory cytopenia with multilineage dysplasia (RCMD), and it comprised a substantial proportion of cases previously grouped in the low-grade RA and RARS categories. Although the recognition of RCMD as a relatively more aggressive MDS served to de-emphasize the importance of the blast percentage for prognosis, the new classification subdivided the RAEB category into 2 types, with 5% to 9% blasts (RAEB-1) and 10% to 19% blasts (RAEB-2), paradoxically emphasizing the prognostic significance of blast percentage in this category.[12]

A further significant change in the WHO 2001 classification scheme for MDS included the exclusion of CMML from the MDS category and the development of a separate nosologic group for CMML and other diseases in which there were features of both myelodysplasia and myeloproliferation.[13] These "overlap" disorders are called myelodysplastic syndromes/myeloproliferative neoplasms and include CMML, "atypical CML," and an unclassifiable category, which includes a provisional entity called RARS-T, a disorder that resembles RARS, but has associated thrombocytosis.

Further refinements in the WHO classification scheme for MDS were made most recently in 2008 (see **Table 1**).[14,15] These included expanding low-grade MDSs from refractory anemia to refractory cytopenia with unilineage dysplasia, in which there is involvement of only 1 cell line. The 2008 WHO classification scheme also placed emphasis on the key role of cytogenetic analysis in the diagnosis of MDS, particularly in cases in which there is otherwise insufficient morphologic evidence to substantiate a diagnosis of MDS. This is reflected in the inclusion of the subtype, myelodysplastic syndrome unclassified, defined by the presence of cytopenia, less than 1% peripheral blasts, less than 10% dysplasia, and less than 5% bone marrow blasts with the presence of a cytogenetic abnormality commonly seen in MDS (**Table 2**). In addition, the WHO 2008 classification now includes "MDS with an isolated del(5q)" as a separate entity. This entity, sometimes referred to as the 5q− syndrome[16] had been well known for some time and is characterized typically by its presentation in middle-aged women with macrocytic anemia, splenomegaly, normal-to-elevated platelet counts, hypolobated megakaryocytes in the bone marrow, and an isolated del(5q).

Prognosis

The heterogeneity in outcome within the various morphologic categories identified by the FAB and WHO classification systems has led to a proliferation of prognostic tools and scoring systems that attempt to predict outcomes of patients with MDS more accurately. The ability to achieve greater precision in prognostication in MDS is of paramount importance, because therapeutic options vary from supportive care and growth factor use to more intensive approaches, such as epigenetic modulators, and to approaches associated with significant potential for morbidity and mortality, such as intensive chemotherapeutic strategies and allogeneic stem cell transplantation. Currently, the higher-intensity approaches are reserved for patients with high-risk disease.[17] All of the contemporary prognostic systems incorporate the cytogenetic pattern as a key element.[18–21]

The most widely used, and validated, prognostic scoring system in current use is the International Prognostic Scoring System (IPSS), which incorporates karyotype, bone marrow blasts, and number of cytopenias and identifies these factors as being the most critical in prognostication (**Table 3**).[18] Nonetheless, there are a number of limitations that have led to the development of other scoring systems as well as

Table 2
Recurring chromosomal abnormalities in the myelodysplastic syndromes

Disease	Chromosome Abnormality[a]	Frequency	Involved Genes[b]	Consequence
MDS Unbalanced	+8	10%		
	−7/del(7q)[a]	10%		
	del(5q)/t(5q)[a]	10%		
	del(20q)	5%–8%		
	−Y	5%		
	i(17q)/t(17p)[a]	3%–5%	TP53	Loss of function, DNA damage response
	−13/del(13q)[a]	3%		
	del(11q)[a]	3%		
	del(12p)/t(12p)[a]	3%		
	del(9q)[a]	1%–2%		
	idic(X)(q13)[a]	1%–2%		
Balanced	t(1;3)(p36.3;q21.2)[a]	1%	MMEL1	Deregulation of MMEL1—Transcriptional activation?
	t(2;11)(p21;q23)/t(11q23)[a]	1%	MLL	MLL fusion protein—altered transcriptional regulation
	inv(3)(q21q26.2)/t(3;3)(q21;q26.2)[a]	1%	RPN1 MDS1/EVI1	Altered transcriptional regulation by EVI1
	t(6;9)(p23;q34)[a]	1%	DEK NUP214	Fusion protein—nuclear pore protein
Therapy-related MDS	−7/del(7q)[a]	50%		
	del(5q)/t(5q)[a]	40%–45%		
	dic(5;17)(q11.1-13;p11.1-13)[a]	5%	TP53	Loss of function, DNA damage response
	der(1;7)(q10;p10)[a]	3%		
	t(3;21)(q26.2;q22.1)[a]	3%	RPL22L1 RUNX1	RUNX1 fusion protein—altered transcriptional regulation
	t(11;16)(q23;p13.3)/t(11q23)[a]	2%	MLL CREBBP	MLL fusion protein—altered transcriptional regulation
CMML	t(5;12)(q33.1;p13)	~2%	PDGFRB ETV6/TEL	Fusion protein—altered signaling pathway

[a] Cytogenetic abnormalities considered in the WHO 2008 Classification as presumptive evidence of MDS in patients with persistent cytopenias(s), but with no dysplasia or increased blasts.

[b] Genes are listed in order of citation in the karyotype, eg. for the t(11;16), MLL is at 11q23 and CREBBP at 16p13.3.

Table 3
International prognostic scoring system

Prognostic Variable	0	0.5	1.0	1.5	2.0
BM Blasts (%)	<5	5–10	—	11–20	21–30
Karyotype	Good	Intermediate	Poor		
Cytopenias[a]	0/1	2/3			

Risk Group	IPSS Score	Median Survival (y)	Time Until 25% of Patients Had AML (y)
Low	0	5.7	9.4
Intermediate-1	0.5—1.0	3.5	3.3
Intermediate-2	1.5—2.0	1.2	1.1
High	>2.5	0.4	0.2

[a] Cytopenias were defined as: Hemoglobin < 10 g/dL, ANC < 1500/μL, Platelet count < 100,000/μL.

ongoing attempts to refine the IPSS. Limitations of the IPSS include the fact that it was validated in previously untreated patients with de novo MDS, which limits the ability to use this tool to predict outcomes in patients with MDS treated using contemporary approaches. In addition, although the numbers of cytopenias are factored into the IPSS, the severity of cytopenias is not taken into account; in particular, transfusion dependency, which has been identified as a poor prognostic marker in recent scoring systems, is not considered. Furthermore, the IPSS includes a limited number of cytogenetic abnormalities (**Table 4**) and there are concerns that high-risk cytogenetic aberrations are not accorded sufficient emphasis.

To address some of the concerns associated with the IPSS, newer systems, such as the WHO classification–based prognostic scoring system (WPSS) have emerged.[20] The WPSS is dynamic, can be applied at diagnosis and during follow-up, and is now being validated in patients with MDS undergoing contemporary treatment modalities, such as allogeneic stem cell transplantation.[22] Prognostic factors of import included in this model are WHO subtype, transfusion dependency, and karyotype subgroup, as defined by the IPSS. Five risk groups are recognized in the WPSS, with median survival times ranging from 12 months to 103 months.

The MD Anderson Cancer Center prognostic scoring system was also proposed recently to address some of the limitations associated with the IPSS.[19] This model is also dynamic, can be applied at any time during the disease course, and encompasses a

Table 4
Cytogenetic abnormalities in the International Prognostic Scoring System

	Cytogenetic Abnormalities	Time until 25% of Patients Had AML (y)	Median Survival (y)
Favorable risk	Normal karyotype	5.6	3.8
	Isolated del(5q)		
	Isolated del(20q)		
	Isolated –Y		
Intermediate risk	Other abnormalities	1.6	2.4
Poor risk	–7/del(7q)	0.9	0
	Complex karyotypes		

Table 5
Proposed 4-Tier cytogenetic risk stratification system

Risk Group	Karyotype	Median Survival (mo)	Time Until 25% of Patients Had AML (mo)
Good	Normal, del(5q), double abnormality including del(5q), der(1;7)(q10; p10)/t(1;7), del(11q), del(12p), +19, del(20q), −Y	50.6	71.9
Intermediate-1	Any other double abnormality (not including del(5q) or −7/del(7q), +8, i(17)(q10), +21, any other single abnormality	25.7	14.7
Intermediate-2	Double abnormality including −7/ del(7q), t(3q26.2), complex with 3 abnormalities	16	9.8
High	Complex (>3 abnormalities)	5.7	3.4

broader patient population, including patients with therapy related MDS (t-MDS) and CMML. Four risk categories are identified that predict overall survival, ranging from a median of 54 months in low-risk patients to 6 months in high-risk patients.

Despite the development of newer systems, there continues to be significant heterogeneity in outcome, particularly in patients identified by current models as being in the lower-risk category, emphasizing the need for continued refinement of these models based on a broader range of anomalies of emerging prognostic significance.[23] An updated cytogenetic system has been proposed that involves an international collaborative effort using data sets originating from the German-Austrian Working Group, the International Risk Analysis Workshop, the Spanish Cytogenetics Workshop, and the International Cytogenetics Working Group of the MDS Foundation. This 4-tiered cytogenetic risk stratification system (**Table 5**) involves 20 cytogenetic subgroups; median survival ranged from 5.7 months to 50.6 months, and time until 25% of patients evolved to AML ranged from 3.4 months to 71.9 months.[23]

There is also ongoing concern that the IPSS accords more prognostic weight to an increase in bone marrow blasts compared with poor-risk karyotypes, for example, 2 points are assigned for bone marrow (BM) blasts in the 21% to 30% range, and 1.5 points for the 11% to 20% range, whereas poor-risk karyotypes are assigned 1 point (see **Table 3**). In a recent retrospective study of 2351 patients with MDS, the prognostic impact of a poor-risk karyotype was as unfavorable as the presence of a significant increase in blasts greater than 20% blasts.[24]

In addition to the broad prognostic variables incorporated in the various systems outlined above, it is clear that gene mutations[25] and epigenetic aberrations play a critical role in the pathobiology of MDS [26,27] including the determination of prognosis. These genetic and epigenetic determinants, described in more detail in the following sections, deserve consideration for inclusion in a contemporary prognostic model developed for 21st century use.

Cytogenetic Analysis

Clonal chromosome abnormalities can be detected in marrow cells of 40% to 100% of patients with primary MDS at diagnosis (see **Tables 1 and 2**).[5,18] The proportion

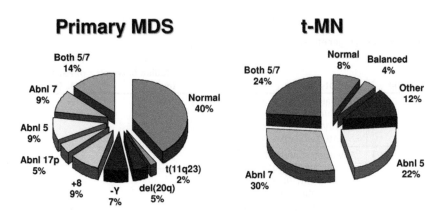

Fig. 2. Recurring chromosomal abnormalities in MDS. Relative frequencies are depicted in the pie chart.

varies with the risk that a subtype will transform to AML, which is highest for RCMD and RAEB. Most recurring cytogenetic abnormalities found in MDS are unbalanced, most commonly the result of the loss of a whole chromosome, a deletion of part of a chromosome, or an unbalanced translocations (**Fig. 2**). The most common cytogenetic abnormalities encountered in MDS, del(5q), −7, +8, and del(20q), have been incorporated into the more robust prognostic scoring systems of MDS outlined above. The recurring translocations characteristic of acute leukemia without prior MDS, such as the t(15;17), inv(16), and t(8;21), are almost never seen. With the exception of MDS with isolated del(5q), the chromosome changes show no close association with the morphologic subtypes of MDS. Clones with unrelated abnormalities, one of which typically has +8, are seen at a greater frequency in patients with MDS (5% vs 1%), than in patients with AML.

Serial cytogenetic evaluations can be informative, particularly when there is a change in the clinical features of a patient. Cytogenetic evolution is the appearance of an abnormal clone in which only normal cells have been seen previously, the acquisition of additional abnormalities within an abnormal clone, or the progression from the presence of a single clone to multiple related, or occasionally unrelated, abnormal clones. Karyotypic evolution in MDS is associated with transformation to acute leukemia in about 60% of cases and reduced survival, particularly for those patients who evolve within a short period of time (<100 days).[5,18]

Fluorescence In Situ Hybridization Analysis

In the last decade, molecular cytogenetic techniques, such as fluorescence in situ hybridization (FISH) have become a powerful adjunct to classical cytogenetic analysis.[28] FISH can be performed on marrow or blood smears or fixed and sectioned tissue because it does not require dividing cells. Advantages of FISH include (1) the rapid nature of the method and the ability to analyze large numbers of cells, (2) its high sensitivity and specificity, (3) the ability to obtain cytogenetic data from samples with a low mitotic index or terminally differentiated cells, and (4) the application to histologically stained cells allowing a direct correlation of the status of the genetic target within morphologically characterized cells. The major disadvantage is the inability to interrogate more than a few abnormalities and to identify the full spectrum of abnormalities in each clone, the presence of multiple clones, and clonal evolution.[28] In a clinical setting, cytogenetic analysis could be performed at the time of diagnosis to identify the chromosomal abnormalities in bone marrow cells from an individual with MDS. Thereafter, FISH with the appropriate probes could be used to detect residual disease or early relapse and to assess the efficacy of therapeutic regimens. Commercially available probes have been developed for the detection of 11q23/*MLL* translocations, −Y, del(5q)/t(5q), −7/del(7q), +8, del(20q), del(13q), del(11q), and −17/loss of 17p. In MDS, FISH analysis of cases with a normal karyotype by cytogenetic analysis detected recurring abnormalities in 10% to 15% of cases.[29]

CYTOGENETIC FINDINGS IN MDS
Normal Karyotype

A normal karyotype is found in approximately 50% of patients with MDS. This group of patients is almost certainly genetically heterogeneous, where technical factors precluded the detection of chromosomally abnormal cells, or where leukemogenic alterations occur at the molecular level and are not detectable with standard cytogenetic methods. Nonetheless, these cases are a standard reference for comparison of outcomes. The IPSS found that patients with a normal karyotype fall within the favorable risk group (see **Table 4**).[18]

−Y

The clinical and biological significance of the loss of the Y chromosome, −Y, is unknown. Loss of the Y chromosome has been observed in a number of malignant diseases but is also associated with aging in healthy men.[30] Patients with a hematologic disease have a significantly higher percentage of cells with a −Y (52% vs 37%, $P=.036$), and −Y in greater than 75% of metaphase cells accurately predicted a malignant disease.[30] Although loss of a Y chromosome may not be diagnostic of MDS, once the disease is identified by clinical and pathologic means, the IPSS found that −Y as the sole cytogenetic abnormality conferred a favorable outcome.[18]

+8

A gain of chromosome 8 in MDS is observed in all MDS subgroups in approximately 10% of patients.[18,31,32] Determining the significance of the gain of chromosome 8 in MDS patients is complicated in that +8 is often associated with other recurring abnormalities known to have prognostic significance, for example, del(5q)t(5q) or −7/del(7q), and may be seen in isolation as a separate clone unrelated to the primary clone in up to 5% of cases. The IPSS,[18] as well as the time-dependent WPSS[20] ranked this abnormality in the intermediate-risk group; however, several subgroups found that +8 as a sole abnormality had a poorer outcome than expected for an intermediate IPSS risk group.[31,33] Hematopoietic cells with trisomy 8 express higher levels of many genes that localize to chromosome 8, including the *MYC* gene, and antiapoptotic genes.

del(20q)

A deletion of the long arm of chromosome 20, del(20q), is seen in approximately 5% of MDS cases and 7% of t-MDS cases.[5,31] Features characterizing MDS patients with a del(20q) include low-risk disease (usually RA), low rate of progression to AML, prolonged survival (median of 45 months vs 28 months for other MDS patients), and prominent dysplasia in the erythroid and megakaryocytic lineages.[34] The IPSS noted that patients with a del(20q) in the context of a complex karyotype identified a poor-risk group (median survival, 9.6 months), whereas the prognosis for patients with

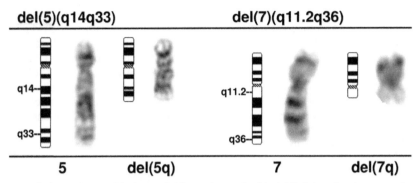

Fig. 3. Deletions of 5q and 7q in myeloid neoplasms. In this del(5q), breakpoints occur in q14 and q33 resulting in interstitial loss of the intervening chromosomal material. In this del(7q), breakpoints occur in q11.2 and q36. In both cases, the critical commonly deleted segments are lost. Normal chromosome 5 and 7 homologs are shown for comparison.

an isolated del(20q) was favorable.[18] Although a commonly deleted segment (CDS) has been identified on 20q, containing 19 genes, there is no definitive evidence linking these genes to the pathogenesis of myeloid neoplasms.[35,36]

Deletions of Chromosome 5

A deletion of the long arm of chromosome 5, del(5q), or an unbalanced translocation leading to loss of 5q are observed in 10% to 20% of MDS patients, more commonly in RAEB-1 and -2 in association with a complex karyotype, and 40% of patients with t-MDS (**Fig. 3**).[37] Abnormalities of 5q are associated with a significant occupational exposure to potential carcinogens as well as previous exposure to standard and high-dose alkylating agent therapy, including use in immunosuppressive regimens.[38,39] Clinically, the patients with del(5q) coupled with other cytogenetic abnormalities have a high frequency of *TP53* mutations, a poor prognosis with early progression to leukemia, resistance to treatment, and short survival.[40,41] MDS with an isolated del(5q) represents a distinct clinical syndrome, "the 5q- syndrome." These patients have a favorable outcome, in fact, the best of any MDS subgroup, with low rates of transformation to AML and a relatively long survival of several years' duration.[16,18] The immunomodulatory agent, lenalidomide, has been associated with significant responses in IPSS low or intermediate-1 risk MDS with the del(5q), including red cell transfusion independency (67% of patients), and complete cytogenetic responses.[42]

A recent study found that minor subclones of *TP53*-mutant cells were present in some patients before lenalidomide therapy and were associated with lenalidomide resistance and trend toward a higher risk of evolution to AML.[43] The molecular mechanisms underlying the clinical effectiveness of lenalidomide in del(5q) MDS remain obscure, but haploinsufficiency of 2 dual-specificity cell cycle phosphatases encoded by genes on 5q, *CDC25C*, and *PP2A* have been implicated in the sensitivity to lenalidomide.[44] However, treatment with lenalidomide is unlikely to be curative because del(5q) malignant stem cells persist in remission, and clinical and cytogenetic progression was associated with recurrence or expansion of the del(5q) clone.[45]

Several groups of investigators have defined a CDS (**Fig. 4**) on the long arm of chromosome 5, band 5q31.2, predicted to contain a myeloid tumor suppressor gene (TSG) that is involved in the pathogenesis of the more aggressive forms of MDS and

Commonly Deleted Segments of 5q

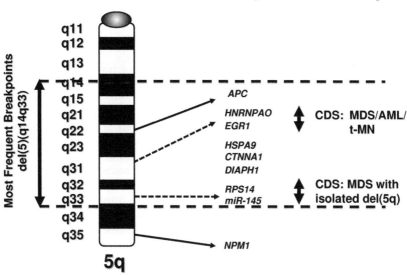

Fig. 4. Ideogram of the long arm of chromosome 5 shows candidate genes within CDSs as reported by various investigators. The proximal CDS in 5q31.2 was identified in MDS, AML, and therapy-related myeloid neoplasm, whereas the distal CDS in 5q33.1 was identified in MDS with isolated del(5q).

AML.[46,47] A second, distal CDS of 1.5 Mb within 5q33.1 has been identified in MDS with an isolated del(5q).[48] Despite intense efforts, the identification of TSGs on chromosomes 5 has been challenging because the deletions of 5q are typically large and encompass both of these regions. Molecular analysis of the 19 candidate genes within the CDS of 5q31.2 and 44 genes in the 5q33.1 CDS did not reveal inactivating mutations in the remaining alleles, nor was there evidence of transcriptional silencing[48–50] (Godley and Le Beau, unpublished data, 2002). Moreover, copy-neutral loss of heterozygosity (also known as acquired uniparental disomy) is not seen on 5q in MDS or AML. These observations are compatible with a haploinsufficiency model in which loss of 1 allele of the relevant gene(s) on 5q perturbs cell fate, rather than the biallelic inactivation of a TSG.[51] A number of genes and several miRNAs located on 5q, including *RPS14*,[52] miRNA-145,[53,54] *EGR1*, [55] *APC*,[56] *CTNNA1*,[57] *HSPA9*,[58] and *DIAPH1*,[59] have been implicated in the development of myeloid disorders caused by a gene dosage effect, and several of these are reviewed below. Together, these studies support a haploinsufficiency model in which loss of a single allele of *more than one gene* on 5q act in concert to alter hematopoiesis, promote self-renewal of hematopoietic stem and progenitor cells (HSPCs), induce apoptosis of hematopoietic cells, and disrupt differentiation.

RPS14
The gene encoding RPS14, which is required for the processing of 18S pre-rRNA, is located at 5q33.1, and is involved in MDS with an isolated del(5q).[52] Downregulation of *RPS14* in CD34+ bone marrow cells blocks the differentiation and increases apoptosis of erythroid cells via a TP53-dependent mechanism.[60] Of interest, the ribosomal processing

defect caused by haploinsufficiency of RPS14 in MDS is highly analogous to the functional ribosomal defect seen in Diamond-Blackfan anemia. Other studies have found that haploinsufficiency of 2 micro-RNAs, miR-145 and miR-146a, encoded by sequences near the *RPS14* gene, cooperate with loss of RPS14.[53,54] The Toll-interleukin-1 receptor domain–containing adaptor protein and *FLI1* are targets of these miRNAs. Haploinsufficiency of miR-145 may account for several features of MDS with an isolated del(5q), including megakaryocytic dysplasia; however, neither *RPS14* nor miR-145 haploinsufficiency is predicted to confer clonal dominance.

APC

APC is a multifunctional TSG involved in the pathogenesis of colorectal cancer via regulation of the *WNT* signaling cascade. The *APC* gene is located at 5q22.2, and is deleted in greater than 95% of patients with a del(5q).[47] Conditional inactivation of a single allele of *APC* in mice leads to the development of severe macrocytic anemia, a block in erythropoiesis at the early stages of differentiation, and an expansion of the short-term and long-term HSCs.[56] *APC* heterozygous myeloid progenitor cells display an increased frequency of apoptosis, and decreased in vitro colony-forming capacity, recapitulating several characteristic features of myeloid neoplasms with a del(5q).

EGR1

The early growth response 1 gene (*EGR1*) encodes a member of the WT-1 family of zinc finger transcription factors, and mediates the cellular response to growth factors, mitogens, and stress stimuli.[61] Recently, Egr1 has been shown to be a direct transcriptional regulator of many known TSGs, for example, *Tp53, Cdkn1a/p21, tgfbeta (Tgfb)* and *Pten,* and acts as a TSG in several human tumors, including breast non–small cell lung cancer.[61] *Egr1*-null mice show spontaneous mobilization of HSPCs into the periphery, identifying Egr1 as a transcriptional regulator of stem cell migration.[55,62] Moreover, loss of a single allele of *Egr1* cooperates with mutations induced by an alkylating agent in the development of malignant myeloid diseases (myeloproliferative diseases [MPD] with ineffective erythropoiesis) in mice, indicating that Egr1 is a haploinsufficient myeloid suppressor gene.[55]

Loss of Chromosome 7 or del(7q)

A –7/del(7q) is observed as the sole abnormality in approximately 5% of adult patients, in approximately 50% of children with primary MDS, and in approximately 55% of patients with t-MDS (see **Fig. 3**).[33,37,39,63] As with del(5q), occupational or environmental exposure to mutagens, including chemotherapy, radiotherapy, benzene exposure, and smoking, as well as severe aplastic anemia (regularly treated with immunosuppressive agents alone), have been associated with –7/del(7q).[18] The IPSS considers the –7/del(7q) to be a poor prognostic cytogenetic finding.[18] "Monosomy 7 syndrome" has been described in young children and is characterized by a preponderance of males (approximately 4:1), hepatosplenomegaly, leukocytosis, thrombocytopenia, and a poor prognosis.[63] Juvenile myelomonocytic leukemia is an MDS/MPD disease in the WHO classification and shares many features with this entity.[63] An emerging paradigm is that –7/del(7q) cooperates with deregulated signaling via the RAS pathway as a result of mutations in the *NRAS* or *KRAS* gene, inactivating mutations in the gene encoding NF1, a negative regulator of RAS proteins, or activating mutations in the gene encoding the PTPN11/SHP2 phosphatase, a positive regulator of RAS proteins, as well as *RUNX1* mutations and methylation silencing of the *CDKN2B (p15^{INK4B})* gene.[41,64,65]

To date, 3 CDSs have been identified on 7q; however, the molecular mutations underlying the development of MDS and AML with del(7q) are poorly understood[66–68] We previously identified 2 distinct CDSs, a 2.52-Mb CDS within 7q22 spanning the interval containing *LRCC17* and *SRPK2*, and a second, less frequent, region in q32-33.[68] Each of the candidate genes within the CDS at 7q22 has been evaluated for mutations[69]; however, no inactivating mutations have been identified in the remaining allele. Mice with a conditional heterozygous deletion of this region in murine HSPCs had no alterations of hematopoiesis, suggesting that this region does not contain a haploinsufficient myeloid TSG, or that mutations in cooperating genes are required.[70] Recently, Dohner and coworkers[71] reported the analysis of a large series of patients with abnormalities of 7q using FISH. Whereas most patients had large deletions, they identified an approximately 2-Mb deleted segment in proximal q22 that overlaps with the proximal portion of the CDS defined by Le Beau and coworkers, but extends more proximally, and includes the *CUTL1*, *RASA4*, *EPO*, and *FBXL13* genes in 7q22.1.[68] The recent recognition of mutations in *EZH2*, a gene located at 7q36.1, is intriguing; however, myeloid neoplasms with *EZH2* mutations typically do not have –7/del(7q), and the del(7q) does not always result in loss of one *EZH2* allele.[72,73]

Rare Recurring Translocations

In MDS, several recurring translocations have been identified, which result in fusion proteins. Translocations involving the *MLL* gene on 11q23 are noted in 3% to 5% of MDS and t-MDS cases. The most common translocations are the t(9;11)(p22;q23) and t(11;16)(q23;p13.3). The t(11;16) occurs primarily in t-MDS, but rare cases have presented as t-AML.[74] *MLL* is fused with the *CREBBP* (CREB binding protein) gene on chromosome 16. The MLL protein is a histone methyltransferase that assembles in protein complexes that regulate gene transcription, for example, *HOX* genes during embryonic development, via chromatin remodeling. CREBBP is a histone acetyltransferase involved in transcriptional control via histone acetylation.

The t(5;12)(q33.1;p13) is observed in approximately 1% of patients with CMML and results in fusion of the protein encoded by the beta chain of the platelet-derived growth factor receptor (*PDGFRB*) on 5q and a novel transcriptional repressor gene, *ETV6* (also known as *TEL*) on 12p. Alterations in the PDGFRB kinase activity and function of the ETV6 repressor contribute to the transformed phenotype. The t(5;12) predicts for a response to imatinib mesylate, a selective inhibitor of the PDGFRB kinase activity.[75] *PDGFRB* participates in several other rare translocations in myeloid neoplasms (reviewed in Olney and Le Beau[76]); a unifying feature is the presence of eosinophilia.

Complex Karyotypes

Complex karyotypes are variably defined but generally involve the presence of >3 chromosomal abnormalities. Complex karyotypes are observed in approximately 20% of patients with primary MDS and in as many as 90% of patients with t-MDS.[37] Abnormalities involving chromosomes 5, 7, or both are identified in most cases with complex karyotypes. There is general agreement that a complex karyotype carries a poor prognosis.[18,20,31]

ALTERATIONS IN GENE FUNCTION

A growing body of evidence suggests that mutations of multiple genes mediate the pathogenesis and progression of MDS. The involved genes fall into two main classes, namely, genes encoding hematopoietic transcription factors or proteins that regulate

Table 6
Frequency and significance of mutated genes in MDS

Mutated Gene	Frequency[a]	Biological Features and Clinical Significance
ASXL1	10%–15%	Polycomb group protein involved in transcriptional regulation Prevalence of frameshift mutations suggest a dominant-negative function Clinical significance unknown
ATRX	Rare	Involved in epigenetic modifications of DNA Loss of expression leads to decreased expression of alpha-globin Associated with acquired alpha-thalassemia, often with severe anemia
CEBPA	2%–5%	TF involved in hematopoiesis, loss of function impairs granulopoiesis Bi-allelic (N-terminal and C-terminal mutations) No apparent effect on time to progression to AML or overall survival
CSF1R	2%–5%	Constitutive activation of the macrophage colony-stimulating factor receptor tyrosine kinase Karyotype predominantly normal Associated with advanced MDS and progression to AML
EZH2	5%	Encodes a histone 3 lysine 27 methyltransferase-regulating transcription Mutations result in loss of function Associated with a poor prognosis
FLT3 ITD	5%–10%	Receptor tyrosine kinase involved in cytokine signaling, critical in hematopoiesis Associated with progression to AML and a poor prognosis
IDH1/2	Rare	Metabolic enzymes catalyzing oxidative decarboxylation of isocitrate to alpha-ketoglutarate. Missense mutations alter catalytic function converting alpha-KG to 2 hydroxyglutarate, while consuming NAPDH Associated with advanced MDS and progression to AML
JAK2	5% of RA 60% of RARS-T	Encodes a tyrosine kinase component of various cytokine signaling pathways Mutations result in constitutive activation of the tyrosine kinase Mutated in 60% of RARS with thrombocytosis, an unclassified MDS/MPD Clinical significance unknown, does not appear to alter prognosis
MPL	5% of RARS-T	Encodes the thrombopoietin receptor Mutations result in constitutive activation of the tyrosine kinase and are associated with dysmegakaryocytopoiesis Higher expression in advanced MDS is associated with a poor prognosis

(continued on next page)

Table 6
(continued)

Mutated Gene	Frequency[a]	Biological Features and Clinical Significance
NPM1	Rare	Nuclear-cytoplasmic shuttling protein with pleiotropic functions Terminal frameshift mutations disrupt the nuclear localization signal leading to redistribution to the cytoplasm Unknown clinical significance in MDS
NRAS/KRAS	5%	Encodes a GTPase component of multiple cytokine signaling pathways Activating mutations result in constitutive signal transduction Increased risk of progression to AML
PTPN11	Rare	Encodes the nonreceptor SHP2 tyrosine phosphatase, a positive regulator of RAS proteins Mutations result in protein activation Mutated in 30% of JMML Mutations in NRAS/KRAS, NF1, and PTPN11 are mutually exclusive
RUNX1	10%–15%	Encodes the DNA-binding subunit of the heterodimeric core binding factor transcription factor required for hematopoiesis Point mutations in the RUNT (DNA-binding) domain result in loss of function and a dominant negative effect Associated with mutations of the RAS pathway and −7/del(7q) Increased risk of progression to AML
TET2	20%	Epigenetic regulator Clinical significance unknown
TP53	5%–10% (25% in t-MDS)	Encodes a checkpoint protein that monitors integrity of the genome, arrests the cell cycle in response to DNA damage Associated with chromosomal instability, del(5q), loss of 17p, and complex karyotypes Associated with rapid progression and poor outcome Significantly differentiates worse prognosis within each IPSS subgroup

Abbreviation: TF, transcription factor.
[a] Rare mutations occur at a frequency of less than 2%.

cytokine signaling pathways. There is an increase in the frequency of molecular mutations from low-risk to high-risk MDS or AML evolving from MDS, emphasizing the role of these mutations in disease progression. A detailed review of these genes is beyond the scope of this article and has been provided elsewhere.[25,76] **Table 6** provides a partial list and overview of some of the salient features of genes implicated in the pathogenesis of MDS.

Recently, Bejar and colleagues[25] found that the integration of mutation analysis into diagnostic classification and prognostic scoring systems in MDS has the potential to stratify a diverse disease into discrete subsets with more consistent clinical phenotypes and prognosis.[25,77] For example, mutations in RUNX1, TP53, and NRAS were associated with severe thrombocytopenia and blast percentage. In multivariate analysis, mutations in 5 genes, occurring in one-third of patients, retained independent prognostic significance (*TP53, EZH2, ETV6, RUNX1,* and *ASXL1*) and predicted poor overall survival. Mutations of these genes stratified low- and intermediate-1, and intermediate-2 IPSS risk groups into 2 risk groups each, identifying patients within these subgroups with a poorer prognosis who may require a more intensive therapeutic approach. The genes most commonly mutated in MDS are *TET2, ASXL1, EZH2, RUNX1,* and *TP53,* which are described briefly below.

An emerging paradigm in MDS is the high frequency of mutations in genes involved in the regulation of transcription via chromatin modifications (*IDH1/2, TET2, EZH2, ASXL1*) and the intriguing observation that mutations often occur in more than 1 gene in the same patient, implying functional cooperation (note that *IDH1/2* and *TET2* mutations are mutually exclusive). The most frequently mutated gene in MDS is *TET2* (20%); point mutations are observed in all cytogenetic subsets.[25,77] TET2 converts 5-methylcytosine to 5-hydroxymethylcytosine, thereby altering the epigenetic mark created by DNA methyltransferases.[78] Recent findings suggest no impact of *TET2* mutations on overall survival in MDS.[77,79]

ASXL1 mutations are observed in 10% to 15% of MDS.[25,80] ASXL1 is a member of the polycomb family of chromatin-binding proteins and is involved in the epigenetic regulation of gene expression (typically repression). Mutated proteins are predicted to function as dominant negative proteins inhibiting the function of the wild-type proteins as well as other members of the polycomb complex. The prognostic significance of ASXL1 mutations in MDS is not yet known.

EZH2 (enhancer of zeste homolog 2) mutations occur in 5% of MDS.[25,72,73] EZH2 encodes a histone methyltransferase that trimethylates histone 3 lysine 27, an epigenetic mark that confers gene silencing. In MDS, the mutations lead to loss of the catalytic activity and are predicted to increase HSC expansion.[81] Although *EZH2* is located at 7q36.1, loss or mutation of *EZH2* does not appear to be the sole driver of myeloid neoplasms associated with –7/del(7q).

Point mutations in the runt-related transcription factor 1 (RUNX1) have been reported in AML and MDS (12%), particularly in MDS secondary to treatment with cytotoxic therapy, and increase with the severity of the disease.[82] RUNX1, also known as CBFA2 or AML1, encodes the DNA-binding subunit of the heterodimeric core-binding factor (CBF) complex, which is essential for definitive hematopoiesis.[83] *RUNX1* mutations impair DNA binding and act as dominant negative proteins and are associated with activating mutations of the RAS pathway, –7/del(7q), and a shorter overall survival.[82] Germline mutations of RUNX1 cause a rare human disease called familial platelet disorder; affected individuals have an MDS-like phenotype with thrombocytopenia or dysfunctional platelets and a predisposition to progress to AML.[84]

The *TP53* TSG encodes an essential checkpoint protein that monitors the integrity of the genome and arrests cell cycle progression in response to DNA damage. Mutations of *TP53* (exons 4-8) or loss of an allele, typically as a result of a cytogenetic abnormality of 17p, are observed in MDS (5%–10%) and t-MDS (25%–30%), particularly in patients who have received alkylating agent therapy.[40] *TP53* mutations may occur as either an early or late event in the course of the disease and are associated with rapid progression and a poor outcome. In t-MDS, *TP53* mutations are associated with –5/del(5q) and a complex karyotype.

JAK2^{V617F} is a constitutively active cytoplasmic tyrosine kinase that is able to activate JAK-STAT signalling and mediate transformation to cytokine-independent growth in myeloproliferative neoplasms, and has been identified in rare cases of MDS (2%–5%) and CMML (3%).[85] An exception is RARS-T, in which 60% of patients have the $JAK2^{V617F}$ mutation.[86] RARS-T patients with $JAK2^{V617F}$ mutations present with higher white blood cell counts and platelet counts.

The role of epigenetic changes in the pathogenesis and treatment of MDS is becoming increasingly important. Transcriptional silencing via DNA methylation of the $CDKN2B$ ($p15^{INK4B}$) gene increases with progression from RA to RAEB-T, is observed in a high percentage of patients with t-MDS, and is associated with -7/del(7q) and a poor prognosis.[64] Recent genome-wide studies have shown that increases in promoter hypermethylation are predictive of survival in MDS, even when age, sex, and IPSS risk groups are considered. Moreover, increases in promoter methylation are seen during progression to AML.[27] These observations form the rationale for use of demethylating agents in MDS. Similarly, inhibition of histone-modifying enzymes represents another rational target for MDS therapy.

EMERGING TECHNOLOGIES

Recent advances in microarray technology have enabled high-resolution genome-wide genotyping using single nucleotide polymorphisms (SNPs) for the identification of disease susceptibility loci, acquired genetic imbalances, and loss of heterozygosity (LOH) that occurs without concurrent changes in the gene copy number, which can be attributed to somatic mitotic recombination (referred to as copy-neutral LOH or acquired uniparental disomy). Gondek and colleagues[87] used high-density 250-K arrays to examine 174 patients (94 with MDS, 33 with AML after MDS, 47 with MDS/MPD).[87] Acquired, copy-neutral LOH was identified in 20% of MDS, 23% of MDS->AML, and 35% of MDS/MPD (particularly CMML). Collectively, abnormalities were detected in a higher proportion of cases compared with those detected with conventional cytogenetic analysis (78% vs 59% for MDS). New lesions detected by microarray analysis included copy-neutral LOH of 6p21.2-pter, 11q13.5-qter, 4q23-qter, 7q11.23-qter, and 7q22.1. When the presence of newly identified SNP array lesions were factored into the IPSS classification, the survival curves diverged for patients originally classified as IPSS intermediate-1, suggesting that SNP arrays provide additional information, allowing for better prognostic resolution (median survival 28 vs 9 months, $P=.03$). Thus, the results of these studies suggest that SNP array analysis may have future diagnostic application and may complement conventional cytogenetic analysis in risk stratification and the selection of therapy.

SUMMARY

Cytogenetic analysis in MDS remains a critical genetic test for establishing diagnosis and prognosis and for therapeutic decision making. The IPSS and the WHO classification systems incorporate only the most common chromosomal abnormalities. An international effort is underway to develop a comprehensive cytogenetic scoring system for MDS that incorporates rare cytogenetic subsets, which will inform an ongoing revision of the IPSS.[23] With the advent of more sensitive techniques already available in the research setting, including next-generation genome and transcriptome sequencing and SNP arrays, the rate of discovery will accelerate, and the compendium of genetic alterations in MDS will undoubtedly expand. Defining the genetic complexity of MDS holds tremendous promise for elucidating the pathogenesis of these diseases, refining the prognostic scoring systems, and identifying novel therapeutic targets.[88]

REFERENCES

1. Brunning RD, Orazi A, Germing U, et al. Myelodysplastic syndromes/neoplasms, overview. In: Swerdlow SH, Campo E, Harris NL, et al, editors. WHO classification of tumors of haematopoietic and lymphoid tissues. Lyons: Agency for Research on Cancer (IARC) 2008.
2. Cazzola M, Malcovati L. Myelodysplastic syndromes—coping with ineffective hematopoiesis. N Engl J Med 2005;352(6):536–8.
3. Sekeres MA, Schoonen WM, Kantarjian H, et al. Characteristics of US patients with myelodysplastic syndromes: results of six cross-sectional physician surveys. J Natl Cancer Inst 2008;100(21):1542–51.
4. Haase D, Germing U, Schanz J, et al. New insights into the prognostic impact of the karyotype in MDS and correlation with subtypes: evidence from a core dataset of 2124 patients. Blood 2007;110(13):4385–95.
5. Olney HJ, Le Beau MM. Evaluation of recurring cytogenetic abnormalities in the treatment of myelodysplastic syndromes. Leuk Res 2007;31(4):427–34.
6. Lichtman MA. Myelodysplasia or myeloneoplasia: thoughts on the nosology of clonal myeloid diseases. Blood Cells Mol Dis 2000;26(6):572–81.
7. Bennett JM, Catovsky D, Daniel MT, et al. Proposals for the classification of the myelodysplastic syndromes. Br J Haematol 1982;51(2):189–99.
8. Germing U, Gattermann N, Minning H, et al. Problems in the classification of CMML—dysplastic versus proliferative type. Leuk Res 1998;22(10):871–78.
9. Voglova J, Chrobak L, Neuwirtova R, et al. Myelodysplastic and myeloproliferative type of chronic myelomonocytic leukemia—distinct subgroups or two stages of the same disease? Leuk Res 2001;25(6):493–9.
10. Jaffe ES, Harris NL, Stein H, et al, editors. WHO Classification of tumours of haematopoietic and lymphoid tissues. Third Edition. Lyon: International Agency for Research on Cancer (IARC). 2001.
11. Rosati S, Mick R, Xu F, et al. Refractory cytopenia with multilineage dysplasia: further characterization of an 'unclassifiable' myelodysplastic syndrome. Leukemia 1996; 10(1):20–6.
12. Germing U, Strupp C, Kuendgen A, et al. Prospective validation of the WHO proposals for the classification of myelodysplastic syndromes. Haematologica 2006;91(12): 1596–1604.
13. Foucar K. Myelodysplastic/myeloproliferative neoplasms. Am J Clin Pathol 2009; 132(2):281–9.
14. Swerdlow SH, Campo E, Harris NL, et al, editors. WHO classification of tumours of haematopoietic and lymphoid tissues. Fourth Edition, Lyon: IARC Press. 2008.
15. Vardiman JW, Thiele J, Arber DA, et al. The 2008 revision of the World Health Organization (WHO) classification of myeloid neoplasms and acute leukemia: rationale and important changes. Blood 2009;114(5):937–51.
16. Boultwood J, Lewis S, Wainscoat JS. The 5q-syndrome. Blood 1994;84(10): 3253–60.
17. Garcia-Manero G, Fenaux P. Hypomethylating agents and other novel strategies in myelodysplastic syndromes. J Clin Oncol 2011;29(5):516–23.
18. Greenberg P, Cox C, LeBeau MM, et al. International scoring system for evaluating prognosis in myelodysplastic syndromes. Blood 1997;89(6):2079–88.
19. Kantarjian H, O'Brien S, Ravandi F, et al. Proposal for a new risk model in myelodysplastic syndrome that accounts for events not considered in the original International Prognostic Scoring System. Cancer 2008;113(6):1351–61.

20. Malcovati L, Germing U, Kuendgen A, et al. Time-dependent prognostic scoring system for predicting survival and leukemic evolution in myelodysplastic syndromes. J Clin Oncol 2007;25(23):3503–10.

21. Morel P, Declercq C, Hebbar M, et al. Prognostic factors in myelodysplastic syndromes: critical analysis of the impact of age and gender and failure to identify a very-low-risk group using standard mortality ratio techniques. Br J Haematol 1996;94(1):116–19.

22. Alessandrino EP, Della Porta MG, Bacigalupo A, et al. WHO classification and WPSS predict posttransplantation outcome in patients with myelodysplastic syndrome: a study from the Gruppo Italiano Trapianto di Midollo Osseo (GITMO). Blood 2008; 112(3):895–902.

23. Schanz J, Tuechler H, Sole F, et al. Cytogenetic risk features in MDS—update and present state [abstract]. Blood 2009;114;A2772.

24. Schanz J, Steidl C, Fonatsch C, et al. Coalesced multicentric analysis of 2,351 patients with myelodysplastic syndromes indicates an underestimation of poor-risk cytogenetics of myelodysplastic syndromes in the international prognostic scoring system. J Clin Oncol 2011;29(15):1963–70.

25. Bejar R, Levine R, Ebert BL. Unraveling the molecular pathophysiology of myelodysplastic syndromes. J Clin Oncol 2011;29(5):504–15.

26. Figueroa ME, Skrabanek L, Li Y, et al. MDS and secondary AML display unique patterns and abundance of aberrant DNA methylation. Blood 2009;114(16):3448–58.

27. Shen L, Kantarjian H, Guo Y, et al. DNA methylation predicts survival and response to therapy in patients with myelodysplastic syndromes. J Clin Oncol 2010;28(18):3098.

28. Gozzetti A, Le Beau MM. Fluorescence in situ hybridization: uses and limitations. Semin Hematol 2000;37(4):320–33.

29. Cherry AM, Brockman SR, Paternoster SF, et al. Comparison of interphase FISH and metaphase cytogenetics to study myelodysplastic syndrome: an Eastern Cooperative Oncology Group (ECOG) study. Leuk Res 2003;27(12):1085–90.

30. Wiktor A, Rybicki BA, Piao ZS, et al. Clinical significance of Y chromosome loss in hematologic disease. Genes Chromosomes Cancer 2000;27(1):11–16.

31. Hasle H. Myelodysplastic and myeloproliferative disorders in children. Curr Opin Pediatr 2007;19(1):1–8.

32. Paulsson K, Sall T, Fioretos T, et al. The incidence of trisomy 8 as a sole chromosomal aberration in myeloid malignancies varies in relation to gender, age, prior iatrogenic genotoxic exposure, and morphology. Cancer Genet Cytogenet 2001;130(2):160–5.

33. Sole F, Espinet B, Sanz GF, et al. Incidence, characterization and prognostic significance of chromosomal abnormalities in 640 patients with primary myelodysplastic syndromes. Grupo Cooperativo Espanol de Citogenetica Hematologica. Br J Haematol 2000;108(2):346–56.

34. Kurtin PJ, Dewald GW, Shields DJ, et al. Hematologic disorders associated with deletions of chromosome 20q: a clinicopathologic study of 107 patients. Am J Clin Pathol 1996;106(5):680–88.

35. Bench AJ, Nacheva EP, Hood TL, et al. Chromosome 20 deletions in myeloid malignancies: reduction of the common deleted region, generation of a PAC/BAC contig and identification of candidate genes. UK Cancer Cytogenetics Group (UKCCG). Oncogene 2000;19(34):3902–13.

36. Wang PW, Eisenbart JD, Espinosa R III, et al. Refinement of the smallest commonly deleted segment of chromosome 20 in malignant myeloid diseases and development of a PAC-based physical and transcription map. Genomics 2000; 67(1):28–39.

37. Godley LA, Larson R. The syndrome of therapy-related myelodysplasia and myeloid leukemia. In: Bennett JM, editor. The myelodysplastic syndromes: pathobiology and clinical management. New York: Marcel Dekker Inc; 2002. p. 136-76.

38. Allan JM, Travis LB. Mechanisms of therapy-related carcinogenesis. Nat Rev Cancer 2005;5(12):943–55.

39. Smith SM, Le Beau MM, Huo D, et al. Clinical-cytogenetic associations in 306 patients with therapy-related myelodysplasia and myeloid leukemia: the University of Chicago series. Blood 2003;102(1):43–52.

40. Christiansen DH, Andersen MK, Pedersen-Bjergaard J. Mutations with loss of heterozygosity of p53 are common in therapy-related myelodysplasia and acute myeloid leukemia after exposure to alkylating agents and significantly associated with deletion or loss of 5q, a complex karyotype, and a poor prognosis. J Clin Oncol 2001;19(5):1405–13.

41. Side LE, Curtiss NP, Teel K, et al. RAS, FLT3, and TP53 mutations in therapy-related myeloid malignancies with abnormalities of chromosomes 5 and 7. Genes Chromosomes Cancer 2004;39(3):217–23.

42. List A, Dewald G, Bennett J, et al. Lenalidomide in the myelodysplastic syndrome with chromosome 5q deletion. N Engl J Med 2006;355(14):1456–65.

43. Jadersten M, Saft L, Smith A, et al. TP53 Mutations in low-risk myelodysplastic syndromes with del(5q) predict disease progression. J Clin Oncol 2011;29(15): 1971–9.

44. Wei S, Chen X, Rocha K, et al. A critical role for phosphatase haplodeficiency in the selective suppression of deletion 5q MDS by lenalidomide. Proc Natl Acad Sci U S A 2009;106(31):12974–9.

45. Tehranchi R, Woll PS, Anderson K, et al. Persistent malignant stem cells in del(5q) myelodysplasia in remission. N Engl J Med 2010;363(11):1025–37.

46. Fairman J, Chumakov I, Chinault AC, et al. Physical mapping of the minimal region of loss in 5q- chromosome. Proc Natl Acad Sci U S A 1995;92(16):7406–10.

47. Zhao N, Stoffel A, Wang PW, et al. Molecular delineation of the smallest commonly deleted region of chromosome 5 in malignant myeloid diseases to 1-1.5 Mb and preparation of a PAC-based physical map. Proc Natl Acad Sci U S A 1997;94(13): 6948–53.

48. Boultwood J, Fidler C, Strickson AJ, et al. Narrowing and genomic annotation of the commonly deleted region of the 5q- syndrome. Blood 2002;99(12):4638–41.

49. Graubert TA, Payton MA, Shao J, et al. Integrated genomic analysis implicates haploinsufficiency of multiple chromosome 5q31.2 genes in de novo myelodysplastic syndromes pathogenesis. PLoS One 2009;4(2):e4583.

50. Lai F, Godley LA, Joslin J, et al. Transcript map and comparative analysis of the 1.5-Mb commonly deleted segment of human 5q31 in malignant myeloid diseases with a del(5q). Genomics 2001;71(2):235–45.

51. Shannon KM, Le Beau MM. Cancer: hay in a haystack. Nature 2008;451(7176): 252–3.

52. Ebert BL, Pretz J, Bosco J, et al. Identification of RPS14 as a 5q- syndrome gene by RNA interference screen. Nature 2008;451(7176):335–9.

53. Kumar M, Narla A, Nomami A, et al. Coordinate loss of a microRNA mir145 and a protein-coding gene RPS14 cooperate in the pathogenesis of 5q-Syndrome. Blood 2009;114:947.

54. Starczynowski DT, Kuchenbauer F, Argiropoulos B, et al. Identification of miR-145 and miR-146a as mediators of the 5q- syndrome phenotype. Nat Med 2010;16(1):49–58.

55. Joslin JM, Fernald AA, Tennant TR, et al. Haploinsufficiency of EGR1, a candidate gene in the del(5q), leads to the development of myeloid disorders. Blood 2007; 110(2):719–26.

56. Wang J, Fernald AA, Anastasi J, et al. Haploinsufficiency of Apc leads to ineffective hematopoiesis. Blood 2010;115(17):3481–8.

57. Liu TX, Becker MW, Jelinek J, et al. Chromosome 5q deletion and epigenetic suppression of the gene encoding alpha-catenin (CTNNA1) in myeloid cell transformation. Nat Med 2007;13(1):78–83.

58. Chen TH, Kambal A, Krysiak K, et al. Knockdown of Hspa9, a del(5q31.2) gene, results in a decrease in hematopoietic progenitors in mice. Blood 2011;117(5): 1530–9.

59. Eisenmann KM, Dykema KJ, Matheson SF, et al. 5q- myelodysplastic syndromes: chromosome 5q genes direct a tumor-suppression network sensing actin dynamics. Oncogene 2009;28(39):3429–41.

60. Barlow JL, Drynan LF, Hewett DR, et al. A p53-dependent mechanism underlies macrocytic anemia in a mouse model of human 5q- syndrome. Nat Med 2010;16(1): 59–66.

61. Baron V, Adamson ED, Calogero A, et al. The transcription factor Egr1 is a direct regulator of multiple tumor suppressors including TGFbeta1, PTEN, p53, and fibronectin. Cancer Gene Ther 2006;13(2):115–24.

62. Min IM, Pietramaggiori G, Kim FF, et al. The transciption factor EGR1 controls both the proliferation and localization of hematopoietic stem cells. Cell Stem Cell 2008;10: 380–91.

63. Luna-Fineman S, Shannon KM, Lange BJ. Childhood monosomy 7: epidemiology, biology, and mechanistic implications. Blood 1995;85(8):1985–99.

64. Christiansen DH, Andersen MK, Pedersen-Bjergaard J. Methylation of p15INK4B is common, is associated with deletion of genes on chromosome arm 7q and predicts a poor prognosis in therapy-related myelodysplasia and acute myeloid leukemia. Leukemia 2003;17(9):1813–19.

65. Loh ML, Vattikuti S, Schubbert S, et al. Mutations in PTPN11 implicate the SHP-2 phosphatase in leukemogenesis. Blood 2004;103(6):2325–31.

66. Fischer K, Frohling S, Scherer SW, et al. Molecular cytogenetic delineation of deletions and translocations involving chromosome band 7q22 in myeloid leukemias. Blood 1997;89(6):2036–41.

67. Johnson EJ, Scherer SW, Osborne L, et al. Molecular definition of a narrow interval at 7q22.1 associated with myelodysplasia. Blood 1996;87(9):3579–86.

68. Le Beau MM, Espinosa R III, Davis EM, et al. Cytogenetic and molecular delineation of a region of chromosome 7 commonly deleted in malignant myeloid diseases. Blood 1996;88(6):1930–5.

69. Curtiss NP, Bonifas JM, Lauchle JO, et al. Isolation and analysis of candidate myeloid tumor suppressor genes from a commonly deleted segment of 7q22. Genomics 2005;85(5):600–7.

70. Wong JC, Zhang Y, Lieuw KH, et al. Use of chromosome engineering to model a segmental deletion of chromosome band 7q22 found in myeloid malignancies. Blood 2010;115(22):4524–32.

71. Dohner K, Habdank M, Rucker FG, et al. Molecular characterization of distinct hot spot regins on chromosome 7q in myeloid leukemias. Blood 2006;108

72. Ernst T, Chase AJ, Score J, et al. Inactivating mutations of the histone methyltransferase gene EZH2 in myeloid disorders. Nat Genet 2010;42(8):722–6.

73. Nikoloski G, Langemeijer SM, Kuiper RP, et al. Somatic mutations of the histone methyltransferase gene EZH2 in myelodysplastic syndromes. Nat Genet 2010;42(8): 665–7.

74. Rowley JD, Reshmi S, Sobulo O, et al. All patients with the t(11;16)(q23;p13.3) that involves MLL and CBP have treatment-related hematologic disorders. Blood 1997; 90(2):535–41.

75. Apperley JF, Gardembas M, Melo JV, et al. Response to imatinib mesylate in patients with chronic myeloproliferative diseases with rearrangements of the platelet-derived growth factor receptor beta. N Engl J Med 2002;347(7):481–7.

76. Olney HJ, Le Beau MM. Myelodysplastic syndromes. In: Heim S, Mitelman F, editors. Cancer cytogenetics. 3rd edition. Hoboken (NJ): John Wiley & Sons, 2008.

77. Langemeijer SM, Kuiper RP, Berends M, et al. Acquired mutations in TET2 are common in myelodysplastic syndromes. Nat Genet 2009;41(7):838–42.

78. Ko M, Huang Y, Jankowska AM, et al. Impaired hydroxylation of 5-methylcytosine in myeloid cancers with mutant TET2. Nature 2010;468(7325):839–43.

79. Kosmider O, Gelsi-Boyer V, Cheok M, et al. TET2 mutation is an independent favorable prognostic factor in myelodysplastic syndromes (MDSs). Blood 2009; 114(15):3285–91.

80. Gelsi-Boyer V, Trouplin V, Adelaide J, et al. Mutations of polycomb-associated gene ASXL1 in myelodysplastic syndromes and chronic myelomonocytic leukaemia. Br J Haematol 2009;145(6):788–800.

81. Majewski IJ, Ritchie ME, Phipson B, et al. Opposing roles of polycomb repressive complexes in hematopoietic stem and progenitor cells. Blood 2010;116(5):731–9.

82. Chen CY, Lin LI, Tang JL, et al. RUNX1 gene mutation in primary myelodysplastic syndrome—the mutation can be detected early at diagnosis or acquired during disease progression and is associated with poor outcome. Br J Haematol 2007; 139(3):405–14.

83. Speck NA, Gilliland DG. Core-binding factors in haematopoiesis and leukaemia. Nat Rev Cancer 2002;2(7):502–13.

84. Song WJ, Sullivan MG, Legare RD, et al. Haploinsufficiency of CBFA2 causes familial thrombocytopenia with propensity to develop acute myelogenous leukaemia. Nat Genet 1999;23(2):166–75.

85. Steensma DP, Dewald GW, Lasho TL, et al. The JAK2 V617F activating tyrosine kinase mutation is an infrequent event in both "atypical" myeloproliferative disorders and myelodysplastic syndromes. Blood 2005;106(4):1207–9.

86. Zipperer E, Wulfert M, Germing U, et al. MPL 515 and JAK2 mutation analysis in MDS presenting with a platelet count of more than 500 x 10(9)/l. Ann Hematol 2008;87(5): 413–15.

87. Gondek LP, Tiu R, O'Keefe CL, et al. Chromosomal lesions and uniparental disomy detected by SNP arrays in MDS, MDS/MPD, and MDS-derived AML. Blood 2008; 111(3):1534–42.

88. Odenike O, LeBeau MM. The dawn of the molecular era of the myelodysplastic syndromes. N Engl J Med, in press.

Solid Tumor Cytogenetics: Current Perspectives

Gouri Nanjangud, PhD, Ina Amarillo, PhD, P. Nagesh Rao, PhD*

KEYWORDS

- Cytogenetics • Chromosome • Solid tumor
- Fluorescence in Situ Hybridization (FISH) • Prognosis
- Diagnosis • Clinical • Review

Following the discovery in 1956 that the human complement comprises 46 chromosomes (23 pairs of autosomes, XY sex chromosomes),[1,2] the development of human cytogenetics has been one of continuous discovery with impressive advances in the underlying methodologies. The translocation t(9;22) or the Philadelphia chromosome identified by conventional cytogenetics in chronic myeloid leukemia in 1960[3] and the ERG-TMPRSS2 fusion transcript identified by high-throughput expression analysis in prostate cancer in 2009[4] are the paradigms of this remarkable journey and technological advances. The limitation of conventional cytogenetics (requirement of dividing cells and limited resolution) was the driving force to develop alternate molecular methods that enable the analyses of nondividing cells along with offering better genome resolution. Fluorescence in situ hybridization (FISH) was the first such molecular method to be developed,[5] followed by several others techniques such as Multicolor FISH (mFISH)/Spectral Karyotyping (SKY), metaphase comparative genomic hybridization (mCGH), Bacterial Artificial Chromosome (BAC), or oligonucleotide/single-nucleotide polymorphism (SNP)-based comparative genomic hybridization (aCGH). All of these molecular methods are based on the principles of in situ hybridization in which single stranded complementary sequences of DNA are hybridized to genomic targets under appropriate conditions to form stable hybrid complexes, which are then visualized usually by a fluorescence detection system.[6-8] As expected, with the advent of every new methodology, the role of conventional karyotyping in routine clinical practice is debated and its utility questioned. Despite its recognized limitations, conventional cytogenetics in conjunction with FISH continues to remain an important and integral component in the diagnosis and management of neoplastic conditions. The ability to effectively detect the vast majority of clinically relevant chromosomal aberrations with a rapid to acceptable turnaround time makes

The authors have nothing to disclose.
Department of Pathology and Laboratory Medicine, David Geffen School of Medicine, University of California Los Angeles, 2-226 Rehab Center, 1000 Veteran Avenue, Los Angeles, CA 90024, USA
* Corresponding author.
E-mail address: nrao@mednet.ucla.edu

Clin Lab Med 31 (2011) 785–811
doi:10.1016/j.cll.2011.07.007
0272-2712/11/$ – see front matter © 2011 Elsevier Inc. All rights reserved.

labmed.theclinics.com

chromosome analysis the most cost-effective detection/screening tool currently available in modern pathology.

Over the past 4 decades, the karyotypes of more than 60,000 neoplasms have been published.[9] Because of the ease with which chromosome preparations can be obtained, leukemias lead the way, with lymphomas and solid tumors following behind. Conventional chromosomal analysis has been extremely crucial in establishing the principle that cancer is a genetic disease and that tumor development is a multistep process driven by accumulation of microscopic and molecular genomic changes. The recognition of recurrent chromosomal changes in specific disease entities has been the basis for the reclassification of many hematopoietic and solid tumors by the World Health Organization (WHO). Over the past decade, an increasing number of solid tumors have been rigorously analyzed by molecular methods, and these studies have revealed additional novel chromosomal alterations (translocations, deletions, gains, and amplifications). Routine karyotyping of solid tumors is still performed in many laboratories but, for clinical purposes, many of the genomic changes identified by conventional and molecular methods are primarily detected by DNA-based FISH assays. It is more sensitive and specific, has a rapid turnaround time, allows for a direct correlation with morphology/histology, and the analyses can be performed both retrospectively and prospectively on a variety of tissue types. An improvement in the quality of FISH probes, microscopy, and standardization of fluorescent signal guidelines has allowed routine FISH testing in formalin-fixed paraffin embedded sections. However, the protocols must be validated in individual laboratories, and parameters such as fixative times, section thickness, quality of the tissue preservation, probe hybridization conditions, areas of malignant cells, and number of abnormal cells scored must be appropriately considered prior to reporting, as these factors are known to affect results and, consequently, clinical management. Commercial FISH probes are now available for all the major rearrangements, and amplifications of clinically relevant genomic regions and new probes or multicolor probe panels continue to be developed. Given the usefulness of both the specific and the global chromosomal profile, our laboratory routinely performs conventional chromosomal analysis and/or FISH on sarcomas and renal cell carcinomas. The other solid tumors are primarily assayed by FISH.

In this review, we address some of the methodological considerations that are important in obtaining a diagnostically useful cytogenetic result, briefly describe the types of chromosomal abnormalities observed in solid tumors, and—because FISH is now the primary detection tool—discuss a representative set of malignant solid tumors in which cytogenetic and/or FISH analyses play, or can play, an important role in routine clinical management.

METHODOLOGICAL CONSIDERATIONS

Most malignant solid tumors exhibit chromosomal abnormalities. The success of obtaining an abnormal karyotype depends to a large extent on the pre-analytical and culture protocols adapted by the laboratory.[10] Factors that contribute to failure or only normal karyotypes (from non-malignant cells) include: (1) microbial contamination—this is very common and generally occurs when specimens are placed on unclean cutting boards when dissecting the tumors, use of nonsterile blades or transport media without antibiotics, or poor handing of the specimens prior to setting up the culture. Tumor specimens from regions that are inherently colonized by bacteria (eg, gastrointestinal tract, lung, and cervix) require special attention; (2) tumor necrosis—many solid tumors are composed of necrotic or fibrotic regions containing very few viable cells or cells useful for short or long-term culture. For cytogenetic analysis, it is crucial to select a maximally viable tumor region(s); (3) overgrowth of neoplastic cells by non-neoplastic or reactive cells—most solid tumor biopsies, depending on the type, stage, and location of the tumor, contain a mixture of neoplastic and non-neoplastic cells (fibroblasts, normal epithelial cells, or endothelial cells). If the culture is not monitored and harvested in a timely manner, the non-neoplastic cells usually overgrow and, sometimes, inhibit—by using up resources and space—the slower growing tumor cells. This is the most likely explanation for a normal-diploid karyotype in solid tumor cytogenetics; and (4) unpredictable growth of neoplastic cells in vitro—cancer cells often do not recapitulate the in vivo growth (doubling time) pattern in vitro. Many solid tumors, particularly those of epithelial origin, are difficult to grow in culture and require optimal culture conditions (seeding density, media, and growth factors), and it is prudent to be aware of the appropriate conditions required by the different tumor types. In general, tumors of soft tissue and bone, renal cell carcinomas, and certain benign tumors harboring recurrent chromosomal alterations are relatively easy to grow; therefore, the cytogenetic data in these tumors predominate in the literature. For certain cancers like ocular melanoma, fine-needle aspirate (FNA) approaches with the cells smeared on slides and their analyses by targeted FISH probes are very useful.[11]

CHROMOSOMAL CHANGES IN SOLID TUMORS: AN OVERVIEW

The vast majority of chromosomal changes in cancer are acquired (somatic). Consistent with a multistep pathogenesis, most solid tumors exhibit multiple chromosomal abnormalities, and it is these changes that lead to an abnormal proliferation (clonal expansion) and, ultimately, to invasion of the surrounding tissues and metastasis to distant sites.[12] The accumulation of chromosomal changes, which in most cases occur over a period of years, underlies both the process of tumorigenesis (the transition from normal cells to invasive cancer) and tumor progression (the transition to a metastatic, and often treatment-resistant, cancer). The karyotypes of many solid tumors (epithelial tumors in particular) are complex, and distinguishing "drives" (causative changes) from "passengers" (bystanders, victims of genomic instability) is often difficult. For example, in breast carcinomas, patients often exhibit heterogeneous karyotypes with multiple numerical and structural abnormalities (mostly unbalanced), and it is not possible to identify the primary aberration. Such complex karyotypes can be resolved and the breakpoints (balanced and unbalanced translocations) mapped by array painting, a method in which individual derivative chromosomes are purified using a fluorescence-activated cell sorter, amplified and hybridized to DNA microarrays. A study of 3breast cancer cell lines has shown that, contrary to the general view, a substantial proportion of translocation breakpoints are actually balanced.[13]

In solid tumors, 3 major types of chromosomal changes can be identified: (1) numerical changes (aneuploidy)—loss or gain of whole chromosomes; (2) structural changes—balanced and unbalanced translocation, deletion, insertion, or inversion of specific chromosomal regions; and (3) amplification—high-level gain of specific chromosomal regions which manifest as double minutes (dm), homogenously staining regions (hsr), or ring (r) chromosomes. In general, whole chromosome gains and losses contribute to the malignancy through increased and decreased gene dosage, respectively. Balanced translocations and inversions lead to fusion proteins with oncogenic potential or deregulation of target gene(s) at the breakpoints, thereby making them oncogenic. Deletions result in loss of tumor suppressor gene(s) and/or contribute through haplo-insufficiency. Unbalanced chromosomal rearrangements (translocations, inversions, and duplication) often result in increased or decreased gene dosage, or potentially activate proto-oncogenes-to-oncogenes or inactivate tumor suppressor genes. Gene amplification (usually >8 copies of specific genes material) leads to activation of proto-oncogenes and are the hallmark of some solid tumors.

CHROMOSOMAL CHANGES IN SOLID TUMORS: CLINICAL SIGNIFICANCE
Sarcomas: Classification, Diagnosis, and Prognosis

Sarcomas comprise a heterogeneous group of mesenchymal neoplasms that arise in the bones and soft tissues. More than 100 distinct diagnostic subtypes, that range from benign, intermediate (locally aggressive), intermediate (rarely metastasizing), to malignant have been described.[14] Such remarkable diversity always poses a challenge in the diagnosis, prognosis, and proper management of the disease. Over the past 2 decades our understanding of the pathobiology and genetics of the different subtypes of sarcomas has increased significantly. Cytogenetic analyses of over 2000 cases has revealed numerous chromosomal alterations that can be broadly classified into 4 categories[9,14]: (1) specific translocations that result in oncogenic fusion products or ectopic expression of proto-oncogenes (**Figs. 1A–C, 2A–C; Table 1**); (2) amplification of specific genomic loci/genes, such as amplification of MDM2/CDK4 in well differentiated liposarcomas, dedifferentiated liposarcomas, and intimal sarcomas. The amplified regions characteristically present as giant marker chromosomes and/or ring chromosomes (**Fig. 3A–C**); and (3) complex heterogeneous karyotypes with multiple structural and numerical abnormalities, such as in leiomyosarcoma, pleomorphic sarcomas, and giant cell tumors (**Fig. 4A–B**).

In addition to providing crucial clues to the genomic regions/genes involved in the development of sarcomas, these abnormalities serve as valuable markers in routine clinical practice in their classification, diagnosis, and prognosis (see **Table 1**). The classic example of classification/diagnosis is the small round blue cell tumors which includes the primitive neuroectodermal tumor (PNET) family, neuroblastoma, rhabdomyosarcoma, and lymphoblastic lymphoma of the bone. Although the majority of cases can be identified by morphology and immunohistochemistry, some of the undifferentiated cases continue to pose a diagnostic dilemma. The finding of t(11;22)(q24;q12)-EWS-FLI1 or its variants (EWS-ERG,EWS-ETV), observed in more than 95% of cases, confirms the diagnosis of PNET/Ewing's sarcoma (see **Fig. 1A**). Similarly, the t(11;22)(p13;q12)/EWS-WT1 points to the diagnosis of small desmoplastic round cell tumors (see **Fig. 1B**), and the t(12;16)(q13;p11.2)/FUS-CHOP or its variants to the diagnosis of myxoid liposarcoma among the mixoid sarcomas (see **Fig. 1C**). The poorly differentiated or monophasic forms of synovial sarcoma can sometimes be challenging to distinguish from tumors such as malignant peripheral nerve sheath tumor, fibrosarcoma, primitive peripheral neuroectodermal tumor, or hemangiopericytoma. Similarly, the detection of t(X;18)(p11.2;q11.2)/SYT-SSX1 (see **Fig. 2A**) is required to make a diagnosis of synovial sarcoma. Other examples include the t(2;13)(q25;q14)/PAX3-FOXO1 (see **Fig. 2B**) and t(1;13)(p36;q14)/PAX7-FOXO1, found only in alveolar rhabdomyosarcoma. Histologically, rhabdomyosarcomas are divided into alveolar and embryonal subtypes, and it is important to distinguish the two. This is because the alveolar subtype carries an unfavorable prognosis and any attempt to improve longterm survival may require more intensive chemotherapy. The identification of specific translocations can also assist in the diagnosis of metastatic tumors whose origin cannot be established with certainty. Several other examples where chromosomal findings are clinically useful are listed in **Table 1**.

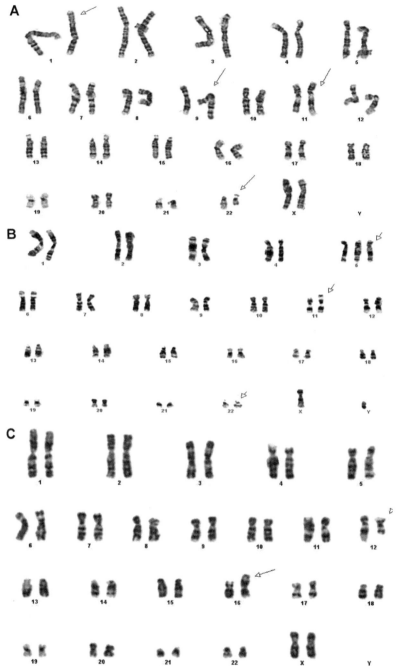

Fig. 1. Representative G-banded karyotypes showing specific translocations and other secondary abnormalities observed in tumors of the soft tissue. Arrows point to the abnormal chromosomes. (*A*) Ewing's sarcoma with the characteristic t(11;22)(q24;q12) and a secondary rearrangement t(1;9)(q21;q22). (*B*) small desmoplastic round cell tumor with the commonly observed t(11;22)(p13;q12) and trisomy 5. (*C*) Myxoid/round cell liposarcoma specific t(12; 16)(q13;p11.2).

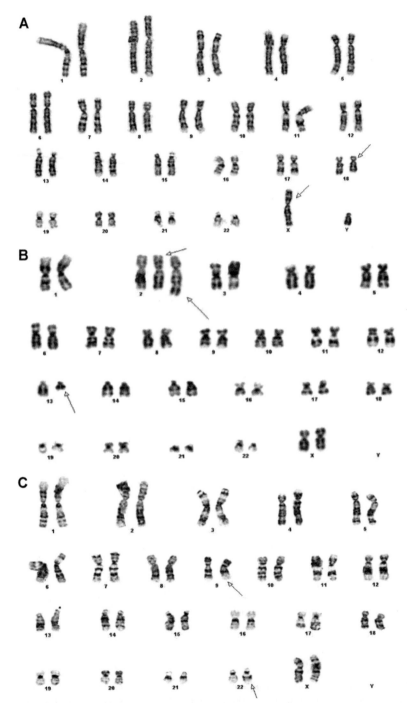

Fig. 2. Representative G-banded karyotypes showing specific translocations and other abnormalities observed in tumors of the soft tissue and bone. Arrows point to the abnormal chromosomes. (*A*) Synovial sarcoma with t(X;18)(p11.2;q11.2). (*B*) Alveolar rhabdomyosarcoma with t(2;13)(q35;q14) and trisomy 2. (*C*) Extraskeletal myxoid chondrosarcoma with t(9;22)(q22;q11.2).

Table 1
Recurrent chromosomal alterations in tumors of soft tissue and bone

Disease	Chromosomal Abnormality	Genes Involved	Histologic or Clinical Association
Ewing Sarcoma/PNET	t(1;22)(p36.1;q12)	*ZNF278-EWSR*	Diagnosis
	t(2;22)(q31;q12)	*SP3-EWSR*	
	t(2;22)(q33;q12)	*FEV-EWSR*	
	t(6;22)(p21;q12)	*POU5FI-EWSR*	
	t(7;22)(p22;q12)	*ETV1-EWSR*	
	t(11;22)(q24;q12)	*FLI1-EWSR*	
	t(17;22)(q12;q12)	*E1AF-EWSR*	
	t(20;22)(q13;q12)	*NFATC2-EWSR*	
	t(21;22)(q22;q12)	*ERG-EWSR*	
Angiomatoid Fibrous Histiocytoma	t(12;16)(q13;p11.2)	*FUS-ATF1*	Diagnosis
	t(2;22)(q33;q12)	*CREB1-EWSR*	
	t(12;22)(q13;q12)	*ATF1-EWSR*	
Clear Cell Sarcoma	t(2;22)(q34;q12)	*CREB1-EWSR*	
	t(12;22)(q13;q12)	*ATF1-EWSR*	Diagnosis
Desmoplastic Round Cell Tumor	t(11;22)(p13;q12)	*WT1-EWSR*	Diagnosis
	t(21;22)(q22;q12)	*ERG-EWSR*	
Myxoid-round Cell Liposarcoma	t(12;16)(q13;p11.2)	*FUS-DDIT3*	Diagnosis
	t(12;22)(q13;q12)	*DDIT3-EWSR*	
Extraskeletal Myxoid Chondrosarcoma	t(9;22)(q22;q12)	*NR4A3-EWSR*	Diagnosis
	t(3;9)(q12;q22)	*TFG-NR4A3*	
	t(9;15)(q22;q21)	*TCF12-NR4A3*	
	t(9;17)(q22;q11.2)	*TAF15-NR4A3*	
Alveolar Rhadomyosarcoma	t(1;13)(p36;q14)	*PAX7-FOXO1A*	Diagnosis and prognosis
	t(2;13)(q36;q14)	*PAX3-FOXO1A*	
	t(2;2)(p23;q36)	*PAX3-NCOA1*	
	t(X;2)(q13;q36)	*PAX3-FOXO4*	
Inflammatory Myofibroblastic Tumor	t(1;2)(q21;p23)	*TPM3-ALK*	Diagnosis
	t(2;2)(p23;q13)	*RANBP2-ALK*	
	t(2;4)(p23;q21)	*SEC31A-ALK*	
	t(2;11)(p23;p15)	*CARS-ALK*	
	t(2;17)(p23;q23)	*CLTC-ALK*	
	t(2;19)(p23;p13)	*TPM4-ALK*	
	inv(2)(p23q35)	*ATIC-ALK*	
Infantile Fibrosarcoma	t(12;15)(p13;q25)	*ETV6-NTRK3*	Diagnosis
Low grade fibromyxoid sarcoma	t(7;16)(q33-34;p11)	*FUS-CREB3L2*	Diagnosis
	t(11;16)(p11;p11.1)	*FUS-CREB3L1*	
Synovial sarcoma	t(X;18)(p11.2;q11.2)	*SS18-SSX1, SS18-SSX2, or SS18-SSX4*	Diagnosis
	t(X;20)(p11.2;q13)	*SS18L1-SSX1*	

(continued on next page)

Table 1
(continued)

Disease	Chromosomal Abnormality	Genes Involved	Histologic or Clinical Association
Alveolar Soft Part Sarcoma	t(X;17)(p11.2;q25)	*ASPSCR1-TFE3*	Diagnosis
Well differentiated/de-differentiated liposarcoma	Ring & Giant marker chromosome (Amplification)	*MDM2, CDK4, HMGA2, GLI, SAS*	Diagnosis in conjunction with morphology.
Dermatofibrosarcoma Protuberans	t(17;22)(q12;q12), der(22)t(17;22), ring(7;22)	*COL1A1-PDGFB*	Diagnosis

Renal Cell Carcinoma: Classification and Diagnosis

Renal cell carcinoma (RCC) is a heterogeneous group of diseases and conventional cytogenetic analyses have played an important role in the diagnosis and classification of this entity. Based on the pathologic and genetic features, the current WHO classification recognizes 2 broad categories, malignant and benign, and each has distinct histologic subtypes.[15] The 3 main histologic subtypes are clear cell, papillary, and chromophobe, and respectively account for 80% to 90%, 10% to 15%, and 4% to 5% of all RCCs. The remaining histologic subtypes are rare. As shown in **Table 2**, each histologic subtype is associated with a unique combination of numerical gains and losses, deletions, and/or translocations. These alterations are extremely useful in the differential diagnosis of RCC.

Cytogenetic and molecular studies have established that deletions of chromosome 3p (VHL and/or FHIT), resulting through monosomy 3 or various unbalanced aberrations, define the clear cell subtype (**Fig. 5A–D**). In up to 35% of the cases, an unbalanced translocation between chromosome 3p and 5q, resulting in the partial loss of 3p and gain of 5q, can be seen; it is reported to have a favorable outcome. Other frequent abnormalities include loss of 6q, 8p, 9p, and 14q, and these appear to be more common in advanced-stage disease. Deletions of 9p have also been associated with an unfavorable prognosis.[16] The papillary subtype is defined by the simultaneous gains of chromosomes 7 and 17 with or without the loss of the Y chromosome. Additional numerical gains include chromosomes 3q, 8, 12, 16, and 20. The chromophobe subtype is defined by a hypodiploid karyotype with monosomies of chromosomes 1, 2, 6, 10, 13, 17, and 21. Loss of the Y chromosome may or may not be observed. The benign oncocytoma is heterogeneous with at least 2 distinct entities identified; one defined by a hypodiploid karyotype with combined loss of chromosomes Y, 1, and 14 and the other by promiscuous translocations of 11q13 resulting in overexpression of CCND1 (Cyclin D1) (**Fig. 6A**). Translocations of Xp11.2 involving the TFE3 gene (see **Fig. 6B** and **Table 2**), accounting for approximately 30% of pediatric and 15% of RCC patients under 45 years of age, identify patients that might benefit from targeted therapy. Several studies have also shown that the different histologic subtypes differ significantly in their clinical outcome and require different treatment approaches, including therapy. Thus, clinically, it is important to diagnose these tumors correctly.[15,16]

Over the last 2 decades, management of RCC has changed significantly. Due to the growing use of new and improved noninvasive abdominal imaging modalities, such as ultrasonography, CT, and MRI, more than 70% of RCC are detected,

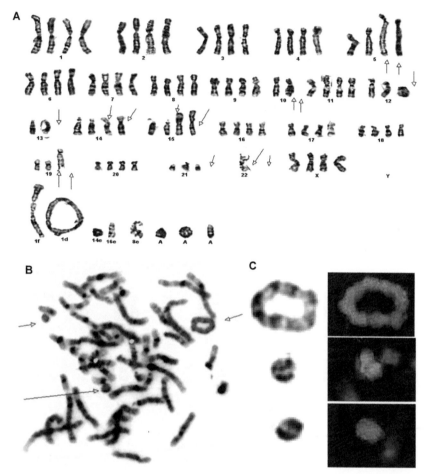

Fig. 3. Well-differentiated liposarcoma. (*A*) G-banded karyotype from a high-grade tumor showing a complex near-tetraploid karyotype with multiple unbalanced structural abnormalities including the characteristic ring and giant marker chromosome. (*B, C*) FISH analysis with probe specific for the *MDM2* gene (*red*) confirms the presence of *MDM2* amplicons in the ring and the two marker chromosomes.

incidentally, as small renal masses in asymptomatic patients. These small asymptomatic masses are more frequently benign or indolent and, following histologic assessment on the biopsy specimen (core or fine-needle aspirate) and other diagnostic work-up, a proportion of patients (elderly and those with significant comorbidity) can enroll in an active-surveillance protocol and avoid the complications and costs of unnecessary surgery.[17] One of the major concerns with core biopsies or fine-needle aspirate of renal masses is the risk of misdiagnosing or undergrading tumors as a result of overlapping histologic features or histologic heterogeneity. In this setting, assessment of histology-specific chromosomal alterations by FISH, along with histopathology, is proving to be useful in classification and treatment decision-making.[18]

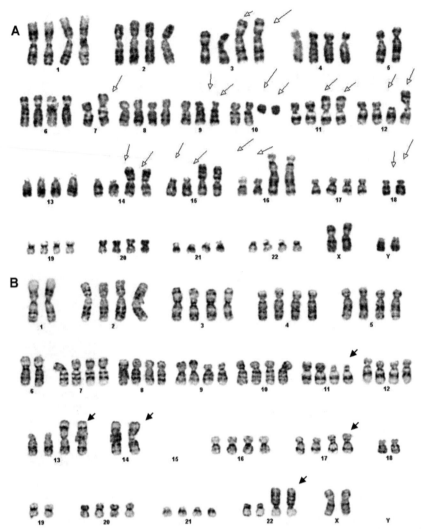

Fig. 4. Representative G-banded karyotype from (*A*) leiomyosarcoma and (*B*) pleomorphic sarcoma showing complex karyotypes with multiple numerical and structural abnormalities (arrows).

Neuroepithelial Tissue Tumors (Gliomas): Diagnosis, Treatment Selection, and Prognosis

FISH analysis plays an important role in the clinical management of gliomas and has become the standard of care in most neuropathology centers.[19-23] Early cytogenetic analyses, followed by molecular studies, have revealed distinct genomic alterations in the various histologic subtypes that are currently classified under 4 main types: astrocytic, oligodendroglial, oligoastrocytic (mixed), and ependymal (see **Table 3**). Co-deletion of 1p/19q (**Fig. 7**A, B) is the genetic hallmark of oligodendroglial tumors, particularly in cases with the classic histologic features. It is an early event and, for unknown reasons, gliomas arising in the cerebral sites are more likely to harbor the

Table 2

Recurrent chromosomal alterations in renal cell carcinoma (RCC) and neuroepithelial tumors (glioma)

Disease	Chromosomal Abnormality	Gene Involved	Histologic or Clinical Association
Renal Cell Carcinoma			
Clear Cell	−3p,+5q22,−6q,−8p −9p,−14q der(3)t(3:5)(p:q)	VHL	Diagnosis (−3p)
Papillary	Hyperdiploidy: +3q,+7,+8,+12,+16,+17, +20,−Y	—	Diagnosis (+7,+17)
Chromophobe	Hypodiploidy: −1,−2,−6,−10,−13,−17,−21	—	Diagnosis (−1,−17)
Oncocytoma	−1,−14,−Y	—	Diagnosis (−1,−14)
	t(11:?)(q13:?)	CCND1	Diagnosis. Distinguish between renal oncocytoma and chromophobe RCC
Collecting Ducts of Bellini	−1q,−6p,−8p,−13q,−21q,−3p (rare)/−14,−15,−22	—	
Mucinous Spindle Cell and Tubular	−1,−4,−6,−8,−13,−14,+7,+11, +16,+17 (absence of −3p, +7, +17)	—	
RCC: Xp11.2 Translocation	inv(X)(p11.2:q12)	TFE3-NONO	Diagnosis
	t(X:1)(p11.2:p34)	TFE3-SFPQ	
	t(X:1)(p11.2:q21)	PRCC-TFE3	
	t(X:3)(p11.2:q23)	TFE3-?	
	t(X:17)(p11.2:q23)	TFE3-CLTC	
	t(X:17)(p11.2:q25)	TFE3-ASPSCR1	
RCC: 6p21 Translocation	t(6:11)(p21:q12)	TFEB-ALPHA	Diagnosis

(continued on next page)

Table 2
(continued)

Disease	Chromosomal Abnormality	Gene Involved	Histologic or Clinical Association
Neuroepithelial Tumors (Glioma)			
Oligodendroglioma	Co-deletion of 1p/19q	?/?	Identifies subset of patients sensitive to treatment. Distinguish high-grade oligodendrogliomas from morphologically similar neoplasm
Glioblastoma	7p12 amplification	EGFR	Distinguish Glioblastoma (small cell phenotype) from morphologically similar neoplasm
	−10q23	PTEN	Poor outcome
Astrocytoma	BRAF duplication/fusion	BRAF	Common in pilocytic astrocytomas.?Diagnosis
Ependymomas	+19	?	Differential diagnosis
Neuroblastoma	2p24 amplification	MYCN	Diagnosis
Schwannomas	−22 or 22q−	NF2	Differential diagnosis
Meningioma	−22 or 22q−	NF2, ?MN1	Differential diagnosis
Medulloblastoma	i(17q10) [−17p/+17q]	TP53	? Poor prognosis

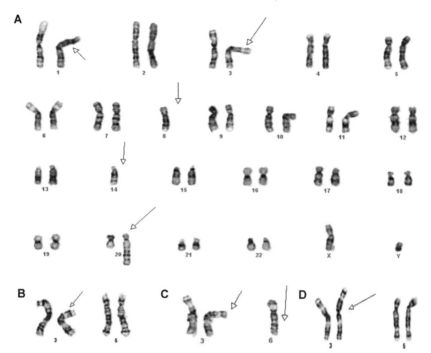

Fig. 5. Renal cell carcinoma (RCC), clear cell subtype: (*A*) A complete karyotype showing 44,XY, der(1;8)(q10;q10), der(3)t(3;5)(p11.2;q11.2),−14,der(20) t(1;20) (q21;q13.3). The der(3)t(3;5) is characteristic of clear cell subtype resulting in loss of 3p and gain of 5q. In addition, the karyotype shows a loss of chromosome 8p through an unbalanced der(1;8) and monosomy 14 which is associated with advanced disease. Partial karyotypes in RCC: (*B*) der(3)t(3;5)(p21;q31). (*C*) der(3)t(3;5)(p11.2;q11.2) illustrate the variable breakpoints on both chromosome 3 and 5. (*D*) der(3;6)(q10;p10) illustrates the loss of chromosome 3p through an unbalanced translocation with chromosomes other than chromosome 5.

1p/19q co-deletion than temporal gliomas. This co-deletion of 1p/19q is uncommon in pediatric gliomas. The most common mechanism through which the co-deletion occurs appears to be through a balanced whole-arm translocation between chromosome arms 1p and 19q, resulting in 2 derivative chromosomes [der(1)t(1;19) and der(19)t(1;19)], followed by the subsequent loss of one of the derivatives.[21] In over 2500 gliomas tested at Washington University School of Medicine (spanning over a decade), the co-deletion was observed in 86% of oligodendroglioma, 17% of oligoastrocytomas, and less than 1% of pure astrocytoma.[20] Overall, it has been observed in 40% to 70% of oligodendroglioma, 20% to 60% of oligoastrocytoma, and 0% to 10% of astrocytoma. In adults, it identifies patients that respond to alkylating chemotherapy and/or radiotherapy and, thus, display significantly longer overall survival even after recurrences. However, the rare pediatric patients that carry the co-deletion do not enjoy the same outcome. It is well recognized that patients can exhibit only deletions of 1p or 19q, or co-deletions can occur via independent interstitial deletions of 1p and 19q, and such variant deletions/co-deletions are not predictive of good prognosis. Histologically, the co-deletion can help distinguish high-grade oligodendrogliomas from morphologically similar neoplasms: oligodendrogliomas central neurocytoma, clear cell ependymomas, and dysembryoblastic neuroepithelial tumors (DNETs).[20]

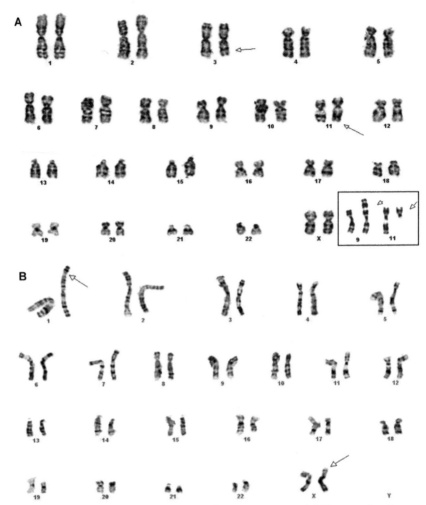

Fig. 6. Translocations of 11q13 (*CCND1*) specific to oncocytoma. (*A*) The complete karyotype shows t(3;11)(q21;q13) and the inset (bottom right) shows t(9;11)(p21;q13). (*B*) Translocation t(X;1)(p11.2;p34) observed in a subset of pediatric and young adults with RCC with Xp11.2 rearrangement.

Amplification of EGFR (7p12) (see **Fig. 7**C), often represented as double minutes, is characteristic of glioblastoma and is of diagnostic value.[19–22] Nearly all primary Glioblastoma Multiforme (GBM) with the small cell phenotype exhibit amplification of the gene. Overall, it is observed in 40% to 70% of the cases and is predominant in primary GBMs and in adults. Secondary GBMs rarely exhibit amplification. Amplification of EGFR and co-deletion of 1p/19q are mutually exclusive, and this renders them useful in distinguishing the small cell variant of GBMs from high-grade oligodendroglial neoplasm. In histologically lowgrade or anaplastic gliomas, amplification is indicative of a high-grade malignancy. The presence of amplification also allows for the selection of patients for targeted therapy with tyrosine kinase inhibitors, but its association with therapeutic response is controversial. More recent studies

Table 3
Recurrent chromosomal alterations in solid tumors

Disease	Chromosomal Abnormality	Gene Involved	Histologic or Clinical Association
Cutaneous Melanoma	+6p25, −6q21, +11q13	RREB1, MYB, CCND1	Metastasis. Distinguish from normal nevi (normal karyotype)
Uveal Melanoma	−3,i(6p),i(8q)		Diagnosis, metastasis
	+6p25, −6q21,+8q,		Metastasis
Lung Carcinoma	5p15.2, 7p12, 8q24	?, EGFR, MYC	Diagnosis in conjunction with cytology
	inv(2)(p21p23)	EML4–ALK	Treatment selection with ALK inhibitors
	7p12 amplification	EGFR	Treatment selection with kinase inhibitors
	−1p31, −3p14, 3p21, −9p21, −17p13	HLJ1, FHIT, SEMA3B, CDKN2A, TP53	
	−4q12−q23	?	? Metastasis
Breast Carcinoma	17q21 amplification of	ERBB2 (HER2)	Anti-HER2 targeted therapy, prognosis
	7p12 amplification	EGFR	
Secretory Breast Carcinoma	t(12;15)(p13;q25)	ETV6–NTRK3	
Gastric carcinoma	17q21 amplification of	ERBB2 (HER2)	Anti-HER2 targeted therapy, prognosis
Bladder cancer (Transitional cell carcinoma)	+3,+7, −9p21,+17 (UroVysion)	CDKN2A	Surveillance, determining therapy of effectiveness
	−13q14	RB1	
	−9p21 (homozygous)	CDKN2A	? Poor outcome
	−10q23	PTEN	
	−17p13	TP53	
	17q21 amplification	ERBB2 (HER2)	? Poor outcome
	−8p, −11/−11p		
Cervical carcinoma	+3q26 or amplification	TERC	Diagnosis
	+5p, +8q24, +20q11or +20q13		? Diagnosis

(continued on next page)

Table 3
(continued)

Disease	Chromosomal Abnormality	Gene involved	Histologic or Clinical Association
Prostate Cancer	inv(21)(q22.2:q22.3)or del(21)(q22.2:q22.3)	*TMPRSS2-ERG*	Early stagedisease,?Clinicaloutcome
	t(7;22)(q21.2;q22.3)	*ETV1-TMPRSS2*	
	t(17;22)(q21.3;q22.3)	*ETV4-TMPRSS2*	
	−8p21	*NKX3.1*	Early stage disease
	+8q24 oramplification	*CMYC*	Metastasis
	−10q23	*PTEN*	Highgrade disease
	−13q14	*RB1*	Highgrade disease
	−17p13	*TP53*	Highgrade disease
	+Xq11−12 oramplification	*AR*	Metastasis

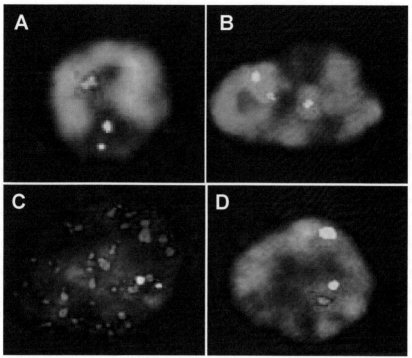

Fig. 7. FISH analysis in neuroepithelial tumors. (*A, B*) Two separate hybridizations identify the co-deletion of 1p36 and 19q in oligodendroglioma on the same tissue section. (*A*) Loss of 1p36 (*TP73*) (*red*) and 2 copies of the control probe at locus 1q25 (*ANGPTL*) (*green*). (*B*) Loss 19q13 (*GLTSCR*) (*red*) and 2 copies of the control probe at locus 19p13 (*ZNF443*) (*green*). (*C*) Interphase nuclei from a patient with glioblastoma showing high level amplification of *EGFR* (7p12) (*red*) and 2 copies of centromere 7 (*green*). (*D*) The same patient also showed loss of *PTEN* (10q23) (*red*) and 2 normal copies of the control probe at centromere 10 (*green*).

have shown a predictive value for the deletion variant EGFRvIII, which results in the constitutive activation of the phosphatidylinositol 3' kinase (PI3K) signaling pathway, but this variant cannot be detected by FISH.[23]

Monosomy 10, deletion 10q (PTEN) (see **Fig. 7**D), or loss of heterozygosity (LOH, which is defined as a loss of normal function of one allele of a gene in which the other allele is already inactivated) of 10q is pathognomic of both primary and secondary GBMs. It occurs in 60% to 90% of cases and, in some studies, is a predictor of poor prognosis in pediatric GBMs. Primary pediatric and secondary GBMs, which usually evolve from pre-existing lowgrade gliomas, are characterized by acquisitions of mutations or deletions of TP53 (17p13). Since the deregulation of TP53 is primarily by mutations, routine evaluation of the deletion status by FISH may not be practical. In cases where grade designation is unclear, testing for hemi- or homozygous deletion of CDKN2A (9p21) can help; deletion of CDKN2A is observed in 30% to 50% of gliomas, but up to 95% of gliomas with high-grade histology (grade III or IV) harbor the deletion.

The potential use of BRAF (7q34) rearrangements in routine clinical practice as a marker of diagnosis, prognosis, and targeted therapy is still under evaluation. Rearrangements of BRAF have been observed in approximately 80% of cerebellar and 40% of noncerebellar pilocytic astrocytomas, respectively. It does not appear to be a reliable differentiator between pilocytic astrocytomas and pilomyxoid astrocytoma. A tandem duplication at 7q34 is the most common mechanism through which the BRAF-KIAA1549 fusion occurs.[20,24]

Cutaneous and Uveal Melanoma: Diagnosis and Prognosis

Cutaneous melanoma is an aggressive cancer with increasing incidence worldwide. Early detection and surgery are keys to improved survival. Once metastatic melanoma is diagnosed, median survival duration of only 6 to 9 months is expected. Based on the clinical, histopathologic, immunopathologic, and cytogenetic features, 5 stages of malignant transformation and tumor progression are recognized: benign melanocytic nevi, atypical nevi, malignant radial growth phase melanoma, malignant vertical growth phase melanoma, and metastatic malignant melanoma. Histopathologic examination is currently the "gold standard" to establish the diagnosis of melanoma, but distinguishing the benign form of malignant melanoma is still a diagnostic challenge. Additionally, at least 17 variant forms of melanomas are known to exist with new variants continuing to emerge. Even among expert dermatopathologists, consensus can be reached in only about 75% to 90% of the cases.[25]

Both environmental and genetic factors drive the pathogenesis of cutaneous melanoma. Several chromosomal and aCGH studies have shown that nearly all malignant melanomas exhibit chromosomal alterations. Losses of chromosomes 6q, 8p, 9p, and 10q and gains of chromosomes 1q, 6p, 7, 8q, 17q, and 20q appear to be the most common. With the exception of Spitz nevus, which exhibits gains of 11p in 10% to 20% of cases, the majority of benign lesions (nevi) tend to be normal. Recently, FISH has emerged as a diagnostic tool in distinguishing benign/variant from malignant melanoma (see **Table 3**).[25–28] In a recent large study of 497 melanocytic lesions, 13 genomic regions on 8 different chromosomes were evaluated and a signal-count based algorithm of 4 genomic regions—6p25 (RREB1), centromere 6, 6q21 (MYB), and 11q13 (CCND1)—provided the highest diagnostic discrimination. The algorithm correctly classified melanoma with 87% sensitivity and 95% specificity, and also identified ambiguous cases with metastatic potential. A 4-color probe set targeting the 4 regions has been commercially developed (Abbott Molecular Inc, Des Plaines, IL, USA) and its effectiveness in conjunction with histopathology remains to be evaluated by additional groups and studies.[27]

Cytogenetic analyses also play an important role in the prognosis of uveal melanoma[29–32] (see **Table 3**). In the early stages of the disease, the karyotypes are either pseudodiploid or near-diploid with relatively simple abnormalities. Disease progression is usually marked by acquisition of multiple abnormalities resulting in complex karyotypes (**Fig. 8**A). The most common abnormalities are monosomy 3 and gain of 8q (through whole chromosome gain, isochromosome, or unbalanced translocation). Other common abnormalities include duplications of 6p/loss of 6q (through isochromosome 6p), loss of 1p, 13q and 16q. Analysis of karyotype patterns suggests that monosomy 3 probably occurs as an early event, while gains of 8q and 6p are secondary. Numerous studies since the 1990s have established the clinical significance of loss of chromosome 3 and gains of chromosome 8/8q identified by conventional cytogenetics (30%–70% of case), and FISH or aCGH studies (11%–40% of cases), as strong predictors of poor outcome and metastasis. Longterm studies have shown that nearly 70% of patients with monosomy 3 in the primary tumor develop metastases within 4 years of initial diagnosis, whereas patients with normal chromosome 3 (2 copies) rarely develop metastatic disease. Since gains of 6p and monosomy 3 are mutually exclusive, gain of 6p is considered to be a marker of

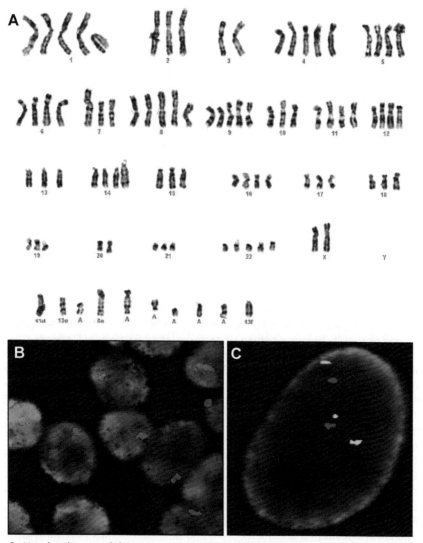

Fig. 8. Uveal melanoma. (*A*) A representative G-banded karyotype showing the characteristic loss of chromosome 3 and gain of chromosome 8q (through isochromosome 8q). (*B, C*) FISH analysis of interphase nuclei obtained from a fine-needle biopsy showing (*B*) monosomy 3 (*red*), which is associated with a poor clinical outcome and (*C*) Gain of 6p (*green*) and 2 normal copies of chromosome 3 (*red*) which is associated with a better clinical outcome.

better prognosis. FISH analysis with probes specific for the centromere of chromosome 3 and a 6p locus is useful in distinguishing patients with poor and good clinical outcome (see **Fig. 8**B, C).

Lung Cancer: Screening and Targeted Therapy

Lung cancer continues to be the most lethal cancer in both men and women worldwide. This is due to detection at an advanced stage, biological aggressiveness of the tumor, and its resistance to therapy. Much of the research in lung cancer is aimed at early detection, understanding the pathogenesis of the disease, and targeted therapy. A combination of environmental, genomic (mutations, deletions, duplication, and amplification), and epigenetic factors initiate and drive the pathogenesis of lung cancer[33,34] (see **Table 3**). Chromosomal abnormalities are thought to precede the development of clinical lung cancer, and the utility of FISH in detection of lung cancer in bronchoscopic brush biopsies, fine needle aspirates, or sputum has been explored since 2002.[35–37] The genomic regions in a commercially developed assay (LaVysion by Abbott Molecular Inc, Des Plaines, IL, USA) include chromosome 5p15.2, the pericentromeric region of chromosome 6 (6p11.1-q11α-satellite DNA), 7p12 (EGFR), and 8q24 (MYC).[35] Nearly all studies show an increased detection of lung cancer when combined with cytology. In the most recent study of sputum samples collected prospectively from 100 incident lung cancer cases, the sensitivity (abnormal for 2 or more of the 4 markers) was substantially higher for samples collected within 18 months (76%) compared to samples collected more than 18 months (31%) before the diagnosis of lung cancer. However, its potential in early-detection needs to be validated in larger prospective screening trials.[37]

Amplification of EGFR or high polysomy as detected by FISH is observed in 10% to 22% of early stage, and 40% to 50% of advanced stage, non-small cell lung carcinoma (NSCLC).[33,34,38] While EGFR FISH status has been useful in selecting patients for treatment with tyrosine kinase inhibitors (TKI) such as gefitinib and erlotinib, its prognostic value is controversial.[33,38] In an attempt to ensure reproducibility and portability between testing laboratories, the University of Colorado Cancer Center (UCCC) has developed a scoring system that stratifies the results into 6 groups based on the copy number of EGFR and centromere 7, and their frequency in tumor cells (disomy, low trisomy, high trisomy, low polysomy, high polysomy, and gene amplification). High polysomy and gene amplification are considered FISH positive.[38] Another study recommends the addition of another control on the 7q31 locus to help interpret complex signal patterns,[39] but these scoring systems remain to be further validated.

The EML4-ALK fusion oncogene is the most recent molecular target in NSCLC.[33,34] The fusion results from a small inversion within chromosome 2p, leading to expression of a chimeric tyrosine kinase in which the N-terminal half of EML4 (echinoderm microtubule-associated protein-like 4) is fused to the intracellular kinase domain of ALK (anaplastic lymphoma kinase). In both EML4 and ALK, the inversion breakpoints do not always occur in the same location, and at least 11 EML4-ALK variants have been described, all reported to be oncogenic. The presence of variable breakpoints and the lack of a robust antibody for the detection of ALK protein make it an attractive detection system by FISH.[40] The fusion defines a distinct subset of NSCLCs— younger age at onset (40 to 50 years), non- or light smokers, and adenocarcinomas with signet ring or acinar histology.[34,40] The incidence of ALK gene rearrangements detected by either RT-PCR or FISH is low (3% to 5%). However, patients with the fusion are candidates for treatment with small-molecule inhibitors of ALK kinase (Crizotinib). The high clinical efficacy in a Phase 1B study has led to Phase 3 studies comparing crizotinib with standard chemotherapy in patients with ALK-rearranged (positive) NSCLC. Routine screening of patients for the ALK translocation is rapidly becoming common practice in the United States. Because the ALK translocation appears to be mutually exclusive with EGFR and KRAS mutations, screening by FISH in non-smokers/light smokers with wild-type EGFR and KRAS mutations is recommended.[34,40]

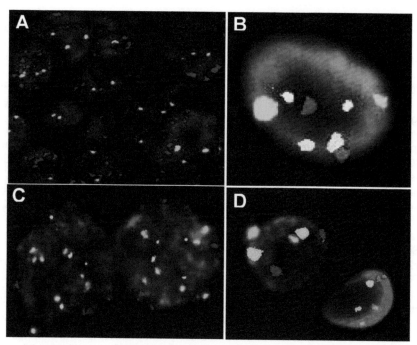

Fig. 9. (A) Amplification of ERBB2 (HER2) gene (*red*) and 2 or more copies of the centromere of chromosome 17 (*green*) in an invasive breast carcinoma. (B–D) FISH analysis on urine specimens from patients with transitional urothelial carcinoma using the multicolor FDA-approved UroVysion kit (Abbott-Vysis) showing (B) normal signal pattern; (C) 3~4 copies of all chromosomes/regions tested (polysomy); and (D) diploid cell with homozygous deletion of 9p (CDKN2B) [centromere 3 (*red*), centromere 7 (*green*), 9p21/CDKN2B (*gold*) and centromere 17 (*Aqua*)].

Breast and Gastric Carcinoma: Targeted Therapy and Prognosis

Amplification of the human epidermal growth factor receptors 2 (ERBB2) (better known as Her2/neu) has been detected in many cancers, including breast cancer (20% to 30%) (**Fig. 9**A) and gastric carcinoma (6% to 35%)[41–46] (see **Table 3**). The gene maps to 17q21, and is 1 of the 4 members of the epidermal growth factor (EGF) receptor family. Trastuzumab (Herceptin; Genentech, San Francisco, CA, USA) is a humanized monoclonal antibody against Her2. Since its approval in women with advanced breast cancer by the US Food and Drug Administration (FDA), targeted therapy with Trastuzumab has become part of standard care for women with amplification and/or overexpression of Her2. All newly diagnosed women with invasive breast cancer, recurrent disease, and metastatic disease are tested for HER2 status (American Society of Clinical Oncology). Women who are Her2 positive, as detected by FISH and/or immunohistochemistry, are eligible for treatment with Trastuzumab in an adjuvant setting, and multiple studies have confirmed the prolonged survival. Additionally, amplification/overexpression of Her2 is predictive of poor clinical outcome and resistance or sensitivity to different types of chemotherapeutic agents.[41–43]

More recently, Trastuzumab was approved by the FDA for Her2-overexpressing metastatic gastric or gastro-esophageal (GE) junction adenocarcinoma without prior treatment for metastatic disease. The approval was based on the results of a single international multicenter open-label randomized clinical trial (ToGA). Although modest, the increase in overall survival was found be clinically significant (13.8 months for trastuzumab + chemotherapy vs 11.1 months for chemotherapy alone, $P = .0002$). Similar to breast carcinoma, HER2 gene amplification in gastric carcinoma is associated with poor outcome and is an independent prognostic factor.[44] Based on the ToGA trial findings, HER2 testing by FISH is now becoming routine in the diagnostic work-up of patients with advanced gastric cancer.

In breast cancer, given the importance of accurate detection of HER2 gene amplification and/or overexpression, the American Society of Clinical Oncology (ASCO) and College of American Pathology (CAP) have outlined reporting guidelines.[42] Amplification appears to be the main mechanism for overexpression and, in general, the concordance between immunohistochemistry (IHC) score 3+ and HER2 gene amplification is high. Discordance is usually observed when the IHC score is 1+ or 2+ and the ratio obtained by FISH (1.8 to 2.2) is equivocal, often due to polysomy 17 and/or intra-tumor genetic heterogeneity.

Some agree that primary tumors with polysomy 17 are histopathologically similar to Her2-negative tumors and may not be predictive of prognosis. Recent studies favor HER2 gene amplification detection by the FISH method over IHC, because it can distinguish amplification from polysomy 17. In addition, since DNA is more stable than protein, it is less sensitive to the pretreatment methods such as type and duration of the fixation.[43] In gastric cancer, the correlation between amplification and overexpression is variable, and currently IHC is recommended as the first testing modality—as in the exploratory analysis in the ToGA study, overexpression was found to have the best predictive value.[45,46]

Bladder Cancer: Surveillance and Prognosis

Since the 1950s, the incidence of bladder cancer has risen by approximately 50%. However, due to the successful use of cystoscopies and bladder wash/urinary cytologic examinations in the surveillance and management of patients with previously treated bladder cancers, mortality has decreased considerably.[47] More than 95% of bladder cancers are transitional cell in origin (TCC) which develops along 2 major routes: muscle-invasive (25%) and muscle noninvasive (superficial), either papillary (70%) or a flat lesion of the urothelium termed carcinoma in situ (CIS) (5%).[48] The natural history of noninvasive urothelial tumors is that of recurrence and, therefore, these patients require longterm surveillance. The gold standard for surveillance has traditionally been cystoscopy and urine cytology. Typically, patients are monitored and cytology is performed every 3 months for 2 years after initial diagnosis, with decreasing frequency thereafter if they remain free of disease. One of the limitations of urine cytology is its low sensitivity (20% to 60%) for detecting low-grade tumors, and this lead to the development of UroVysion Bladder Cancer kit (Abbott Molecular, Des Plaines, IL, USA), a DNA-FISH-based assay [49] that detects gain in copy number of chromosomes 3, 7, and 17, and deletion of 9p21 (CDKN2B) (see **Fig. 9**B–D). The assay was initially approved by the FDA as a surveillance tool for patients with a history of urothelial carcinoma and, later, extended for use as a screening tool in patients with hematuria and risk factors for TCC. UroVysion FISH has a reported sensitivity of 30% to 86% and a specificity of 75% to 90% for TCC detection and, despite the concerns (low sensitivity in low-grade tumors and FISH-positive results in non-TCC carcinoma), FISH in conjunction with cytology is routinely used as a surveillance tool.[47,49,50]

Overall, molecular genetic analyses suggest that the noninvasive (superficial) and invasive lesions develop along distinct molecular pathways.[48,51] Low-grade papillary tumors, which do not tend to invade or metastasize, harbor constitutive activation of the receptor-tyrosine kinase-Ras signal transduction pathway and have a high frequency of fibroblast growth factor receptor 3 (FGFR3) mutations. In contrast, CIS and invasive tumors have a higher frequency of TP53, RB1, and cell cycle gene alterations. Additionally, many potentially prognostic genomic regions and candidate genes have been identified and remain to be evaluated for clinical use (see **Table 3**).

Cervical Cancer: Screening and Risk Stratification

Cervical cancer (CC) is one of the most common causes of death in women. Over the past 40 years, in the developed-world, the mortality rate has decreased by 50% due to widespread screening with the Pap smear.[52] Molecular and epidemiological studies have unequivocally shown that the vast majority of cervical cancer cases worldwide are caused by persistent infections with human papillomavirus (HPV). The high-risk HPV types have been found in approximately 95% of cervical cancers and their precursor lesions worldwide. More than 90% of lesions with mild (cervical intraepithelial neoplasia 1[CIN1]/ low grade squamous intraepithelial lesion [LSIL]) and moderate (cervical intraepithelial neoplasia 2 [CIN2]/ high grade squamous intraepithelial lesion [HSIL]) dysplasia regress spontaneously or resolve over time, and approximately 10% of precancerous lesions, through deregulated expression of the viral oncogenes (E6 and E7) and accumulation of genomic alterations, progress to invasive CC. In the vast majority, progression is extremely slow and the estimated time from cervical intraepithelial neoplasia 2 (CIN3) to invasive carcinoma is 10 to 15 years.[52] This long natural history provides the opportunity to effectively detect precancerous lesions during screening, thus allowing early treatment and cure. However, current screening methods cannot predict which CIN lesions will resolve and which will progress to invasive CC.

Conventional chromosomal analysis and, more recently, aCGH analyses have shown that more than 90% of invasive cervical carcinomas carry specific genomic imbalances, mostly gains and losses[53-57] (see **Table 3**). Among the many described, gain/amplification of 3q26 (TERC) as detected by FISH, has shown a consistent association with disease progression (from precancerous dysplastic lesions to invasive carcinoma).[53-57] Other potential progression associated genomic alterations include gain of chromosomes 5p, 8q24, 20q11 and 20q13 and, in one recent study, gain of 8q24 was predictive of disease progression.[57] Although additional studies are required to validate the utility of FISH in identifying women who are at risk of developing cervical cancer, studies thus far are promising.

Prostate Cancer: Screening and Risk Stratification

The development of prostate cancer proceeds through a series of defined states, including preinvasive disease or prostatic intraepithelial neoplasia (PIN), androgen-dependent cancer, and eventually androgen independent metastasis. Chromosomal alterations play a crucial role in the initiation and progression of this disease.[58-63] Prostate specimens are not amenable to conventional chromosomal analyses, but recent molecular methods have identified reciprocal translocations and genomic imbalances (see **Table 3**). The most common abnormalities include translocations of TMPRSS2 and ERG, deletions of 8p (NKX3-1), 10q23 (PTEN), 13q14 (RB1), 17p13 (TP53), and gains or amplification of 8q24 (MYC) and Xq28 (AR). While TMPRSS2-ERG fusion and deletion of NKX3-1 are early initiating events, the others contribute to disease progression and transformation. A surprising finding in a recent targeted resequencing study of 138 genes was the rarity of somatic point mutations. Genes such as TP53 and PTEN, which are frequently altered by somatic point mutations in other cancers, were primarily altered through copy-number loss (haplo-insufficiency) in prostate cancer.[62]

In the post-Prostate Specific Antigen (PSA) era, one of the biggest clinical challenges is to distinguish between men who have disease destined to progress from those who will not require therapeutic intervention. Clinicians currently depend on serum PSA levels, Gleason score, and clinical stage for risk-stratification and outcome prediction. However, these variables fail to detect a significant proportion of cases that do not require therapeutic interventions resulting in over-treatment of many men.[60–63] Therefore, there is a great need for new biomarkers and/or assays that can independently or, along with other clinical and histologic variables, allow for better risk-stratification. Autopsy data indicate that PIN (precursor lesion) generally precedes prostate cancer by 5 to 10 years, and this allows sufficient time for detection of potentially transforming lesions and subsequent therapeutic intervention. Given the progressive accumulation of specific genomic changes (translocation, losses, and amplifications) from PIN to prostate cancer, and the fact that somatic mutations are rare, DNA-based FISH assays can be potentially useful in screening and risk-stratification.

SUMMARY

By pointing to the genes involved, conventional chromosomal analysis has provided critical insights into the biology of neoplastic transformation of many solid tumors. It is still the most cost-effective way of obtaining a global genomic profile and delineating the clonal and genetic heterogeneity, and these studies have been extremely useful in the diagnosis of sarcomas and renal cell carcinomas. Various molecular cytogenetic methods have significantly expanded the application of genomic analysis in both research and clinical management. Recent array CGH studies have confirmed the involvement of previously suspected pathogenic genomic regions/genes and, in addition, identified novel genomic regions/genes. Although many laboratories still perform conventional karyotyping in solid tumors, FISH has become the method of choice for detecting specific genomic alterations, particularly in archival specimens. In conjunction with cytology, histology, and morphology, conventional karyotyping along with high-resolution cytogenetics (FISH, array CGH) of solid tumors has become a valuable tool in screening, diagnosis, classification, prognosis, risk-stratification, and selection of patients for newly developed or developing targeted therapy.

REFERENCES

1. Tjio JH, Levan A. The chromosome number of man. Hereditas 1956;42:1–6.
2. Ford CE, Hamerton JL. The chromosomes of man. Nature 1956;178:1020.
3. Nowell PC, Hungerford DA. A minute chromosome in human chronic granulocytic leukemia. Science 1960;132:1197.
4. Tomlins SA, Bjartell A, Chinnaiyan AM, et al. ETS gene fusions in prostate cancer: from discovery to daily clinical practice. Eur Urol 2009;56:275–86.
5. Pinkel D, Straume T, Gray JW. Cytogenetic analysis using quantitative, high-sensitivity, fluorescence hybridization. Proc Natl Acad Sci U S A 1986;83:2934–8.
6. Schrock E, du Manoir S, Veldman T, et al. Multicolor spectral karyotyping of human chromosomes. Science 1996;273:494–7.
7. Kallioniemi A, Kallioniemi OP, Sudar D, et al. Comparative genomic hybridization for molecular cytogenetic analysis of solid tumors. Science 1992;258:818–21.

8. Speicher MR, Carter NP. The new cytogenetics: blurring the boundaries with molecular biology. Nat Rev Genet 2005;6:782–92.

9. Mitelman Database of Chromosome Aberrations and Gene Fusions in Cancer (2011). Mitelman F, Johansson B, Mertens F, editors. Available at: http://cgap.nci.nih.gov/Chromosomes/Mitelman. Accessed April 16, 2011.

10. Lukeis R, Suter M. Cytogenetics of Solid Tumors. In: Campbell LJ, editor. Methods in Molecular Biology # 730: Cancer Cytogenetics: Methods and Protocols. New York: Springer Science and Business Media, LLC; 2011. p. 173–87.

11. Burgess BL, Rao NP, Eskin A, et al. Characterization of three cell lines derived from fine needle biopsy of choroidal melanoma with metastatic outcome. Mol Vis 2011;25: 607–15.

12. Ellisen LW, Haber DA. Basic Principles of Cancer Genetics. In: Chung DC Haber DA. Principles of Clinical Cancer Genetics: A Handbook from the Massachusetts General Hospital. New York (NY): Springer Science and Business Media, LLC; 2010. p. 1–22.

13. Howarth KD, Blood KA, Ng BL, et al. Array painting reveals a high frequency of balanced translocations in breast cancer cell lines that break in cancer-relevant genes. Oncogene 2008 27:3345–59.

14. Rosenberg AE. Liposarcoma of Bone. In: Fletcher CDM, Unni K, Mertens F, editors. Pathology and Genetics of Tumours of Soft Tissue and Bone. World Health Organization Classification of Tumours. Lyon (France): IARC Press; 2002.

15. Lopez-Beltran A, Carrasco JC, Cheng L, et al. 2009 update on the classification of renal epithelial tumors in adults. Int J Urol 2009;16:432–43.

16. Klatte T, Rao PN, de Martino M, et al. Cytogenetic profile predicts prognosis of patients with clear cell renal cell carcinoma. J Clin Oncol 2009;27:746–53.

17. Volpe A, Terrone C, Scarpa RM. The current role of percutaneous needle biopsies of renal tumours. Arch Ital Urol Androl 2009;81:107–12.

18. Roh MH, Dal Cin P, Silverman SG, et al. The application of cytogenetics and fluorescence in situ hybridization to fine-needle aspiration in the diagnosis and sub-classification of renal neoplasms. Cancer Cytopathol 2010;118:137–45.

19. Pfister S, Hartmann C, Korshunov A. Histology and molecular pathology of pediatric brain tumors. J Child Neurol 2009;24:1375–86.

20. Horbinski C, Miller CR, Perry A. Gone FISHing: clinical lessons learned in brain tumor molecular diagnostics over the last decade. Brain Pathol 2011;21:57–73.

21. Jenkins RB, Blair H, Ballman KV, et al. A t(1;19)(q10;p10) mediates the combined deletions of 1p and 19q and predicts a better prognosis of patients with oligodendroglioma. Cancer Res 2006;66:9852–61.

22. Riemenschneider MJ, Jeuken JW, Wesseling P, et al. Molecular diagnostics of gliomas: state of the art. Acta Neuropathol 2010;120:567–84.

23. Mellinghoff IK, Wang MY, Vivanco I, et al. Molecular determinants of the response of glioblastomas to EGFR kinase inhibitors. New Engl J Med 2005;353:2012–24.

24. Jones DT, Kocialkowski S, Liu L, et al. Tandem duplication producing a novel oncogenic BRAF fusion gene defines the majority of pilocytic astrocytomas. Cancer Res 2008;68:8673–7.

25. Blokx WA, van Dijk MC, Ruiter DJ. Molecular cytogenetics of cutaneous melanocytic lesions - diagnostic, prognostic and therapeutic aspects. Histopathology 2010;56: 121–32.

26. Morey AL, Murali R, McCarthy SW, et al. Diagnosis of cutaneous melanocytic tumors by four-color fluorescence in situ hybridization. Pathology 2009;41:383–7.

27. Gerami P, Mafee M, Lurtsbarapa T, et al. Sensitivity of fluorescence in situ hybridization for melanoma diagnosis using RREB1, MYB, Cep6, and 11q13 probes in melanoma subtypes. Arch Dermatol 2010;146:273–8.

28. Pouryazdanparast P, Newman M, Mafee M, et al. Distinguishing epithelioid blue nevus from blue nevus-like cutaneous melanoma metastasis using fluorescence in situ hybridization. Am J Surg Pathol 2009;33:1396–400.

29. Shields JA, Shields CL, Materin M, et al. Role of cytogenetics in management of uveal melanoma. Arch Ophthalmol 2008;126:416–9.

30. Damato B, Coupland SE. Translating uveal melanoma cytogenetics into clinical care. Arch Ophthalmol 2009;127:423–9.

31. Bonaldi L, Midena E, Filippi B, et al. FISH analysis of chromosomes 3 and 6 on fine needle aspiration biopsy samples identifies distinct subgroups of uveal melanomas. J Cancer Res Clin Oncol 2008;134:1123–7.

32. Lake SL, Coupland SE, Taktak AF, et al. Whole-genome microarray detects deletions and loss of heterozygosity of chromosome 3 occurring exclusively in metastasizing uveal melanoma. Invest Ophthalmol Vis Sci 2010;51:4884–91.

33. Wen J, Fu J, Zhang W, et al. Genetic and epigenetic changes in lung carcinoma and their clinical implications. Mod Pathol 2011;24:932–43.

34. Ramalingam SS, Owonikoko TK, Khuri FR. Lung cancer: new biological insights and recent therapeutic advances. CA Cancer J Clin 2011;61:91–112.

35. Sokolova IA, Bubendorf L, O'Hare A, et al. A fluorescence in situ hybridization-based assay for improved detection of lung cancer cells in bronchial washing specimens. Cancer 2002;96:306–15.

36. Voss JS, Kipp BR, Halling KC, et al. Fluorescence in situ hybridization testing algorithm improves lung cancer detection in bronchial brushing specimens. Am J Respir Crit Care Med 2010;181:478–85.

37. Varella-Garcia M, Schulte AP, Wolf HJ, et al. The detection of chromosomal aneusomy by fluorescence in situ hybridization in sputum predicts lung cancer incidence. Cancer Prev Res (Phila) 2010;3:447–53.

38. Varella-Garcia M, Diebold J, Eberhard DA, et al. EGFR fluorescence in situ hybridization assay: guidelines for application to non-small-cell lung cancer. J Clin Pathol 2009;62:970–7.

39. Casorzo L, Corigliano M, Ferrero P, et al. Evaluation of 7q31 region improves the accuracy of EGFR FISH assay in non small cell lung cancer. Diagn Pathol 2009;4:36.

40. Camidge DR, Kono SA, Flacco A, et al. Optimizing the detection of lung cancer patients harboring anaplastic lymphoma kinase (ALK) gene rearrangements potentially suitable for ALK inhibitor treatment. Clin Cancer Res 2010;16:5581–90.

41. Shah S, Chen B. Testing for HER2 in Breast Cancer: A Continuing Evolution. Patholog Res Int 2010;2011:903202.

42. Wolff AC, Hammond ME, Schwartz JN, et al. American Society of Clinical Oncology/College of American Pathologists. American Society of Clinical Oncology/College of American Pathologists guideline recommendations for human epidermal growth factor receptor 2 testing in breast cancer. Arch Pathol Lab Med 2007;131:18–43.

43. Vranic S, Teruya B, Repertinger S, et al. Assessment of HER2 gene status in breast carcinomas with polysomy of chromosome 17. Cancer 2011;117:48–53.

44. Bang YJ, Van Cutsem E, Feyereislova A, et al. ToGA Trial Investigators. Trastuzumab in combination with chemotherapy versus chemotherapy alone for treatment of HER2-positive advanced gastric or gastro-oesophageal junction cancer (ToGA): a phase 3, open-label, randomised controlled trial. Lancet 2010; 376:687–97.

45. Hofmann M, Stoss O, Shi D, et al. Assessment of a HER2 scoring system for gastric cancer: results from a validation study. Histopathology 2008;52:797–805.

46. Rüschoff J, Dietel M, Baretton G, et al. HER2 diagnostics in gastric cancer-guideline validation and development of standardized immunohistochemical testing. Virchows Arch 2010;457:299–307.

47. Sullivan PS, Chan JB, Levin MR, et al. Urine cytology and adjunct markers for detection and surveillance of bladder cancer. Am J Transl Res 2010;2:412–40.
48. Goebell PJ, Knowles MA. Bladder cancer or bladder cancers? Genetically distinct malignant conditions of the urothelium. Urol Oncol 2010;28:409–28.
49. Sokolova IA, Halling KC, Jenkins RB, et al. The development of a multitarget, multicolor fluorescence in situ hybridization assay for the detection of urothelial carcinoma in urine. J Mol Diagn 2000;2:116–23.
50. Caraway NP, Khanna A, Fernandez RL, et al. Fluorescence in situ hybridization for detecting urothelial carcinoma: a clinicopathologic study. Cancer Cytopathol 2010; 118:259–68.
51. McConkey DJ, Lee S, Choi W, et al. Molecular genetics of bladder cancer: Emerging mechanisms of tumor initiation and progression. Urol Oncol 2010;28:429–40.
52. Apgar BS, Kittendorf AL, Bettcher CM, et al. Update on ASCCP consensus guidelines for abnormal cervical screening tests and cervical histology. Am Fam Physician 2009;80:147–55.
53. Kloth JN, Oosting J, van Wezel T, et al. Combined array-comparative genomic hybridization and single-nucleotide polymorphism-loss of heterozygosity analysis reveals complex genetic alterations in cervical cancer. BMC Genomics 2007;8:53.
54. Wilting SM, Steenbergen RD, Tijssen M, et al. Chromosomal signatures of a subset of high-grade premalignant cervical lesions closely resemble invasive carcinomas. Cancer Res 2009;69:647–55.
55. Heselmeyer-Haddad K, Sommerfeld K, White NM, et al. Genomic amplification of the human telomerase gene (TERC) in pap smears predicts the development of cervical cancer. Am J Pathol 2005;166:1229–38.
56. Li Y, Zeng WJ, Ye F, et al. Application of hTERC in thin prep samples with mild cytologic abnormality and HR-HPV positive. Gynecol Oncol 2011;120:73–83.
57. Policht FA, Song M, Sitailo S, et al. Analysis of genetic copy number changes in cervical disease progression. BMC Cancer 2010;10:432.
58. Sun J, Liu W, Adams TS, et al. DNA copy number alterations in prostate cancers: a combined analysis of published CGH studies. Prostate 2007;67:692–700.
59. Tomlins SA, Bjartell A, Chinnaiyan AM, et al. ETS gene fusions in prostate cancer: from discovery to daily clinical practice. Eur Urol 2009;56:275–86.
60. Liu W, Laitinen S, Khan S, et al. Copy number analysis indicates monoclonal origin of lethal metastatic prostate cancer. Nat Med 2009;15:559–65.
61. Shen MM, Abate-Shen C. Molecular genetics of prostate cancer: new prospects for old challenges. Genes Dev 2010;24:1967–2000.
62. Taylor BS, Schultz N, Hieronymus H, et al. Integrative genomic profiling of human prostate cancer. Cancer Cell 2010;18:11–22.
63. Rosenberg MT, Froehner M, Albala D, et al. Biology and natural history of prostate cancer and the role of chemoprevention. Int J Clin Pract 2010;64:1746–53.

Index

Note: Page numbers of article titles are in **boldface** type.

Clin Lab Med 31 (2011) 813–827
doi:10.1016/S0272-2712(11)00108-9
0272-2712/11/$ – see front matter © 2011 Elsevier Inc. All rights reserved.

United States Postal Service

Statement of Ownership, Management, and Circulation
(All Periodicals Publications Except Requestor Publications)

1. Publication Title	2. Publication Number	3. Filing Date
Clinics in Laboratory Medicine	0 0 0 - 7 1 1 3	9/16/11

4. Issue Frequency	5. Number of Issues Published Annually	6. Annual Subscription Price
Mar, Jun, Sep, Dec	4	$225.00

7. Complete Mailing Address of Known Office of Publication (Not printer) (Street, city, county, state, and ZIP+4®)

Elsevier Inc.
360 Park Avenue South
New York, NY 10010-1710

Contact Person
Amy S. Beacham

Telephone (Include area code)
215-239-3687

8. Complete Mailing Address of Headquarters or General Business Office of Publisher (Not printer)

Elsevier Inc., 360 Park Avenue South, New York, NY 10010-1710

9. Full Names and Complete Mailing Addresses of Publisher, Editor, and Managing Editor (Do not leave blank)

Publisher (Name and complete mailing address)

Kim Murphy, Elsevier, Inc., 1600 John F. Kennedy Blvd. Suite 1800, Philadelphia, PA 19103-2899

Editor (Name and complete mailing address)

Katie Hartner, Elsevier, Inc., 1600 John F. Kennedy Blvd. Suite 1800, Philadelphia, PA 19103-2899

Managing Editor (Name and complete mailing address)

Sarah Barth, Elsevier, Inc., 1600 John F. Kennedy Blvd. Suite 1800, Philadelphia, PA 19103-2899

10. Owner (Do not leave blank. If the publication is owned by a corporation, give the name and address of the corporation immediately followed by the names and addresses of all stockholders owning or holding 1 percent or more of the total amount of stock. If not owned by a corporation, give the names and addresses of the individual owners. If owned by a partnership or other unincorporated firm, give its name and address as well as those of each individual owner. If the publication is published by a nonprofit organization, give its name and address.)

Full Name	Complete Mailing Address
Wholly owned subsidiary of	4520 East-West Highway
Reed/Elsevier, US holdings	Bethesda, MD 20814

11. Known Bondholders, Mortgagees, and Other Security Holders Owning or Holding 1 Percent or More of Total Amount of Bonds, Mortgages, or Other Securities. If none, check box ☐ None

Full Name	Complete Mailing Address
N/A	

12. Tax Status (For completion by nonprofit organizations authorized to mail at nonprofit rates) (Check one)
The purpose, function, and nonprofit status of this organization and the exempt status for federal income tax purposes:
☐ Has Not Changed During Preceding 12 Months
☐ Has Changed During Preceding 12 Months (Publisher must submit explanation of change with this statement)

PS Form 3526, September 2007 (Page 1 of 3) (Instructions Page 3) PSN 7530-01-000-9931 PRIVACY NOTICE: See our Privacy policy in www.usps.com

---

13. Publication Title	14. Issue Date for Circulation Data Below
Clinics in Laboratory Medicine	September 2011

15. Extent and Nature of Circulation		Average No. Copies Each Issue During Preceding 12 Months	No. Copies of Single Issue Published Nearest to Filing Date
a. Total Number of Copies (Net press run)		606	496
b. Paid Circulation (By Mail and Outside the Mail)	(1) Mailed Outside-County Paid Subscriptions Stated on PS Form 3541. (Include paid distribution above nominal rate, advertiser's proof copies, and exchange copies)	193	182
	(2) Mailed In-County Paid Subscriptions Stated on PS Form 3541 (Include paid distribution above nominal rate, advertiser's proof copies, and exchange copies)		
	(3) Paid Distribution Outside the Mails Including Sales Through Dealers and Carriers, Street Vendors, Counter Sales, and Other Paid Distribution Outside USPS®	85	96
	(4) Paid Distribution by Other Classes Mailed Through the USPS (e.g. First-Class Mail®)		
c. Total Paid Distribution (Sum of 15b (1), (2), (3), and (4))	▲	278	278
d. Free or Nominal Rate Distribution (By Mail and Outside the Mail)	(1) Free or Nominal Rate Outside-County Copies Included on PS Form 3541	69	50
	(2) Free or Nominal Rate In-County Copies Included on PS Form 3541		
	(3) Free or Nominal Rate Copies Mailed at Other Classes Through the USPS (e.g. First-Class Mail)		
	(4) Free or Nominal Rate Distribution Outside the Mail (Carriers or other means)		
e. Total Free or Nominal Rate Distribution (Sum of 15d (1), (2), (3) and (4))	▲	69	50
f. Total Distribution (Sum of 15c and 15e)	▲	347	328
g. Copies not Distributed (See instructions to publishers #4 (page #3))	▲	259	168
h. Total (Sum of 15f and g)	▲	606	496
i. Percent Paid (15c divided by 15f times 100)		80.12%	84.76%

16. Publication of Statement of Ownership

☐ If the publication is a general publication, publication of this statement is required. Will be printed in the **December 2011** issue of this publication. ☐ Publication not required.

17. Signature and Title of Editor, Publisher, Business Manager, or Owner

[signature] Amy S. Beacham — Senior Inventory Distribution Coordinator

Date: September 16, 2011

I certify that all information furnished on this form is true and complete. I understand that anyone who furnishes false or misleading information on this form or who omits material or information requested on the form may be subject to criminal sanctions (including fines and imprisonment) and/or civil sanctions (including civil penalties).

PS Form 3526, September 2007 (Page 2 of 3)

Moving?

Make sure your subscription moves with you!

To notify us of your new address, find your **Clinics Account Number** (located on your mailing label above your name), and contact customer service at:

Email: journalscustomerservice-usa@elsevier.com

800-654-2452 (subscribers in the U.S. & Canada)
314-447-8871 (subscribers outside of the U.S. & Canada)

Fax number: 314-447-8029

Elsevier Health Sciences Division
Subscription Customer Service
3251 Riverport Lane
Maryland Heights, MO 63043

*To ensure uninterrupted delivery of your subscription, please notify us at least 4 weeks in advance of move.

Printed and bound by CPI Group (UK) Ltd, Croydon, CR0 4YY

03/10/2024

01040442-0011